THE
FIBROMYALGIA
CONTROVERSY

M. CLEMENT HALL

THE FIBROMYALGIA CONTROVERSY

Prometheus Books

59 John Glenn Drive
Amherst, New York 14228–2119

Published 2009 by Prometheus Books

Inquiries should be addressed to
Prometheus Books
59 John Glenn Drive
Amherst, New York 14228–2119
VOICE: 716–691–0133, ext. 210
FAX: 716–691–0137
WWW.PROMETHEUSBOOKS.COM

13 12 11 10 09   5 4 3 2 1

Library of Congress Cataloging-in-Publication Data

Hall, M. Clement
    The fibromyalgia controversy / M. Clement Hall.
        p. cm.
    Includes bibliographical references and index.
    ISBN 978–1–59102–681–5 (pbk. : alk. paper)
    1. Fibromyalgia. 2. Fibromyalgia—diagnosis. 3. Fibromyalgia—psychology.
4. Fibromyalgia—therapy. 5. Sick Role.

RC927.3 .H328 2008
616.7/42—dc22

2008033995

Printed in the United States of America on acid-free paper

To family

The truth is never pure and rarely simple.
—**Oscar Wilde**

CONTENTS

INTRODUCTION

The book is constructed as a notional research project to explore the diversity of strongly held opinions on the reality or otherwise of the fibromyalgia syndrome and to explore the issues involved.

It is postulated that a university medical school has been awarded a grant by an interested private donor to test this hypothesis: "The symptoms of fibromyalgia can be abolished or at least alleviated by a program of therapy when combined with an expertly conducted self-realization project."

The pilot study in this program is reported as it applied to the first six participants. The protocol for the research project calls for *fully informing* the participants of their condition, its origin, diagnosis, management, and outcome.

Instruction will progress serially from the most simple to quite complex, consistent with the differing educational levels of the participants.

THE AMERICAN COLLEGE OF RHEUMATOLOGY CRITERIA FOR DIAGNOSIS OF FIBROMYALGIA (1990)

There are only two diagnostic requirements—one is based on the history, and the other is based on a specific and limited physical examination. First: A history of continuous pain in all four quadrants of the body and the axial skeleton for the previous three months. Second: Pain to firm pressure must be elicited in at least eleven of eighteen designated tender points.

CHAPTER ONE

PERSONAL NARRATIVES

ANNA

Hello! My name is Anna.

I'm forty-five years old. I was born in the South. I never knew my father. I hold but the vaguest memory of a man in the house when I was very young. If that were my daddy, then my mom never told me so, and I chose never to ask her. My mom has been ailing all my life, and I don't know for how long 'fore that. Seems to me, most of her life, she's just stood in bed.

I started to earn when I couldn't have been more than six—running errands, fetching, and carrying. All I earned went into the earthenware pot on the kitchen dresser. I never spent a penny on myself. My clothes were all hand-me-downs from neighbors or charity ladies or maybe some of them were relations. It was never explained to me—I suppose they thought it were none of my business—when all was said and done, I was just the kid who got to wear them, and it truly weren't none of my affair who'd worn them 'fore me.

I did go to school. But they never learnt me much. My fault I'm sure. Not theirs. I spent too much time in the junior grades thinking of food and too much time in the middle grades thinking of when was a boy gonna get me out of there—and which boy would it be?

Well, I got out the same way as most of the girls. Going to have a baby 'fore I was seventeen. I didn't give too much thought to how I'd manage to feed him and clothe him—I just knew he'd be a boy—but I so much wanted to have something to love that'd be my very own.

I left school. My boy was taken away from me. They let me see him and hold him for a few minutes—and then no more. Where he is now—who he is now—I have no notion.

Without a school-leaving certificate, all you can get is minimum-wage work. And with minimum-wage work, some days they offer you work, an' other days you're told you're not needed. So you get two jobs to make sure you got one.

I did get married. Same trouble as the last one. He seemed kind, Joseph did. Probably he was. But three babies in thirty months was too much for him. I never heard from him after the third one was on the way. He went to his work one December morning, and I never saw hide or hair of him since.

So what with never knowing I was going to get work or be sent away, and what with the cost of my mom's medicines and the three children's care, I took three jobs to make sure I had one.

P'raps it was really because I was a good worker, like they said, or more like they couldn't get no one else—even the illegals were in short supply! Anyways, my three jobs to make sure I had one turned into three jobs most all the time. Working seven by fourteen I was, and sometimes sixteen. Not surprising I felt tired all the time, even though I fell asleep the moment my bed saw me.

And then I was aching. The muscles at the top of my shoulders and back of my neck were what I noticed first. Not surprising, stooped like I was cleaning bathtubs for seven hours at a stretch. Got my friend to massage them—don't misunderstand me. Nothing like that. Nothing so interesting! She did the vacuum, I did the bathtubs.

But I couldn't sleep proper—not like I didn't try. Not like I didn't fall asleep and dream about bathtubs. That I did! Tossed and turned all night dreaming about those grimy bathtubs and sodden towels all over the tiled floors. But come the morning, I felt like I hadn't been to bed at all. Just as tired, aching just as much, and so stiff I could hardly get out of bed. Mind you, my mattress was secondhand—everything I had was at best secondhand—most of it probably third, fourth, or fifth. And it was lumpy. And the springs beneath it were broke. But there was a time I were able to sleep on it just fine. What had changed weren't the bed—'twas me.

Then I started getting pains in my elbows. Pain I can stand. After four birthings, you know what pain is. But I couldn't hold the scrub brush on account of my elbows. Had no grip left at all. So even though I had no insurance, I had to get help. Went to a walk-in clinic. The young chit of a girl at the reception was rude when she found I'd no coverage. Pretty much as said she knew I'd rob them. I walked out. Looking over my shoulder, I could see she was back to reading her magazine 'fore I was even through the door.

I couldn't get rested, and the pains got so bad I could do no work. I had to go on the county. They took care of the kids. The pills they gave me were no help. Maybe 'cause I didn't take them. Wasn't going to get addicted. Seen too many like that. It was the welfare lady who sent me to the clinic, and then the clinic that sent me here.

BETTY

Hi, there! My name's Betty. Maybe we've met. I'm the check-out girl at Cyrenberg's Fresh Fruit and Vegetables Market. And let me tell you, that's a heavy job. You lift your one bag of vegetables, and you think it's heavy. I lift them for eight hours. OK, I get a break. Half an hour for lunch, ten minutes for a smoke a couple times a shift. The boss isn't bad. It's his wife who watches us. Take a minute extra, and she's down on you like a ton of bricks. So when my neck was sore and my shoulders hurt from lifting all those bags, "Do your work or get another job" was all the sympathy I got from her. And I told my husband, Bill, I might have to get another job. He'd just got home from the sports bar after midnight, but he fell asleep while I was talking.

The pain got worse, and I did get fired. "Get yourself fixed," Bill said on his way to the big autoshop where he's their lead mechanic. I grew up on a farm and "fixed" doesn't mean to me what it means to him. He's got good medical coverage, and I had no trouble getting seen in the medical clinic. Nice young doctor, had one of those hand computers, typed everything into it, and bingo! Out popped the answer. Soft tissue rheumatism, he'd said. Didn't explain it to me. Wrote it on my sheet and sent me back to the desk, still clutching the back of the gown so I'd not attract those nosy old men sitting in the hallway, holding their walking canes.

The massage hurt, but the heat felt good. Felt good until I went home to mum, who never stopped talking about her pains, "hier und hier," since she came from the old country and thinks I speak the language, which I don't. I left her thinking I'd end up the same if I didn't get better treated. So I got more heat and more massage and then some electric machines they strapped onto me. Every day I went.

At first it was better, then day by day, the pains spread. Down from my neck and over my back. Then I couldn't sleep. Bill snores, lies on his back, makes me think of our pigs. In the morning, I was more tired than when I went to bed. Hardly had the strength to go to the clinic for their treatments. The same young doctor wrote me prescriptions for pills—all they did was leave me confused. Said I shouldn't drive, but Bill has the only car, so it made no difference.

The massage therapist seemed to be getting frustrated when I told her she made me hurt even more. She passed me on to the exercise therapist, who had some crazy idea I should lift weights. I told her that was what started me off in the first place. They sent me to a dietitian. Don't think she'd have kept her man happy, not with the food she suggested. So much vegetables and fruit my stomach never stopped rumbling. Not that Bill would've noticed. Then more pills that did nothing. Then they sold me insoles with magnets to put in my shoes. I didn't tell Bill about those. They made me limp. My legs and back were hurting every bit as much as my neck and arms.

Finally, Bill told me either I get fixed or he'd get out. Couldn't stand me whining like my mother, he said. So here I am. Specialist said he wasn't sure they'd help me, but I was getting nowhere like I was, and the insurance refused the last payment. Said I'd gone over the limit.

CICELY

Good afternoon. My name is Cicely. I'm very pleased to meet you. I think perhaps we share the same problem. I'm very fortunate in life. I don't go out to work, but I work very hard at home. At the old age of fifty-five, I'm an empty nester, but not for much of the time. Our four children were married young— they're following the family traditions and already they've got three children each. But I stayed home and looked after my children. (Young people these days don't seem to think that's necessary. Perhaps they're right. Perhaps they're entitled to some fun while they're still young.) But I do get so tired when they bring the grandchildren. Don't get me wrong—I love them dearly. But chasing after them as they run wild through the house does my pressure no good. And I began to ache very badly when the two girls decided they'd go away together. "Make a foursome" they said, but it was a "sixsome" they left me with, three children each. Then I really started to ache, couldn't sleep, tired all the time. "What do you expect?" my husband said. "At your age?" As if that would make me hurt any less.

I'm lucky with my doctor. Don't have to wait long for an appointment. Always pleased to see me. Always friendly. Always busy, too, so I don't like to take up too much of his time. His nurse takes my pressure. I tell him I feel tired looking after six children. He laughs, doesn't examine me, he's so busy, but he gives me a packet from his drawer. "Latest thing," he says. "Come back next week and tell me how you're doing."

The pills make me drowsy through the day, don't help me sleep at night. The children exhaust me. Seems my good husband is more busy at the office now and never gets home until after I've put the kids to bed. Then I have to get his dinner. Don't have an appetite for anything myself, but he eats like a racehorse.

I couldn't understand my doctor. Every time I went to his office, he had a different sample medication to give me. It wasn't as if I needed anything free. We have a perfectly good insurance, but always it was a new sample. Always it was "the latest thing." But they never helped. None of them.

The more I hurt, the harder it was to get to see him. Finally, I told his nurse I really thought he ought to examine me. Perhaps I had cancer or something. I knew he was busy. I knew he was very kind, but perhaps if he were to examine me, he might find a reason for the pains and the tiredness and that dreadful stiffness.

"He doesn't think there's anything wrong," his nurse said. "If he did, he'd have looked at you."

"So what should I do?" I asked her, totally bewildered.

"Try the herbalist. They're for people like you." And that was where I found the brochure that led to the Web site that led to the specialist who fixed for me to come here. There were quite a few boxes of herbs in between, while the pain got worse and I became more and more desperate.

DELILAH

I can't hide it from you. It's on the sheet in front of you. My name's Delilah. I know how I got it, or at least why I got it, and that's of no account right now. Please call me Dee. What's not on the form, and I won't hide it from you, I used to work as an insurance adjuster. Yeah. I can read your thoughts. I did personal accident. Maybe I handled some of your claims. We deal with paper. We don't deal with faces. Just paper. And so much paper. And so many claims. And the jokes about them. Listening to the managers you wouldn't believe anyone was ever truly hurt in an accident.

This is my story.

I'm forty. I'm a single mom. We've all promised here to be absolutely honest with each other, so I have to tell you, I've always been a single mom. Not like I didn't know who the man was, but I never wanted him as a husband, and he'd never have been much of a father. So I've a child to support, going on ten. Nice polite kid. Does his homework, makes his own bed. Keeps his room tidied. But that's not what you want to hear. Maybe later we'll show pictures?

Why I'm here? I had an accident. Is that God's judgment? I wouldn't know. God and me, we never had much to do with each other. Driving to work, traffic slow, stop and start, then it speeded up a little, and we were moving along at a good pace. I hadn't expected the truck to stop, no lights. No warning. But I managed to stop my car an inch behind him. Didn't touch him. Not until the pickup I saw in the mirror came slamming into me, threw my car partway under the truck, and threw me onto my back. The seat flattened. I couldn't move. Not even when the gentleman whose pickup had hit me came and shouted at me. Won't tell you what he said, but it was in the nature I earned my living like the way I was lying—on my back.

I'm rambling on. The paramedics came. They looked really worried. They asked if I could feel my feet. I could, but it was obvious they thought I was going to be paralyzed. They told me not to move. I knew they thought I'd die if I did. They put a collar 'round my neck. I could hardly breathe. They wrapped, like, a corset around me, lifted me out and laid me on a board, tied me to it, straps all over me, and my head bound to the board with sticky tape. I was scared when it happened. I was terrified when they did all this. I knew my neck and back were broke, or they'd not have gone to so much trouble. They knew there had to be internal bleeding, or they wouldn't have started an IV, would they?

Then the sirens as they rushed me to the emergency room! There they were nice enough. The clerk found what she needed in my purse. The nurse looked sympathetic. The boy who came, wearing jeans and a workshirt, said he was a doctor. I didn't believe him. So young. But the nurse said he was, and gave me his name. Then they took blood. They took x-rays. They shook their heads. They talked out of my sight in low voices. I knew there was something terrible they'd found. They wheeled me back to the ER. The boy who said he was a doctor undid the collar, tossed it onto the shelf under the stretcher, put a piece of paper in my hand, said, "Follow up with your own doctor," and walked away. I hurt like hell. All over. And they said there was nothing wrong! Like I'd imagined the accident!

Then came the paperwork. I'd never thought it was people in pain who filled out all those forms. And my car wasn't worth repairing. A pittance they gave me; wretch of an adjuster said it was all it was worth.

My doctor was kind. She gave me a prescription, ordered another collar, sent me for therapy. Sent me to several places. But I just got worse. I hurt everywhere. My job was held for me. I couldn't go back to it, so they put me on short-term disability. Then I had to see a doctor who specialized in accidents; I could see he didn't believe anything I told him. Didn't seem to care that my usual once-a-month migraine was now every three days, or my periods that'd always hurt were now an agony. And my tummy, you'll excuse me, ladies, sometimes it worked too much, and sometimes it didn't work for days. But my therapist sent me to a lawyer. He sent me to an arthritis doctor, I guess because my neck was on fire and my back no better. She was the one who said I'd got fibromyalgia. And that's why I'm here.

ENOLA

Hi! I'm Enola. Not Enola May. Just Enola. And I guess I'm the same as the rest of you. I hurt.

But I'm tired. I'm just so damn tired I can barely drag myself out of bed. Just as well my husband left me. If he hadn't already, then he would've now.

Like Betty, I work in sales, but at a counter. General office supplies, paper, computers, that kind of thing. The men, they give the advice. Me, I ring in the sales. Just the one job, forty hours a week. Unionized. Good benefits. Clean and warm place. Good boss, and nice guys to work with.

Depression, my doctor called it. He was right. I'm so damn depressed I sit at the table, holding my head and the tears flow. I just can't stop them. Pills he gave me. Helped the sleep a little. The psychiatrist was kind. Told me lots of women are depressed at my age, forty-three, some men, too. "Go on with the pills," he said. "Don't lose hope. Your doctor's got it right." That didn't explain why I hurt so much, just ache right through. Not in any one place, not so I could explain it to my doctor. 'Sides, how many problems am I going to tell him about?

Then they laid me off. Very nice about it, they were. I knew I wasn't doing the work. I had nothing to complain about. Fact, in the long run, it was likely a good thing. I got to get some sleep during the day when the kids were at school. I didn't tell you they both got learning and behavioral problems. Go to a special school. But that doesn't keep them quiet when they're home. Not even the meds they take seem to quiet them. But we've all got our problems. You don't want to hear too much about mine. So I'll tell you the bright bit.

My short-term disability was switched to long-term, and they made me go and see another doctor. Lawyer said his job was to cut me off my benefits. But he asked me more questions than any doctor I'd ever been to. I didn't expect to tell him about my childhood. Not even the psychiatrist had asked about that, and I'm not going to tell you today what I told him then. But he thought it might have something to do with my pains, and my trouble sleeping, and my sitting by myself weeping. Fibromyalgia, he called it. I'd never heard the word before. But that's what led to me coming here.

Guess we'll all have to wait and see what's in store for us. I know I couldn't go on like I was.

FRIEDA

I don't think I belong here. Don't know why they made me come. Least of all why they make me talk to you. I'm twenty-five. I don't think I belong here. It was my mother who took me to the hospital. Sat for hours in the emergency room. She wouldn't let me leave. OK for her—she knew everyone there. Hospital's where she works. But not me. Bored out of my skull.

I knew what was wrong. They'd told me in the university health clinic, irritable bowel, they called it. They had that right. Irritable it was, and then some. On top of my painful periods and my weekly migraine, that was all I needed. So they put their damn telescopes into me. One into my belly, one up my ass, another through my mouth. "Won't bother you," I was told. I was out of school for six weeks. In agony all that time. Lost my chance to enroll in the master's program I'd set my heart on. Stupid jerks. Made my pains worse than they'd ever been. All through my body. Not just with the periods. Not just with the migraines. All the time.

Of course, I've been having pain ever since my periods started. No fun being a woman, is it? Not just my periods, though they're agony enough. Aching all through me. "Growing pains," the stupid doctors said. Not like I wasn't fully grown anyway.

Then, "Need to get some exercise," they said. Exercise killed me. Pains so bad I couldn't move for days. Every time they made me exercise, I missed three days of school. Whole weeks sometimes.

So we sit in the waiting room. Not like it was the first time. My mother thinks she has influence. She hasn't yet learned influence is something you think you've got until you need it. She works in the operating room. Tells the surgeons which tool to use. Doesn't swing much weight in emergency.

They mark a number four on my chart. Lowest priority they've got. Last time we were here, ended up in a visit to the psych. They were happy enough with what I told them. Come to the right place—I was one for them, they said. Problem's all in my head. That's what they deal with. Jerks! Wasn't having that. Neither was my mother. Not often we agree about anything.

Then we sit nearly an hour in an examination room. "Couldn't this have been dealt with by your own doctor?" the young intern asks me. My mother stops my answer. "We need a referral," she said. "I've been looking up her symptoms on the Internet. I think she's got fibromyalgia. She needs to be referred to a specialist."

Must have been years younger than me, that intern. Looked at me. I could swear his nose twitched like a rabbit's. Wrote something on the chart, gave it to my mother, and walked out. Never spoke to me. Never examined me.

That's about enough. I went to the arthritis clinic. Saw a junior resident who stopped talking to me after I asked her how long she'd been out of diapers. Then my mother got me sent here. Doubt they're going to be any better.

And that's the story of my life so far.

CHAPTER TWO

EXPLANATIONS TO PARTICIPANTS

WHAT IS A DIAGNOSIS? HOW IS IT MADE?

Doctors work as individuals—they may work as members of a team, but they are always individuals within that team. Over the years, each doctor develops his own way of conducting his work. Patients become familiar with their usual doctor's manner of meeting, greeting, and examining them. Because another doctor handles things differently does not make one doctor right and the other wrong.

Since this is a research program, however, it's necessary to have a standardized protocol in order that all issues considered significant to the ultimate conclusions are addressed and are recorded for future analysis. The protocol was accepted by all participants including, of course, the patients—the subjects of the research—as well as the investigators.

There are terms used by doctors that should result in a clear separation of fact from supposition. (It's convenient here to use the term "doctor," although it's recognized that an "extended-role nurse" might frequently be the individual involved. Since it is simply too complicated to list all the roles and alphabetical terminology, understanding and forgiveness of the "nondoctor" is requested.)

Symptoms and Signs

A symptom is what the patient tells the doctor. A sign is what the doctor sees, or in some manner elicits, using his eyes, ears, hands, stethoscope, reflex hammer, and so forth.

For example, the patient says, "I have pain right here," pointing to some part of the body (*symptom*) and the doctor feels a lump in the place indicated (*sign*).

The doctor asks, "Does that hurt when I squeeze it?" The patient says, "Yes, it does. Please don't squeeze so hard, that really hurts" (*symptom*). The doctor records, "Mass two inches in diameter (*sign*); pain elicited, increasing with pressure" (*not a sign, but a symptom elicited, meaning caused by the doctor*). It is only a sign if the doctor can see, feel, hear, smell, or otherwise record something physical that goes with the symptom.

Where does the patient's reaction to the doctor's touch fit in? Is it a sign or is it only a symptom?

To explain sign a bit further, it can be thought of as something the doctor has found that does not depend on the patient's voice or behavior, and something an actor on a stage could not pretend to have.

The patient may wince when touched and pull away. Is that a sign or a symptom? Most doctors will record the fact, for instance, "winced when touched," without worrying too much about which category he'll place this finding. However, if pushed, he will probably state that "wincing" may indicate pain was caused, or that his hand was cold, or that the patient was apprehensive and frightened of his touch—therefore, it is a symptom, not a sign. This wincing may be extremely important; it may be the only abnormal feature of the examination, but it requires evaluation and interpretation to determine if it's of significance in making the diagnosis.

Doctors will often use the word "complaint." Their typical opening question to the patient is, "What are you complaining of?" Despite its routine use, this question is not only poor grammar, it's also misleading and likely to be answered by the irritated patient with, "Doctor, I never complain. I'm here because of this pain." There are many, more appropriate opening questions a doctor could use.

Subjective and Objective

Understanding the difference between these terms is essential to understanding the doctor-patient relationship in fibromyalgia.

The patient is the "subject." It is the patient who is talking about herself, using the pronoun "I."

From the viewpoint of all other persons outside the patient, she is viewed (don't take offense!) as an "object." This can most readily, and least offensively, be understood from the now-out-of-fashion grammatical terms in which each clause was required to have a subject and an object as well as a verb. In the sentence, "I lift the box," "I" is the subject, and "box" is the object. In another sense, when the pronoun "I" is in use, the statement is subjective. When the word "you" comes into use, it's no longer subjective.

The absolute essential importance in understanding the differences between subjective and objective is that it provides the key to understanding the controversy over the reality, or otherwise, of the fibromyalgia condition. Doctors expect that when a patient produces a symptom, they can match it with a sign. If the patient says, "This is where I hurt," then there should be a lump or a deformity, a change in temperature or in skin color, something different on the x-ray, or some abnormality in the lab reports. That is to say, diligent examination or testing will produce a sign for the doctor to match against the symptom. The terms "subjective" and "objective" can be married so a conclusion regarding the cause of the symptoms can be made. This is known in our inevitable and all-pervasive jargon as a diagnosis—derived from the Greek, and meaning "through knowledge."

The Importance of Marrying Signs to Symptoms

In attempting to arrive at a diagnosis, the doctor will take a history and perform a physical examination.

"History" involves asking the patient questions about her problem and anything that might be considered important in understanding the problem. Reasonably, it could be called a "verbal examination" and is entirely a word process. It is generally undertaken while the patient is still clothed; there is no touching involved. It is often said, if not for the considerable importance attached to the observation of behavior, the actual details of the history could be taken over the telephone.

"Physical examination" is the part that requires physical contact between the patient and the examiner; some of this is a request for the patient to perform certain activities while being watched, such as movements of the limb and spine, and much of the examination does not require any touching.

There is a tendency for the word "complete" to creep in here. If "complete" is taken to mean "everything," then obviously there is no such thing as a history in which every conceivable question was posed or an examination in which every conceivable test was performed. "Full" is a more appropriate term to use.

When the positive features of the history and the elicited physical signs can be matched, when subjective and objective details can be married, and the doctor is able to make a diagnosis and formulate a treatment plan—everyone has done his part. The patient has provided the doctor with evidence he can use—and the doctor has satisfied the patient and himself because he now responds with a statement of belief that he has subjective, physical, and scientific evidence to support his conclusions.

But what if there are "complaints"—lots of subjective symptoms—but no signs or objective findings to marry up with the subjective? That is our present situation in dealing with fibromyalgia—a multitude of severe subjective symptoms, but a total absence of objective signs.

If Anne Hathaway had suffered fibromyalgia—and who knows, maybe she did—Shakespeare might well have said, "Aye, there's the rub."

WHO HAS PAIN?

Everyone will have his or her own idea of the meaning of the word "pain," but when it comes to a discussion, it's commonly found that each person's ideas, based perhaps on personal experiences, may not be the same as those held by others.

Doctors, professors, biologists, and the like are no different. It has required a conference, or several conferences, to come up with a definition of pain, which still doesn't satisfy everyone. And then, of course, there is a burgeoning multiplicity of subcategories.

The International Association for the Study of Pain, a generally recognized authority, defined pain as "An unpleasant sensory and emotional experience associated with actual or potential tissue damage, or described in terms of such damage" (Merskey 1994). This definition provides for the acceptance of pain related to actual damage of a part of the body (tissue) and that it is also associated with emotions. It is widely accepted by those who research the cause and engage in the treatment of pain, but it is far from being all-encompassing, nor does it satisfy all the people all the time (Mailis-Gagnon 2005).

Much of our problem with fibromyalgia lies in the above definition. This is not due to the definition itself, since the experts who phrased it were well aware of the nature of fibromyalgia, but due to a misreading or misunderstanding.

In most painful conditions, tissue damage is there for the eyes to see—a fracture, a burn, childbirth, rheumatoid arthritis. Then there are those instances where tissue damage is clearly occurring but not visible—such as a heart attack or appendicitis. All these instances are accepted without question by family and the general public as real causes of pain.

Then there are invisible causes where no tissue damage is known to occur, such as a severe, short-term headache or pain with menstrual periods. These are common conditions, everyone is aware of them, and for the most part everyone will accept them as real.

But what about pain that's all over or pain that's not associated with an easily understood, single part of the body, such as the brain or the womb? Pain that's not short term? That has nothing to show for itself? Nothing to help family and friends to explain it? No visible marks? No distortions? That is how we find fibromyalgia.

Some further definitions, or putting pains into categories, are required. It has been common practice to describe pain as either acute or as chronic. Most persons using these terms would know the intended meaning, but those on the other side of the communication barrier might not.

"Acute" is often misinterpreted by the general public as meaning "severe," while, in fact, doctors use it to mean "it has recently happened," without any reference to its severity or danger to the patient. A sudden heart attack is an acute condition, but then, so is a sore throat—they've both recently started and, at the time of first treatment, are of short duration. If the heart attack degenerates into heart failure, the heart failure would also be called acute. If the heart failure persists for months, then it becomes labeled as chronic.

How many months between acute and chronic? It's a matter of personal taste, usually not controversial, generally obvious to all that the condition is not getting better, that it is persisting. For its simplicity of understanding, many clinicians now prefer the use of the concept of "persistent" pain instead of the vagueness of the word "chronic" (Sessle 2007).

But does chronic mean permanent? Does it mean it will never get better?

Yes, that's usually the way the word is used, but it doesn't mean the condition is beyond useful treatment. It doesn't mean the symptoms cannot be suppressed with appropriate therapy. But, in general terms, if the correct diagnosis has been made, it does mean the condition will be with you forever. Perhaps an exception needs to be made to recognize the value of the surgeon. Certain chronic conditions can be removed altogether by an operation, for instance, chronic inflammation of the gallbladder. But despite a surgeon's hard-learned skills, even after surgery, most conditions are ameliorated or relieved but are not abolished by surgical treatment.

Is all pain the same, just happening in different places, at different times, to different degrees? Can all pains be squeezed into one category, as though they have all come out of the same mold? Easy answer—no, they can't. And once we accept that all pains are not the same, then we can begin to understand the basis of some of the less obvious causes of pain. Once again, we resort to categories to explain this.

It's easy to accept that pain can be categorized by how long it's been felt or whether it's acute or chronic. It's also easy to say where it's located, the leg or the head. However, it's a little more difficult to put pain into a "severity" category since doctors rely heavily on what the sufferer says about it. But what about the origin of the pain and its cause? This is where the term "organic" came into use. The pain the doctor heard about was coming from one of the body's organs—the heart, the gallbladder, the uterus—or involved the fracture or the burn. As the Staples slogan goes, "That was easy." But the practice of medicine isn't easy. How should we label the pains that don't come from a specific organ?

The easy solution is to call them "nonorganic," which in its own way seems correct enough, but "easy and obvious" is nearly always the route to perdition, and "nonorganic" became "You're telling me it's all in my head, Doctor?" And so we developed a more complicated set of words to describe the origins of different types of pain (Woolf 1999; Woda 2005).

Organic became either somatic or visceral—somatic from the Greek word for body, and applied to the body's frame, muscles, and bones; visceral from the Latin, implying the entrails and involving pain carried from the inner organs by a set of nerves, different from those transmitting somatic pain.

This brings us to the pain whose cause cannot be seen. Here the term "neuropathic" has been devised for pain that is initiated or caused by an abnormality of function that lies within the nervous system. That is to say, it is not merely pain transmitted by the nervous system from elsewhere in the body, but pain that originates within the nervous system, which is then interpreted by the owner of that nervous system as vaguely located all over the body. "I hurt everywhere," they report.

It is the "all-over," the "everywhere," that is so difficult for the uninitiated to understand but that is fundamental to the clinician arriving at her diagnosis of fibromyalgia.

WHAT IS MEANT BY FIBROMYALGIA SYNDROME?

Defined as "a group of symptoms constantly associated in a particular disease and together presenting a characteristic picture of that disease or condition," the term "syndrome" first appeared in English in 1541 in Copeland's translation of Galen (Skinner 1961).

Syndrome in Terms of Fibromyalgia

There were numerous attempts to define the elusive characteristics and disputed nature of fibromyalgia. It was variously described as a disorder characterized primarily by widespread pain, decreased pain threshold, sleep disturbance, fatigue, and psychological distress.

It was diagnosed on the basis of widespread pain, interpreted by some as a decreased pain threshold to palpation, and by various characterizing symptoms, all of them present at the same time.

Fibromyalgia was called a disorder of "pain modulation" (Smythe 1979; Moldofsky 1982; Simons and Travell 1983; Yunus 1992), a "disorder of pain amplification" (Smythe 1979), and the "irritable everything syndrome" (Smythe 1985). It could be described as a syndrome in which not only pain, but all sensations, appeared to be magnified.

In 1981, Yunus listed some lesser-associated symptoms and required the reporting of at least three of these to confirm the patient's diagnosis as fibromyalgia. They were:

- Symptoms affected by physical activity; and/or climate; and/or anxiety and stress
- Poor sleep; generalized fatigue; chronic headache; irritable colon
- Subjective sensation of edema; sleep derangement

For purposes of research, an involved and experienced group of workers in the fibromyalgia field sought a consensus and arrived at an agreed definition in 1990. Their goal was to have generally accepted criteria for research purposes. It was not their intention to develop an impenetrable barrier between those who did and those who did not have the syndrome. To the expressed regret of specialists in this field, however, that is what it has become (Winfield 2007). Their published consensus, under the aegis of the American College of Rheumatology (ACR), required that to meet the diagnosis, the patient must have suffered widespread pain continuously for three months and had a specified number of specific areas of tenderness.

There is now general agreement that fibromyalgia is a syndrome of widespread pain. Commented on by Yunus and others before the ACR definition, numerous other symptoms are frequently associated with fibromyalgia, which may include sleep disturbance, fatigue, and stiffness. Although separate from widespread, four-quadrant pain, the only other issue considered by the ACR group to be essential to the definition is the "tender point" count. The actual number of painful tender points correlates strongly with the degree of psychologic distress.

It is found, in addition to the wide distribution of pain, there is also a pain magnification process. This results in a pain that in normal health would be considered as only mild, but in fibromyalgia it is often perceived as very severe.

Associated with the change in pain threshold is an unexpected increase in the distribution of pain, which becomes wider and more generalized. The extent of the pain is often surprising and may suggest the diagnosis, but when patients with widespread complaints consult clinicians who are not aware of this diagnostic feature in fibromyalgia, the diagnosis they arrive at may depend on the specific clinician chosen (Wolfe 1995).

At the Temple of Delphi in Greece, there is an obelisk symbolizing the central navel of the earth. Russell (2004) draws an analogy between a statement made by the Delphi oracle and the rigid manner in which this ACR definition has been employed; certainly, the ACR statement has become the center of the world for fibromyalgia definitions. But whereas the Delphic oracular statements were so generalized anything could be read into them, the ACR statement has been so rigid that not enough can be read into it—something never intended by its proponents.

Because of legal, insurance, disability, and various other issues, however, the question of whether a patient has fibromyalgia must be answered with an unhesitating yes or no. This, perhaps, explains why the ACR criteria have been so rigidly employed. Wolfe, a coauthor of the original 1990 research criteria, urged in 2003 to "stop using the ACR criteria in the clinic."

Writing on behalf of a group of physicians actively caring for fibromyalgia patients in the United States and Canada, Russell (2004) drew attention to the original purpose of the ACR 1990 definition, which was created to guide the uniform selection of patients to standardize research in the field of fibromyalgia. The new submission of this group works toward a clinical definition for use in community medical practice. Based on the collective experience gained in the treatment of their twenty thousand fibromyalgia patients, they designated the phrase "Canadian Clinical Working Case Definition of the Fibromyalgia Syndrome." They gave credit to previous work, such as that of Yunus—who suggested attaching importance to the numerous concomitant symptoms experienced by the patient with fibromyalgia and recognizing a wider range of symptoms than merely the "widespread pain," although this was, and remains, an undisputed major criterion to the diagnosis. Additional clinical symptoms are not required for the *research classification* but are important to the clinician, as Yunus had suggested in 1989, and are most certainly important to the patient. The two compulsory pain criteria adopted from the ACR 1990 standards are merged with "Additional Clinical Symptoms and Signs" to expand the classification of the fibromyalgia syndrome into a Clinical Working Case Definition, described in more detail in chapter 3.

HOW IS FIBROMYALGIA DIAGNOSED?

Client versus Patient

For an unknown period, at least as far back as Middle English, medical doctors have referred to the persons for whom they were providing care as "patients." The word is of French origin, referring, initially at least, in both languages, to a person who had patience. Now in French a "patient" is either someone about to be executed or about to undergo a surgical procedure (one has to wonder at the connection). In French, a doctor may refer to those for whom he provides care in his office as his clients, more usually in the hospital as *les malades*. Only recently have Anglophone medical doctors been under pressure to refer to their patients as "clients," a term we have always associated with commerce. But then, we're also being discouraged from allowing ourselves to be addressed as "doctors," instead being encouraged to use the preferred term "health-care providers," perhaps to keep our egos in proportion. Many therapists will use the term "clients," but most medical doctors cling to the old-fashioned "patients," and we will use that term throughout this book.

Complaint

Complaint is a word all doctors use, and many patients, not surprisingly, find objectionable. Probably the word has an origin in "lamentation," and in *doctor-speak,* "What are your complaints?" means "Tell me your troubles." It doesn't mean "Tell me whom you don't like."

Most of us were taught to ask as our leading question, "What's your complaint?" Not unreasonably, we're teaching our students now to phrase their opening question rather differently. We have yet to go to the commercial, "How can I help you?" but perhaps we should. As it stands, the first question posed is going to be directed at the matter concerning the patient, in whatever phraseology it's couched.

Wolfe, an old hand in the world of fibromyalgia, observed (1995) that the patient frequently has many issues (which, in *doctor-speak*, is read "complaints") but knows the specialist he has been sent to consult with deals exclusively in one area of the body or one type of disease and so mentions only that one. As a consequence, the patient gets a treatment program directed only at the one complaint mentioned. The patient needs to be sure the doctor understands, and the doctor should not need to be reminded of this—the first complaint mentioned is not necessarily the only significant one. For this reason, the most significant aspect of the patient-doctor encounter is verbal. Physical signs matter, but the physical can wait. Verbal symptoms matter most.

Who Will Make the Diagnosis?

There is a very wide range of persons involved in medical care, and the more difficult a condition is to diagnose and treat, the more varieties of therapists and caregivers the patient is likely to have sought. A survey of patients with fibromyalgia, employing the medium of a voluntarily completed questionnaire conducted via the Internet, not surprisingly, showed this spectrum. More than four out of ten patients had received the diagnosis of fibromyalgia from a rheumatologist; two out of ten from a family physician; one of ten from a general internist; and the balance of 10 percent from a mix of other practitioners, including psychiatrists, gynecologists, and various non-MDs working in the healthcare field (Bennett 2007).

History

If you're trying to get hired for a job, the process of questioning by the personnel officer, today called human resources (HR), is known as an "interview." If you're at the end of the anatomy or biology course, it's called an "oral." If you're trying to get your doctorate and you're presenting your dissertation, it's called a "defense." If the litigation lawyer wants information, it's known as "discovery." If you're a prisoner, it's called "interrogation." Varying only with the profession, all these terms mean the same thing—a session of systematic and close questioning to uncover the information the professional needs, so he may form his opinion about you.

For the doctor it's called "taking a history" and ideally does not have the intimidating features of an interrogation, nor is it as cold sweat–provoking as defending a thesis. The purpose in taking a history is to have revealed every issue that might be of importance in making the correct diagnosis, perhaps more than one concurrent diagnoses, and to avoid making a wrong diagnosis (Greenhalgh 2001).

The process of arriving at a diagnosis varies slightly, depending on who's sitting on the other side of the table from you, the patient. If it's a family physician who interviews the patient, she may start with no further information than the few words taken by the office receptionist, "Hurts everywhere."

Should it be a consultant rheumatologist, she may have received an extensive report from the referring family physician or from a hospital-based physician.

Although the physician may have an indicator pointing to the diagnosis that she eventually reaches, ideally she will start with an open mind; to jump to conclusions is a sure way to miss important issues. The conclusion might very well be correct. For an experienced doctor it usually will be, but since fibromyalgia is a *syndrome*, there may be a lot more to discover and to uncover than is at first apparent. The skillful examiner draws information from the patient that she had not expected to relate or did not think relevant, or feared might be relevant, but for any number of reasons was reluctant to disclose.

The patient should be allowed to tell her own story but given some guidance to stick to the point. We are all aware of the two extremes: the person who perhaps out of deference, perhaps insecurity, will offer nothing voluntarily, and the opposite, who gushes inconsequential information and consciously or unconsciously skirts around what really matters.

For every issue, the "six little words" must be applied: when, where, why, who, what, and how. It takes time. Each statement the patient makes should be analyzed and the answers broken down fully until the import of each answer is completely understood. It's often aggravating to all concerned, but only by probing is the depth of a considerable problem elucidated. And if the patient does have fibromyalgia, she does have a considerable problem that's both wide and deep.

If the doctor is doing her job correctly, the history-taking process will be lengthy. It will be searching. It will likely reveal more than you ever expected to discuss or even recognize about yourself. For with fibromyalgia, the history has an importance not so essential in conditions that are more self-revealing in their diagnosis, such as chickenpox or a broken leg. Fibromyalgia does not come with any conveniently obvious external features, so diagnosis and treatment are heavily dependent on a painstaking and detailed history.

The term "complete history" is sometimes encountered, and is, of course, nonsense. There is always another question that might have been asked, another canary in the bushes that might have been pursued; the objective is to pursue all issues that are relevant and to leave no stone unturned that might reveal hidden gold.

Sometimes a line of questioning, verging on personal or psychically painful subjects, runs into an obstruction. The experienced physician knows when not to pursue an issue right at that moment, but instead return to the same issue at a later time. Typically, when a patient is reluctant to discuss an issue, it may be the one of maximum relevance and significance to the diagnosis and management of her problem.

Physical Examination—General

When the diagnosis is obvious (let's once more take the example of a broken leg), the examination is of the "relevant part," namely, the broken leg, and whatever else is needed to ensure safe treatment—for instance, the heart and lungs to ensure safety under anesthetic. But fibromyalgia is not an obvious condition.

The physician is presented with a patient who can say nothing more diagnosis defining than, "I hurt everywhere, all the time," and a great deal of effort, for which read time, must be expended in the physical examination.

There are two components to this physical examination, known in abbreviated form as the "PE." The physician must perform both a generalized and a specific examination. Although specific features in the PE point to a diagnosis of fibromyalgia, there is also a large "exclusion" element. The features revealed while taking the history will point to certain parts of the body as the cause of the problem and certain suspicions will be aroused. Nevertheless, the examination must cover all areas, not merely those cited as a concern.

Ancillary Testing

A very clear statement can be made without fear of contradiction. As of now, there are no laboratory tests, no imaging methods, no electrical tests—no tests of any kind—that define fibromyalgia.

Put simply, your physician will order tests, but don't expect these tests to tell you whether you do or do not have fibromyalgia. Your physician will order a number of tests to exclude other conditions, but ruling in or out these other conditions does not rule in or rule out a diagnosis of fibromyalgia.

Is the Diagnosis Easily Made?

Because of the lack of specific characterizing features, and the wide spectrum of medical problems covered by pain and fatigue, it is unusual for a patient to be diagnosed with fibromyalgia the first time she expresses her problems to a health care provider. One self-reported survey showed that a quarter of the patients had sought diagnostic help from more than six persons, half from more than three, before they arrived at the definitive diagnosis of fibromyalgia (Bennett 2007).

Even when the diagnosis of fibromyalgia had been awarded, a quarter of these patients remained in doubt whether their physicians construed the condition of fibromyalgia as truly legitimate.

WHO HAS FIBROMYALGIA?

Demography is the study of human populations and how they change. We turn to it to ask two questions: Who gets fibromyalgia? Who has fibromyalgia?

Chronic Pain

In the United States, the symptoms of chronic pain and chronic fatigue are surprisingly widespread and are reportedly found especially in women and in persons designated as "of lower socioeconomic status" (Winfield 2007). Reported figures are:

- Regional pain (limited to one area of the body): 20%
- Chronic fatigue: 20%
- Widespread pain (throughout the body): 11%
- Fibromyalgia according to ACR criteria: 3–5% in females; 0.5–1.6% in males

The problem of chronic pain is international. Blotman (2006) reports numerous studies from Spaeth and others:

Author	Year	Country	Type of practice	Number of consultations	Pain as reason %	Musculo-skeletal %
Hasselstrom	2002	Sweden	Primary care	6,890	28	66
Mantyselka	2001	Finland	Outpatient	5,646	40	50
Willweber-Strumpf	2000	Germany	Internists	900	36	>50
Gureje	1998	14 countries	Primary care	5,447	22	>50

Blotman refers to a study conducted in South Africa by Lydell (1992) on a simple rural population that had not experienced education. There was little evidence of widespread pain, but over 3 percent were found to have "tender points" as outlined in the ACR criteria.

The Overall Impression of Who Has Fibromyalgia

It is reported as occurring anywhere from four to nine times as frequently in the female sex and the higher figure is the one more commonly given. It is universally agreed that the condition is seen most frequently in women between twenty and fifty years of age. The average age of a woman diagnosed with fibromyalgia is in her late forties, which does not take into account the age of onset of the condition and is much more difficult to specify (Wolfe 1995; Winfield 2007; Gilliland 2007).

It is also known that fibromyalgia is found in adolescence and, in some cases, in childhood (Buskila 1993; Winfield 2007).

What Proportion of the Population Suffer Fibromyalgia?

This is a difficult question to answer intelligently. If a survey was taken to determine the frequency of drivers' accidents, it would make little sense to include persons who never drove a car; to compare the iconic little old lady who drives to church once a week with the commercial traveler who's on the road every day would also make little sense. The figure we need is the "at risk" population, generally considered to be a female who has reached child-bearing age. The figures we have vary from 2 percent (Wolfe 1995) of the whole population to 10 percent of the "at risk" population (Croft 1994).

The National Arthritis Data Workgroup states they have to rely on small studies of uncertain applicability but estimate there are five million persons in the United States with fibromyalgia (Lawrence 2008).

In Ontario, White (1999) reported 3.3 percent of noninstitutionalized adults had diagnostic evidence of fibromyalgia. In a consultant rheumatologist's practice, fibromyalgia is reported as the second most common condition seen, and it may account for as many as half of the patients registered in the office (White 1995). Family physicians may find that approximately 8 percent of their patients have fibromyalgia. In a specialized rheumatology or physiatry practice, however, as many as 15 percent of evaluated patients have fibromyalgia.

This incidence implies that on average one of every ten patients evaluated in a medical practice has fibromyalgia. Over the past twenty years, fibromyalgia has emerged as a leading cause of office visits to rheumatologists, both in its primary form and as an accompaniment of other rheumatic disorders (Bennett 2007).

The condition is increasingly recognized and diagnosed in younger persons (Clark 1998). In a survey in Israel of randomly selected schoolchildren, over 6 percent met the diagnostic criteria for fibromyalgia (Buskila 1993).

To bring the incidence into perspective with a condition that most persons have known in a family member or a friend, fibromyalgia is reported as more common than rheumatoid arthritis by factors of anywhere from two to five times as frequent.

It is increasingly evident that the fibromyalgia syndrome represents a significant challenge in view of its high prevalence, the common occurrence of other conditions found in association with it, and the reported frustration experienced with the inadequacies of currently available treatment.

Fibromyalgia Is an International Condition

If reports of fibromyalgia emanated only from the United States, one might perhaps think it related to the nature of the healthcare system. If they also come from Canada, where there is a totally different healthcare system, then perhaps fibromyalgia is just a North American phenomenon. And, if coming from the United Kingdom, perhaps stretching it now, it's due to heritage. But if fibromyalgia is widely reported from other countries, more than the three mentioned, we have to accept it as an internationally occurring condition, not related to heritage or health systems. It is, in fact, a global condition.

Researchers from around the world have reported the incidence of fibromyalgia (Gilliland 2007), and it's suggested the condition is encountered in Scandinavia even more frequently than in the United States. Epidemiological studies report a fibromyalgia prevalence of between 2 and 7 percent in most nations (Bennett 2007), with the standard female-to-male ratio of approximately nine to one.

No racial predilection has been shown to exist in fibromyalgia. Researchers have reported the condition in all ethnic groups and cultures, but the experience reported by Lydell in rural South Africa where he found tender points, and not widespread pain, is perplexing.

Blotman, referring also to Wolfe (1994), records the international prevalence of fibromyalgia:

- Campbell (1993), Oregon, USA, 5.7% fibromyalgia, consulting internist
- Hartz (1987), Pennsylvania, USA, 2.1% fibromyalgia, general medicine practice
- Miller (1987), Switzerland, 7.5% fibromyalgia, hospital consulting general practice
- Alarcón-Segovia (1993), Mexico, 17.5% fibromyalgia, rheumatology practice
- Calabozo (1990), Spain, 10.7% fibromyalgia, rheumatology practice
- Jacobsson (1989), Sweden, 1.1% fibromyalgia, general population, age 50–70 years
- Mäkelä (1991), Finland, 0.75% fibromyalgia, general population
- Forseth (1992), Norway, 10.5% fibromyalgia, women 20–49 years (questioned)
- Walewski (1992), Poland, 4.4% fibromyalgia, older general population; 13% women
- Lydell (1992), South Africa, 3.2% fibromyalgia, if absence of "widespread pain" is ignored
- Buskila (1993), Israel, 6.2% fibromyalgia, children 9–15 years
- Raspe (1993), Germany, 2.3% fibromyalgia, adults 25–74 years
- Wolfe (1995), Kansas, USA, 3.4% fibromyalgia, women all ages; 7% women aged 60–79 years
- Farooqi (1998), Pakistan, 1.5% overall fibromyalgia

Validity of Statistics

Although the general impression of the fibromyalgia patient is a white, middle-aged female, it's not easy to obtain reliable, meaningful statistics on any subject—medical or any other. In interpreting statistics, it's necessary to consider the source and the means of obtaining the information.

There is no such thing as a "requirement to report" in fibromyalgia, so although we might know who has been documented in a survey and who was included, we have no way of determining who has been missed. This brings to mind the age-old conundrum, "How do you know what you don't know?" Therefore, if anything, the reported prevalence of the condition is likely to be underestimated, due only in part to incorrect medical or psychiatric diagnoses (Russell 2004).

Is the self-reported information in answer to an appeal? Was the appeal limited to those who use a computer? Was the source a university clinic, thereby eliminating all those who don't go to such clinics? Was it taken as a cross-section of a specialist consultant's practice? Or taken in a community where the population is predominantly of one ethnic group or of one socioeconomic group? Were the ACR criteria for diagnosis meticulously observed, or did the diagnostician employ his own set of rules? Broadly speaking, as stated above, it is probable that available numbers are, if anything, underreported since those diagnosed are included and those yet to be diagnosed, or actually misdiagnosed with another condition but in fact suffering from fibromyalgia are, obviously, not going to be included.

Are There Characterizing Features of a Fibromyalgia Patient?

Robert Bennett and his associates (2007) carried out an extensive survey to answer this question. The survey has the strength of representing the private responses of twenty-five hundred persons suffering fibromyalgia. It has, however, the weaknesses (well understood by the authors) of giving information only from persons who used computers to access the Web site of the National Fibromyalgia Association. Responses were received from each state and forty-six responses from a wide range of other countries. Logically, the respondents do not include persons who do not have or cannot use, or do not choose to use, a computer; this may well introduce a socioeconomic bias, and given that the study was predominantly in the United States, "socioeconomic" might translate, to an extent, into "racial." The statistics, therefore, should be considered to represent a cross-section of twenty-five hundred persons with fibromyalgia, and should only with caution be considered to be representative of the condition throughout the world.

- The respondents were predominantly middle-aged Caucasian females (96.8% female), 75% of whom had experienced fibromyalgia symptoms for more than 4 years.
- Only 3.2% of the respondents were male (not representative of the usually reported ratio F:M = 9:1).
- Age distribution was slightly skewed toward older individuals (mean = 47.3 ± 10.68; range: 17 to 77 years).
- Respondents were moderately overweight, having gained approximately 50 pounds since they were 18.
- Just over 50% of the respondents had a household income of between $20,000 and $80,000.

Where Does the Fibromyalgia Patient Find Information?

A purpose of this book is to draw attention to the massive amount of incorrect and otherwise misleading information on the subject of fibromyalgia. Bennett and his associates sought to find where fibromyalgia patients obtained their information, but once again the fount of the survey was a nonprofit organization devoted to the dissemination of correct information.

They found patients obtained information about fibromyalgia from:

- family physicians (45.8%)
- rheumatologists (43.6%)
- internists (23.1%)
- massage therapists (20.3%)
- chiropractors (20.2%)
- physical therapists (14.4%)
- mental health professionals (psychiatrists, psychologists, social workers) (13.1%)
- pharmacists (7.8%)
- nurse practitioners, physician assistants (7.6%)
- nurses (5.3%)
- nutritionists/dietitians (4.4%)
- gynecologists (2.9%)

In addition to healthcare professionals, respondents received information from a number of other sources, including:

- National Fibromyalgia Association (sponsor of the survey) (70%)
- General media (41.6%)

- Arthritis Foundation (35.2%)
- Internet message boards (23.4%)
- Internet chat rooms (12.5%)
- Local support groups (12%)
- Informal sources (e.g., friends) (32.6%)
- Health food store (13.6%)
- Family member (10.7%)

CHAPTER THREE

HOW IS FIBROMYALGIA DIAGNOSED?

WHAT SHOULD BE ASKED IN THE HISTORY AND WHY?

In a remote area of the Canadian north, I received an elementary lesson in opening a conversation with a patient.

"What are you complaining of?" Standard opening question, as taught in the best medical schools.

"Never complain, Doctor. I never likes to complain."

Rethink the exercise. "Well, what brought you here?"

"Came in a boat, Doctor. Jim Petty's dory. He brung me. 'Long with the fish."

Rethink again. "Are you sick?"

"No, Doctor. Thanks be to God, I've not been troubled by that for goin' on four year. That don't bother me no more." *Sick* turns out to be a local euphemism for menstrual periods.

And so it went on. Until at last the right question was asked, "How can I help you?"

"You gotta to fill this up, Doctor," and the welfare form was pushed across the desk.

Taking a history is asking the patient questions about her problem and anything that might be considered important in understanding her problem—it could be called a "verbal examination." It is generally undertaken while the patient is still clothed and the discussion must be structured.

Although we are dealing with fibromyalgia, to retain a balanced point of view, one should consider the taking of the history as it would, under ideal circumstances, be conducted by the first contact physician. Wolfe (1995) described the patient who said, "When I go to see a doctor I tell them about the pain that's worst. If I tell them about everything, they think I'm nuts," which led Wolfe to suppose that if facial pain is the worst today, then the patient is diagnosed with a temporomandibular joint disorder; if neck or back pain is worst, he's sent to a neurosurgeon or an orthopedist.

This is exactly what happens when the patient is rushed (the usual state of affairs in any medical office), doesn't want to "bother" the doctor, and is embarrassed about the seemingly vague nature and the multiplicity of her problems. An experienced examiner will sense this.

But you can't count on the doctor pushing the questions, and you must be prepared to tell all. Warn the receptionist when you schedule the appointment that this is not an emergency, but you do need enough face time with the doctor so that she can elicit the full details of your history. And come with your story organized. It's a two-way street!

Patients with fibromyalgia do significantly better when they receive a comprehensive, individualized treatment regimen than when they do not, and a thorough history is the first step toward developing one. Although insurance reimbursement and the other infrastructures are often barriers to giving patients the necessary time, a thorough and detailed history saves time in the long run, reduces the potential for litigation, helps prevent incorrect diagnosis, and eliminates inappropriate or unnecessary treatments. Without a thorough history, it is impossible to develop a complete list of the comorbid (simultaneous) illnesses. Inevitably, an inadequate history results in incomplete and often inappropriate treatment (Gilliland 2007).

The Essential Questions

Why
Who
When
Where
How
What

Why is the history taken?
Who asks the questions?
When does it occur?

Where is it taken?
How is it conducted?
What are the questions?

Who answers the questions?

How long does it last?

Who else is present?

Dressed or undressed?

Why Is the History Taken?

Fibromyalgia is a condition with the most widespread physical, emotional, and social ramifications, and there is little about the patient that would not be relevant to the full understanding of her condition. The underlying purpose of the history is to reveal every issue that might be relevant to:

- making the correct primary diagnosis
- diagnosing other concurrent conditions
- initiating treatment and further care.

In summary, the hallmark of the history is a gathering of essential and accurate information that can be used together with the findings of the physical examination to make decisions about diagnostic and therapeutic interventions (Hills 2006).

Who Asks the Questions?

The depth of inquiry, the mechanism of obtaining information, the time spent, and the personnel involved will alter from place to place and practitioner to practitioner.

In our research project, we have the luxury of time. We can spend as much time with each patient as needed. We have the luxury of appropriate ancillary personnel who can, as required, assist in taking the details of the history. You cannot expect this in a solo practitioner's office. In a university clinic, you don't get face time with the head honcho until lots of lesser fry have talked to you. Clinic staff may be as well trained and organized as one could hope to find, or the world being what it is, there may be some lesser level of perfection. It's probable that giving your history will start with a nurse, medical student, or junior resident. They may be wonderful, caring persons, or they may be working against the clock. It's your responsibility as a patient to see that your problems are not brushed aside and that they get recorded in as much detail as you believe relevant. But stand in the other guy's shoes and be reasonable.

Should There Be an Initial Self-Report?

We have all experienced the medical office where the receptionist, with one eye still on the computer monitor, says, "Here! Fill this out," as she hands you a form and you look for a place to sit in the overcrowded waiting room. Forms are best used for developing a brief, general overview and for research purposes when particular issues are to be documented and numerical comparisons required; statistics, unfortunately, are numerical, and attempts must be made to reduce the body's sensations to numbers. To keep in step with other workers and with no intention of reinventing the wheel, we will use the standardized forms and then expand on them.

If a diagnosis has not been established, a preliminary questionnaire might capture such routine information as the patient's address, age, workplace, insurance, and so on. It might briefly go into previous illnesses, childbirth, and operations; medications currently and recently taken; and any allergies to medications, foodstuffs, and so forth.

For a tentative diagnosis of fibromyalgia, all the questions relevant to every condition must be posed, but the patient may fill out more specific questionnaires. Doctors should acknowledge that patients easily get put off by extensive detail and demands. Forms should not be so detailed that a patient feels harried and wishes she'd never come to the doctor. Standardized forms applicable to fibromyalgia are a self-report form that incorporates visual analog (0–10) scales for pain and fatigue, the Modified Health Assessment Questionnaire, and the Fibromyalgia Impact Questionnaire (checklist of current symptoms). Obtained at the first visit, this information will be invaluable for the psychosocial assessment of pain and will aid with monitoring the response to therapy (Winfield 2007).

Who Answers the Questions?

If the patient is an adult, able to speak for herself, and of clear mind, then she should be the one to answer the questions posed on the form or by the doctor. If she is an adult and doesn't meet these stipulations, then whoever accompanies her (and she shouldn't have come alone) will *assist* in providing, rather than give directly, the answers. If the patient is a child, the same holds. She should be assisted to answer, but care should be taken to avoid putting answers in her mouth.

There are occasions when a husband will insist on answering all the questions for his wife, although she's the patient and of sound, if downtrodden, mind. I've been told at times, "She's my woman. I speak for her." This is not acceptable. In itself it may be a triggering factor in the fibromyalgia. Each case has to be dealt with tactfully on its own merits, but "I speak for her" is not acceptable.

Who Else Is Present?

Not only does it make good sense, but it may be a requirement of some registration bodies, that a female patient should be accompanied by another person of her choice. The physician doesn't have much choice after the fact in whom this might be. She, the physician, is not in a position to say, "I don't want you to bring that person with you."

To preempt an unpleasant situation, a routine should be arranged with the receptionist, or whoever books the appointments, so that the patient knows she is welcome to have another person to accompany her throughout the process, but it would be constructive if that other person were there to support the patient and not one who wished to dominate her.

Situations arise in which mothers won't let daughters speak for themselves, or husbands their wives; from time to time, there are well-meaning friends who believe it is their role to harass the doctor. Should such a situation arise, the interview should be terminated with tact and rearranged in a different manner.

That was the negative side. The plus side is the patient gains confidence in the presence of a trusted friend or relative and, particularly during the physical examination, is more at ease than she would be if this physician had never previously been visited. There are advantages in having at the interview the person with whom the patient sleeps, since several questions are directed at sleeping or issues that occur while sleeping. Possibly the more intimate details of sexual history and family relationships should be asked in a one-on-one interview at a later time when confidence and trust have been gained.

When? Where? How?

Every clinic and every physician has his or her own routine, but it would be highly unusual for a physical examination to occur prior to taking the history. Ideally, a fairly short, generalized history should be taken by a primary contact physician who doesn't suspect fibromyalgia until the physical examination and further general discussion that reveals fibromyalgia as a possibility; a second, longer interview would then be scheduled to take a full history. It cannot be overemphasized that, the more time spent taking the history, the more understanding will be gained of the patient's issues and the more value can be attached to her treatment program.

Solo practitioner? Primary care physician? Tertiary-level consultant? Community hospital clinic? University hospital clinic? Each will have a different routine. You may experience the luxury of sitting in a comfortable armchair, with your expensive physician on the other side of the coffee table, or you may be in a small cubicle talking to a young resident whose command of English is less than your own. Some degree of acceptance of a less-than-perfect ambience may be necessary on the patient's part, and she can comfort herself knowing that the medical staff of the not-very-opulent building would be just as happy as she if it were to be improved. Ambience is of less significance than warmth of interest and quality of care.

As a patient, you're entitled to a degree of warmth and interest from your physician. If you have fibromyalgia, you have a long road ahead of you and must walk it with someone who exhibits interest in what you have to say about yourself and a warmth of feeling about it. If you're convinced this is lacking, better go elsewhere. On the other hand, do not mistake the false enthusiasm of the professional salesperson—yes, Virginia, there are doctors who are selling themselves 24/7—for a real interest in you and your problems.

In all circumstances, taking the history is essentially question-and-answer time. It helps everyone if the patient answers the questions. All doctors run into patients who seem unable to focus—ask about their back, and they tell you about their foot; ask about their menstrual history, and they tell you about the pains of their first childbirth. It's frustrating. It's time consuming. It's a fact of life!

How Long Does It Last? Dressed or Undressed? What?

One thing you will know: it's not going to be over quickly, not if it's done properly. There's a lot to find out, one of the several reasons for employing a questionnaire.

Traditionally the interview, the taking of the history, is conducted before the patient is asked to undress and put on the skimpy gown with the ties missing. If you're told to undress before anyone has spoken to you, you might wonder about how much time is going to be spent on history taking. It's not an absolute no-no but would require an explanation.

A well-trained and experienced physician will start with an explanation of why the questions are posed, letting the patient understand that, with fibromyalgia, only a full understanding of the patient's medical and social background will suffice.

History of the Present Illness—The Presenting (Chief) Complaint

Traditionally the history starts with what is known to doctors either as the "chief complaint," or the "presenting complaint" (Hall 1998). It's hard to avoid that word "complaint," it's so ingrained, but bear with it.

There may well be coequal complaints. The patient may be uncertain which to her is the more prominent, but what's really important is that the history should not stop at the chief complaint (usually pain)—it should be extended to search for others (Wolfe 1995). The physician must, however, avoid treating the patient based only on this chief complaint, since a fluctuating pattern of the symptoms is common (Gilliland 2007). Premature decisions regarding treatment plans may lead to symptom chasing and render treatment ineffective.

In cases involving chronic pain, the consulting physician is often the last in a long string of healthcare professionals to encounter the patient. Although it may be complex and convoluted, the history often sheds light on the problems and may provide insight on how best to treat a patient with overwhelmingly complex medical issues (Hills 2006).

The questions should explore in depth the chief complaint by asking specific points about the patient's pain:

- Date of onset of the pain? Sudden or gradual? (A sudden onset may be associated with an incident and remembered exactly; a gradual onset is more difficult to place in time.)
- Trigger or causing event, including trauma?
- Location of the pain? Regional? Generalized? All over?
- If the pain is widespread, further questioning is appropriate: Right and left sides of the body? Above and below the waist? Along the axial skeleton?
- Progression of symptoms? Duration of pain? More than three months? (An ACR criterion for fibromyalgia diagnosis.)
- Character of the pain (without suggesting the words)? Migratory? Constant? Burning? Tender? Sore? Aching? Sharp? All of the above?
- Aggravating factors? Alleviating factors?

Major Secondary Complaints

Few patients with fibromyalgia have only one major problem—their difficulty lies in choosing which to discuss first. The physician should not attempt to force a list of "most important" and should be prepared for "coequals"; some attempt to determine relative severity and quality of symptoms is appropriate.

Each secondary complaint must be dissected as fully as the primary complaint. When did it start? Duration of these symptoms? Coexistence of symptoms?

And so on. It's important to get listed all the significant problems that the patient will volunteer and then to explore them. These are the issues brought to light by repeating the question, "Is there any other physical problem bothering you?"

Complete Search of All Systems for Other Physical Complaints— Systems Review

Once the patient's volunteered complaints are exhausted, the physician sets about a systematic inquiry to ensure the patient has not forgotten to mention other physical problems. Some problems the patient may have thought irrelevant; some may have been put aside because she thought the list was already too long; some she may have thought were too personal to discuss with a stranger. In medical jargon, the doctor makes a "systems inquiry." The word "system" implies various parts of the body, for instance, the cardiovascular system (heart and blood vessels), the respiratory system (windpipe and lungs), the alimentary system (gullet, stomach, intestine), and so on. It might equally well be interpreted as a systematic, all-embracing, nothing-overlooked inquiry, for that's what it's intended to be.

Solicited Symptoms (By Direct Questioning)

These are worded like a Senator McCarthy inquiry: "Do you have, or have you ever had, problems with . . . ?"

- fatigue
- head: headaches, memory, processing thoughts, etc.
- eyes, ears, mouth, teeth, jaw joint, face
- neck, upper back, lower back; morning stiffness
- arms, hands, legs, feet; pains in muscles or joints; morning stiffness
- heart and pulse
- chest and breathing
- stomach and digestion
- bowels and bowel habits
- urination
- menstruation; vaginal discharge or discomfort
- autonomic system: episodes of fainting, lightheadedness

Sleep

How long does it take you to fall asleep? How many times do you waken? Is it pain that causes you to waken? What do you do when you awaken? How do you feel when you first wake in the morning? (Your sleeping partner, if available, will be asked if you snore or kick while asleep.)

Emotional Issues

Fear, anger, guilt in relation to the condition
Psychological problems, for example, depression, anxiety, panic attacks

Social Issues

Alcohol, smoking, recreational drugs
Sexual activities
Exercise history, current exercise or other physical activities

Nutrition

Diet, weight gain or loss, measures taken to control weight
Caffeine, carbohydrates

Current Medications

Specifically, medications directed against fibromyalgia-type symptoms
Other medication (e.g., for diabetes, hypertension, etc.)

Allergies

To medication, to foodstuffs, seasonal, and so on
Precautions taken against allergies

Current Physical or Other Treatments Specifically Directed at Symptom Relief

Medication, prescribed and self-arranged
Therapy, prescribed and self-arranged

Activities of Daily Living

Feeding, grooming, bathing, dressing, and toileting; driving ability; and all activities fundamental to independence from the assistance of others

Past History as Related Directly to Current Issues

Consultations sought: From whom? When? Advice given? Whether followed? With what benefit?

Treatments given: When? By whom? With what benefit?

Diagnostic studies: Which? Where? When? What results?

Functional History

Characterizes the extent to which a disability may have resulted from an illness or a chronic disease; questions start at the beginning of your life, asking about childhood rearing and illnesses, then progress

Medical treatments, hospitalizations; surgical procedures

Pregnancy, childbirth experience(s); unintended miscarriages; intended abortions

Abuse (physical and/or mental), in childhood and/or as an adult

Accidents; comprehensive trauma history and response to earlier trauma

Emotional Stability

Do you still have self-confidence? Or have you surrendered to a feeling of helplessness?

Do you believe with help your situation can be improved? Or do you believe "I can't go on, I'm overwhelmed"?

Do you sincerely want to improve your situation? Or do you prefer the effects of secondary gain?

No longer having to look after others—it's their turn to look after me?

Family History

Was yours a happy childhood?

Siblings: How many? Health? Any with similar medical issues?

Parents: Relationship to parents? Their health? Any with similar medical issues?

Social History

Domestic situation (e.g., married, children)—the medical history and general health of individuals close to you (e.g., spouse) become important in planning treatment

Description of your home (e.g., ranch-style versus colonial); floor surfaces (e.g., carpet, rugs)

Degree of support at home, how much requested, how much needed, how much provided

Are there members in the household who don't believe in your pain?

Do you have support from outside the home?

Visit friends or a club? Do they come to visit you?

Education History

Was school a happy experience?

Do you have employable skills? Do you employ them?

Work History

These give a better understanding of the effects of your disability

What marketable skills do you possess? Remunerated employment and non-remunerated employment? Still possess? Still marketable?

Your competence with activities of daily living (ADL)

Your competence with instrumental activities of daily living (IADL), such as the preparation of meals, grocery shopping, household chores

Recreation History

Physical and nonphysical

Avocation: Your avocational pursuits may have no immediate bearing on rehabilitation services; however, the information obtained about your hobbies, recreation, and amusements may be turned to benefit in rehabilitation

What the History Reveals

I once heard a social worker explaining the true meaning of disability. "It's like a stone thrown into a pond," she said. "The medical problem is the stone. And then there are all the ripples it causes to spread over a previously tranquil surface—that's the disability."

The history of widespread pain will point to the diagnosis of fibromyalgia. Unlike most medical conditions, the objective is less a question of finding out what is wrong than finding out the effect of what is wrong. Attention must be given to what effect fibromyalgia has on the patient and her family. Therapy will be directed not only at relief of symptoms but also at alleviating the effect of those symptoms.

An attempt to start on a level playing field will be made by ascertaining what you, the patient, think about your own status:

- How do you view the various diagnoses you've previously been given?
- What confidence do you still have in the medical profession?
- What are your expectations?
- Will you accept anything less than total resolution of your problems?

THE PHYSICAL EXAMINATION

There are two aspects of the examination, an initial generalized total examination and one specific to fibromyalgia. Since so frequently other conditions are found accompanying fibromyalgia, and since it's always possible there may be present a totally unrelated and unexpected condition, a very thorough and extensive physical examination is required.

This begins in an informal manner from the time the physician (let's just accept him as a physician) first sees the patient and throughout the interview, the history-taking process. During this time, the physician gains an impression of the type of person he is dealing with, her attitude to her own life and her problems, her attitude to the health professions, and most important of all, her attitude toward recovery.

The formal part of the physical examination searches for diagnostic features and physical signs and intends to rule out various explanations for what is wrong. Although the physical examination is something that could be delegated to a person who had no knowledge of the patient's history that had just been given, it is more usual for the person who took the history also to perform the examination. In that way, clues given in the history toward diagnosis will be confirmed or refuted. The physician, of course, keeps his mind open to finding the totally unexpected and, for that reason, follows a time-honored routine in order that the unexpected will not be the unfound.

The normal findings are here passed over briefly, and the abnormal or the unusual are explored in greater depth; you know your doctor has found something unusual when he keeps going back to it. Gasps of surprise, muttered "Wow"s and "How about that!"s are expected to have been left behind in medical school.

General Examination

An explanation of terms in traditional use: "inspection" is looking at the patient, preferably not as in a meat market; "palpation" is feeling with the hands; "percussion" is tapping with the fingers; "auscultation" is listening with the ear, these days usually at a distance from the body aided by a stethoscope. What are known in the trade as vital signs (VS) may be taken by the doctor, but in most offices and clinics, they will have been noted by a nurse or an assistant. They compose the standard measurements of height, weight, temperature, blood pressure, pulse, and breathing. With "inspection," the physician initially gains an overall impression, pretty much what you'd get sitting in your own home, looking at a friend across the table. What is her appearance? Does she look ill? Worried? Frightened? Aggressive? Angry? How is she dressed? Her makeup? All of which may or may not be relevant, and none of it goes to a judgment of character or personality, only to medical issues. This is sometimes misjudged by a dissatisfied patient (yes, they do exist), but the prudent physician knows not to record anything that could in hindsight be considered an adverse or a derogatory judgment.

Questions the Physician Asks Himself about His Patient

What is her behavior? Is she brisk and cooperative? Does she have difficulty following directions? Does she seem to understand or not understand what is explained to her? Is she in tears when she talks about herself? Is she willing to talk about personal issues in a forthright manner, or does she evade them? How briskly does she move?

Who is with her in the waiting room? Does she have a bevy of friends running around her? Is she alone? Does she have her husband with her? How does she interrelate with the staff and the other patients in the waiting room?

Does she wear or use aids? A neck collar? Crutches? Walking canes? Does she spread her crutches across the floor so everyone trips over them?

What is her posture, seated and standing? Does it indicate pain? Does she show what we call "pain behaviors"? Does she limp? Does she seem to have trouble with balance?

There are innumerable details that the physician observes in his first appraisal, all of which go to create an impression, none of which make an irrevocable judgment.

Mental Status

While taking the history, the physician will have formed an opinion on your mental status. If there appear to be difficulties with memory or thought processing, a common problem in fibromyalgia, he might have you undertake a few additional simple tests, and there is a rapid "mini-mental" set of questions that he might use.

Neurologic Examination

Once again, an opinion on much of normal neurologic functioning is obtained by observation, but if there appears to be a problem with gait, balance, or stability, or if problems have been ascertained in taking the history, the physician might ask you to perform a few simple tricks, much as a sheriff's officer will do with a suspected drunk; you might be surprised to be asked to close your eyes while he tries to push you off your feet!

Regional Examination

To an experienced observer, the skin tells the patient's life history. It also is subject to a number of specific medical conditions, and quite apart from any tenderness, scars and tattoos tell a story in themselves. Nails are affected by many medical conditions and are an indicator of personal hygiene and grooming, which a severely depressed person might have let slip.

Head

The general shape of the head is not of importance, but the quality of hair deteriorates in chronic ill health, and grooming may be significant.

Eyes are subject to a number of medical conditions, some associated with fibromyalgia. Acuity of vision is not of consequence unless recently changed. The internal pressure of the eyeball will be measured (there are relevant conditions that affect it), and the retina at the back of the eye will be examined with the ophthalmoscope; it's the only place in the body where a direct view of the arteries can be obtained. The eyelids are remarked and should be symmetrical.

Ears are of less importance in what the physician can see, but she will notice whether you use a hearing aid, whether you can hear her deliberately quieted voice, whether you cock your head if one ear isn't working as well as the other.

The mouth, and what little can be seen of the throat, has not too much importance, apart from the teeth, whose general state of care does matter. The traditional "put out your tongue" is impressive in the cinema but tells the physician very little. The most relevant issue in the mouth is: how does it open? The jaw joints will be palpated as you open and close the mouth to determine whether the joint is tender and whether both sides move smoothly.

The face will be examined lightly to assure the sensation of touch is normal. Then the muscles at the side of the jaw are scrupulously palpated to determine whether they contain trigger points.

Cranial Nerves

There are twelve nerves that (mostly) pass through holes in the base of the skull and may be indicators of significant medical problems, but whose function would be expected to be normal in fibromyalgia. Each is known by its function and a designated Roman numeral; their functions can be rapidly tested:

I—Olfactory, sense of smell
II—Optic, vision, and visual fields
III, IV, and VI—Oculomotor, trochlear, abducens, pupil and eye movements
V—Trigeminal, face sensation
VII—Facial, muscle symmetry and strength
VIII—Auditory, hearing
IX—Glossopharyngeal, palate movement
X—Vagus, functions in heart assumed by normal pulse
XI—Spinal-accessory, action of trapezius muscles visible
XII—Hypoglossal, tongue protrusion

Neck

There's a front and a back to the neck. The throat will be examined by inspection from the front and by palpation while you are seated and the examiner stands behind you. She looks to see if the trachea (windpipe) is central, whether the thyroid is visible, and to what extent the veins stand out; she feels to determine whether there are enlarged lymph nodes, an abnormally enlarged thyroid, an abnormal "thrill" in the carotid artery, and any tender areas, in particular, any trigger points in the sternomastoid and trapezius muscles.

Movement of the neck is important in whether it provokes pain. The range of movement varies from person to person and is important only if it has changed. The young and the double jointed can turn their heads like ostriches; even the old should be able to look along their shoulders. Chiropractors, plaintiffs' lawyers, and kinesiologists are in love with all those gadgets that give a numerical measurement to a fraction of a degree for each time-consuming tested movement, but there is no real value in this type of examination.

Movements should be actively performed under observation. There is no benefit but there is substantial hazard in testing passive movement, that is, movement forced by the examiner's hands.

Back

Inspection reveals posture, the curve of the spine, the protuberance of the abdomen. Normally, the lumbar spine is concave, and the thoracic (chest) spine is convex. Curves become exaggerated with poor posture. A lateral curve (scoliosis) is not necessarily a source of pain but may become a problem in later life. It is not associated with fibromyalgia or with its concomitant conditions.

Active movements are observed. There is no inherent value in being able to touch your toes or put your hands flat on the floor. What matters is whether the range of movement has changed, whether the rhythm of movement is normally executed, whether movement is painful, whether muscle spasm is provoked.

Palpation searches for tender points in the muscles; trigger points are located if present; and any pain when compressing individual vertebrae is noted.

Upper and Lower Limbs

We've each been given four limbs, and they should be symmetrical. Muscle development and ranges of joint movement should be in balance. The physician expects symmetry of function and needs to know from you if there has been any change.

Skin sensation can be adequately tested with the fingers; if there are questionable abnormalities, more complicated testing can be performed; none are expected in fibromyalgia.

Joints will be inspected for ranges of movement and palpated for abnormal temperature, thickening, or tenderness, which might indicate an arthritis. Muscles will be systematically palpated for trigger points. Pulses at the wrist and ankle will be assessed and should be easily found and equal in volume.

Reflexes will be sought at elbows, wrists, knees, and ankles and should be symmetric in briskness. You're not a better person if they're really sharp or a worse person if they can't be found, just so long as all reflexes in all four limbs are similar. Don't be surprised when the doctor scratches the bottom of your foot to see if your big toe flexes down. (If it bends up, you've got a problem!)

Don't be surprised when she puts the butt of the tuning fork to your ankle to see whether you feel the vibrations expire before she does. This tests a vital and relevant function of your spinal cord, despite it being carried out at the ankle. She might even ask if you know which way your toe is pointing, which seems absurd, but this tests the same important spinal cord function.

Chest

The organs in your chest will be examined by percussion and auscultation. No abnormality in heart and lung structure or function is to be expected, but the possibility must be eliminated. The exterior of the chest will be palpated to determine whether there are trigger points in the muscles. A careful physician never misses the opportunity to perform an examination of the breast and lymph glands in the armpits to eliminate the possibility of unrecognized cancer.

Abdomen

While you are lying comfortably, the abdomen will be inspected, palpated, percussed, and auscultated. Here, there is substantial possibility of positive findings, given the frequency of irritable bowel disease accompanying fibromyalgia. The physician will determine whether spleen (patient's upper left) or liver (upper right) are enlarged; tenderness elsewhere within the abdomen will be sought, as well as the possibility of trigger points in the muscles of the abdominal wall, most particularly the rectus muscles, the vertical bands down the middle. The possibility of hernia in the groins will be eliminated; the usually palpable lymph glands in the groin will be sought.

Perineum

The possibility of conditions accompanying fibromyalgia, as well as the general status of health, mandates examination of the perineal structures, that region lying in front of the tailbone and between the thighs.

Palpation of the muscles at the floor of the pelvis will be performed to eliminate the possibility of trigger points. Rectal examination will be performed, in part for what can be felt, in part for what it contains. In a man, the prostate gland is important; in a woman, the uterus can partially be felt by one finger in the rectum and the other hand on the lower abdomen (called "bimanual examination"). What's on the gloved finger after removal from the anus is important and is routinely tested in the office for blood—a simple test, important to eliminate forms of gastrointestinal pathology that cause bleeding, but possibly not enough bleeding for you to have noticed it (occult blood).

The external aspect of the female genitalia, the vulva is inspected and tenderness sought, very gently, with a cotton-tipped stick if needed. The glands contained there are examined. The interior, the vagina, is at first blindly palpated, usually with two fingers, permitting a search for tender areas, palpation of the cervix, and determination whether movement of the cervix provokes pain.

Using the bimanual technique described, the uterus (womb) and the adnexae (tubes and ovaries) are palpated; depending on the size of the abdomen and the patient's ability to tolerate the examination, these may or may not be felt.

Next comes the part the patient was least looking forward to, the reason why it's left to the last, but must nevertheless be performed. The device inserted into the vagina is called a "speculum"; originally this was a mirror, but today the physician looks through it at you, not at herself. Be grateful it has only two blades (duck-bill)—the one found in Pompeii has four (Skinner 1961). It allows direct observation of the walls of the vagina, specific spot palpation with an instrument to seek tender areas or trigger points, examination of the orifice of the cervix, and the required swabs to be taken for lab testing of the infections to which women are subject.

WHAT TELLS HER IF I HAVE FIBROMYALGIA?

There is essentially only one set of tests required in the physical examination for fibromyalgia. All the preceding is to eliminate other possible explanations for your problems or to diagnose the numerous conditions found with fibromyalgia.

The two criteria set by the American College of Rheumatology (ACR) in 1990 for the diagnosis of fibromyalgia were displayed in shortened form in an earlier part of this book. One is based on the patient's history, the other on a very specific, focused, and limited examination for what are termed "tender points."

The history criterion requires:

a.   continuous pain for a minimum of three months in all regions to be described
b.   that the pain must have been felt in all four quadrants of the body, which means symmetrically in both arms and both legs, and/or the regions of shoulders and buttocks, or alternatively described as right and left sides, above and below the waist
c.   that pain must also have been present in the axial skeleton for the same period. "Axial skeleton" is explained as the spine and anterior chest.

To meet the physical examination criterion, pressure on eighteen designated areas had to provoke pain at a minimum of eleven points.

Some explanations are required.

The ACR criteria deal with widespread pain, attempting to distinguish this from regional pain. Without disparaging the severity of pain limited an entire side of the body, or both legs or similar limited distribution, it was decided this was regional pain and not the same condition as widespread pain; therefore, it was excluded from the diagnosis of fibromyalgia.

The members of the ACR committee designated eighteen discrete points in the body where experience had taught them their patients found pain to pressure. These were not in themselves sites of complaint of pain, because the complaint was, by definition, widespread and not discrete. In my opinion, the choice of the word "tender," when "painful" was expressly intended, has been the cause of much confusion and has led to some physicians' disparaging remarks such as, "Press hard enough, on any part of the body, and of course it's tender!"

The eighteen designated points come in nine pairs, four on the anterior and five on the posterior aspects of the body. The anterior bilateral sites are:

- at the side of the neck, between the transverse processes of the mid-cervical spine
- at the second rib where it meets the chest bone (sternum)
- at the outer side of the elbow, just above the joint line
- at the inner knee, just above the joint line

The posterior bilateral sites are:

- at the base of the skull, close to the midline
- over the shoulder blade, near its upper inner margin
- at the middle of the upper border of the trapezius muscle, above the shoulder blade
- at the upper outer margin of the buttock muscle (gluteus maximus)
- at the back of the hip prominence (greater trochanter)

The ACR committee designated the amount of force to be used as four kilograms, which can be applied either by an instrument known variously as an "algometer" or a "dolorimeter," and in use since 1949 (Staud 2005), or by the thumb with enough force to blanche the nail. It's been suggested that trainees should practice this pressure against a weight scale. It is also expected that the patient will declare this pressure to cause her pain, possibly severe pain, and that a declaration of "Hey! That's tender!" doesn't get her a pass mark.

Gilliland (2007) describes her technique for evaluating tender points and suggests it should be carried out in a standard systematic manner at each examination of each patient. She further suggests it should be the first item on the agenda in the physical examination, which is appropriate once the diagnosis has been established, but questionable if it has not.

In addition to the eighteen ACR designated tender points, she adds three control sites, points that would not be expected to cause pain, against the possibility the examiner is dealing with a "Yes to everything—I hurt everywhere you touch me" patient. Gilliland also suggests identifying all points visually before commencing the tests, and the examiner should press once only on each site. What conclusion to reach about the "Yes to everything" patient is not discussed. Is she a fake? Or does she really experience pain everywhere she's touched?

Other problems found with the widespread pain, such as fatigue and unrestorative sleep, were left out of the criteria, not to everyone's satisfaction. Anyone who's served on a committee knows the problem characterized by setting out to design a racehorse and how easy it is to end up with a hippo. One supposes the members of the committee must have concluded a sleek definition was preferable to an overloaded one, and it has since been emphasized their intention was for research classification and not for general practice. According to Merskey (1996), "There are those who don't quite fit the criteria; some patients have all the pain and few or no tender points; other individuals have a qualifying number of tender points but no pain." Crofford (2005) asks, "Do patients with widespread pain and only ten tender points have a different syndrome?"

To make a more user-friendly guide, a second consensus took the two compulsory pain criteria adopted from the ACR 1990 standards and merged them with "Additional Clinical Symptoms and Signs" to expand the classification of the fibromyalgia syndrome into the Clinical Case Definition for Practitioners (Russell 2004):

- history of **widespread pain**, for three months, in four quadrants of the body and axial
- **pain on palpation** over at least eleven of the eighteen designated tender points
- additional clinical **symptoms and signs** categorized as:
  — neurological manifestations, neurocognitive manifestations
  — fatigue, sleep dysfunction
  — autonomic and/or neuroendocrine manifestations, stiffness

WHAT LABORATORY AND OTHER TESTS WILL HELP DETERMINE IF I HAVE FIBROMYALGIA?

There are no chemical, blood, or urine tests that will prove or disprove fibromyalgia. The condition is not unique in that regard, but combined with the absence of physical signs, the lack of supporting laboratory evidence makes it difficult for the Doubting Thomases of the world to accept the condition as real.

On first assessment, a battery of routine laboratory studies will be ordered to assess your general health and to eliminate the possibility of other conditions. These tests will be extended in proportion to the variety of complaints and the need to exclude other conditions affecting the various regions of the body, revealed in the history-taking process and described in a later chapter.

Imaging Studies

The same issue applies to imaging studies, what used to be called x-rays, but pictures are now made with ultrasound and magnets (MRI), neither of which use x-rays. (CAT scans use a lot of x-rays, the reason why practitioners don't mind repeating MRIs but hesitate to repeat CAT scans.)

There are no specific areas that absolutely need to be imaged. Studies may be ordered to eliminate the possibility of other diagnoses, and this will depend on the patient's presented concerns (polite euphemism for complaints). But such imaging studies are used, in medical jargon, to rule out other conditions and cannot rule in fibromyalgia except by a process of elimination.

The Use and Abuse of Tests

Lab tests come back with a set of blunt numbers. Unfortunately, the well-disposed laboratory will also provide the doctor with the usual range in which those numbers should fall. The doctor looks at them, decides the test is "borderline normal," and repeats it. And so it may go on, ad infinitum.

Imaging studies will come back with no positive findings. But the radiologists who read them often make helpful suggestions about another type of study to be performed in their establishment that could help, or possibly they may suggest how soon in their view it would be appropriate to repeat this normal study.

"Maybe the MRI last week was read wrong?" the disappointed patient asks. "Maybe it didn't show anything that day, so let's repeat it at another hospital. See if their doctors are better at finding what's wrong?"

Once again, the imaging goes on ad infinitum, searching the haystack for needles that aren't there and never were. Popular belief in technology is so strong, the patient finds it impossible to believe no one can take a picture of her particular problem. "Try the Hubble," she says.

A patient reasonably expects that, when a test is ordered and a needle is stuck in her arm, she will obtain a benefit. It's depressing to be told, test after test, that nothing has been found. She knows there's something wrong—there just has to be a test out there to prove it. It's quite extraordinary in practice to find how often the patient is angry when told a test result is normal. You expect her to be pleased. Instead, she feels frustrated and rejected by medical science and all its representatives. This sets her on the path to the doors of the quack doctors who'll guarantee to her weird and wonderful "tests," facile explanations and certain cures.

The physician has a moral duty to explain his purpose, to explain that what he requests are tests to rule out certain conditions so that his patient does not anticipate positive test results. For these reasons, testing of all kinds should be reduced to the unavoidable minimum.

The same reasons and the same rule applies to consultations with specialists: as few as possible, but as many as are going to help the patient.

Functional Testing

The objective of the program, your goal, is to improve your ability to function in your home and your community. We wish to relieve your pain. We wish to help you sleep better, but we wish to see you restored to an improved level at which you can more comfortably function. Not a question of dragging yourself in agony from pillar to post, but tolerable functioning.

To this end, the consultant occupational therapist supplemented the Lawton-Brody scale, which allows the therapist, with your cooperation, to evaluate numerically your capacity to undertake the activities of daily living (ADL), meaning no more than what you would wish to be able to do in the course of a day looking after yourself.

The assessment is extended (more letters!) into an IADL, the instrumental activities of daily living, to measure your ability to use the routine household equipment to care for your domicile and your family, in addition to your own purely physical requirements.

To be examined for a baseline report and repeated at intervals through the program will be your ability to perform, or the extent you need help to perform:

- bathing and/or showering
- dressing, including tying shoelaces
- entering, using, and exiting the toilet
- transferring in and out of bed, low and high chairs
- feeding with normal utensils
- using a telephone, including remembering numbers
- shopping, including choosing and picking items
- preparing food, including planning and preparation
- keeping house, including use of vacuum cleaners and mops and making beds
- laundry, including carrying and using machines
- transportation, ability to drive, take a taxi, and/or use public transportation

For those who are employed, or wish to be gainfully employed, the work-place and any barriers to work will be assessed, with your cooperation, by the occupational therapist, and, if indicated, suggestions for improvements will be made by the ergonomist.

This baseline report is used to understand your difficulties. Further reporting will be by the Fibromyalgia Impact Questionnaire (FIQ—letters, of course!), which asks similar questions; gives you a choice of numbers to circle, representing a scale from "Never" to "Always"; and is useful for following your progress.

Psychologic Testing

The consultant psychologist for the project suggested that information on each participant should be integrated from multiple sources, including the personal history and physical examination performed at the project site; collateral infor-mation received from family physicians, consultants, and other medical sources; and the results of a battery of psychological tests the psychologist would super-vise and/or conduct. These results will remain private and will be used only for your benefit, or your name would be removed if the results were used collec-tively to report the research benefits of the project.

The basic, objective personality test is the Minnesota Multiphasic Person-ality Inventory, usually known as MMPI, which, unusual in the medical field, remains the copyrighted property of the university where it was devised sev-enty-five years ago. The current version, MMPI-2, requires a response to 567 yes/no questions, and it's estimated a fully alert person will spend two hours to complete it. To reduce emotional strain on our patients, who may have the "fibro fog" discussed elsewhere, the shortened version (only 370 questions!) will be used.

The test is divided into ten parts, numbered as scales with broad, seemingly inappropriate, generic titles: hypochondriasis, depression, hysteria, psycho-pathic deviate, masculinity femininity, paranoia, psychasthenia, schizophrenia, hypomania, and social introversion.

She will not discuss it with her patients, but the psychologist is aware of pre-vious test results using the MMPI on patients with fibromyalgia in which com-parisons were made with patients diagnosed with rheumatoid arthritis (Payne 1982; Dailey 1990; Ahles 1991; Aaron 1996). The fibromyalgia group was, in general, found to be more psychologically disturbed, with highest scores in the depression, hypochondriasis, and hysteria sections of the test. The severity of clinical features did not correlate with psychological status.

Another study has shown what appears to be strata within the overall diag-nosis of fibromyalgia. A group of nearly one hundred patients were tested for the standard fibromyalgia protocol of tender points, for response to painful stimuli and with an overall battery of psychologic profiling tests (Giesecke 2003). The stratification showed:

- Seventeen percent were very tender, but emotionally stable and with a high degree of mental control over their pain
- Fifty percent were not very tender, emotionally stable, and with moderate mental control of their pain
- Thirty-three percent were moderately tender, emotionally unstable, and lacking mental control of their pain

Similar findings, stratifying the patients studied into four groups, the fourth with a somatoform pain disorder (see elsewhere in this book), were described by Müller (2007).

A literature review attempting to evaluate the personality profiles of fibromyalgia patients found, compared with controls, there was a prevalence of depression disorders, reported between 20 and 80 percent, and of anxiety disorders, reported between 13 and 64 percent, compared with a rate of psychiatric disorders of 7 percent in the general population (Fietta 2007).

Cognitive Behavioral Group Therapy

The psychologist explains to the members of the group they will collectively be lectured on the techniques of this form of treatment. They have already explained themselves to the group's members and will continue to meet under guidance to discuss their prior problems, as well as their current issues and how they are tackling them. Meetings will be in a group and, as the therapist sees the indication, on an individualized basis.

The psychologist will continue to emphasize the goal of the project, namely, an improvement in function.

Putting It All Together

The lengthy periods of history taking and physical examination are over. Each of you has been examined. Each of you, unfortunately, has "graduated" with more than the requisite eleven tender points and the widespread four-quadrant-plus-axial pain. Each of you not only has fibromyalgia, but all of you have at least one, and some of you several, concomitant conditions. You've filled out forms. You've had your pep-talk from the psychologist. Now you start your education and your program of treatment. You'll be heartened to know it's based on all the latest world research, and it's been put together by the best brains in Europe and the Middle East (Carville 2007).

CHAPTER FOUR

TREATMENT

HOW SHOULD FIBROMYALGIA BE TREATED?

"**V**ery carefully" is the obvious answer.

As a patient with fibromyalgia, you are part of the group called the "Cinderella of Rheumatology" (Hazelton and Hickey 2003). Remember, Cindy might have gone through a few ups and downs, and perhaps her family wasn't as supportive as they might have been, but eventually good things did happen to Cinderella, and if you work with us, good things will happen to you, too.

In the meanwhile, as you wait in the ashes contemplating your future, much of what needs to be done lies in your own hands. We've passed the hurdles of painstaking, all-revealing history when you surrendered your mind and memories to the physicians. We've passed the hurdle of the physical examination, where you offered up your body to the physicians to pat, push, probe, and insert cold steel, as they saw fit. The surrender of your mind and your body to be examined is evidence of trust. And it's trust on which treatment must be based.

Treatment must have a defined purpose, otherwise known as a "goal," or why you went to the doctor in the first place. The very simple answer is: you had symptoms that you'd prefer to live without. There were issues bothering you that you'd like to have resolved.

All neatly wrapped up in the original question—poorly worded but correctly posed—what are you complaining of?

If attention is not given to the original purpose, what the military training manuals call "the object of the exercise," then the objective, the goal, is forgotten, and you the patient end up in the commercialized world of treatment, getting bounced from one therapist to another, all of whom may be honest persons but many of whom have not had their eyes set on the object of the exercise, which is to relieve you of your complaints—put it another way—to abolish or at the very least, to alleviate your symptoms so you may return to the maximum possible level of functioning in your society.

Provision of treatment is not in itself an objective. Both physician and therapist can be fooled into believing as long as something is being done to the patient, some action seen to occur, then that renders the situation satisfactory—for the time being—for today. I've had arguments in court with lawyers on this very subject (education is not a barrier to illogical thought), their argument being that every treatment known to mankind should be attempted, and sooner or later the right one, by pure chance, will come along. This is the same mentality that believes there's a pill for everything. The cold fact remains—there is not.

So we define our goal first, then we set about devising a plan to reach that goal, reemphasizing all the while that the goal is not the mere provision of treatment.

One can think of treatment as the vehicle you will mount to arrive at your destination. It is the car, the canoe, the parachute, the royal road, the snake-infested path—all of these with the single purpose of employing each and every necessary one to reach your goal. And if they're not bringing you closer to your goal, then you need to rethink why you're using that vehicle on that road.

Think of yourself as Indiana Jones and your goal as the Lost Ark. But unlike Doctor Jones, you're not on your own, you have a team of experts on your side devoted to helping you reach your goal. And the goal must be easily defined in a single short sentence. It is: restoration of function by removal of the barriers inhibiting function. Or if you have a taste for the exotic and like the Latin: restoration to the *status quo ante*. And if you put those together, it means getting you back to the situation you were in before the fibromyalgia overtook you. If you didn't play the piano before fibromyalgia, you won't be playing it now; but if you kept house, enjoyed sexual relations, had a satisfying remunerated job, then the goal is to rehabilitate you to that previous state.

On the other hand, if you couldn't get a job, or perhaps worse had a job you loathed, hated having sex with your husband, and were bored to tears with your life, then rehabilitation will not be a process of restoring you to a status that was unsatisfactory, but by revealing and removing barriers will habilitate you to a status you never before had the opportunity to enjoy.

The reason to discuss this issue is to emphasize there are psychosocial aspects to habilitation or rehabilitation, and that it is not a purely physical issue.

Nor is it a passive process. It is one in which you will be guided, but one where you make the effort yourself. Think of Harrison Ford searching for whatever his current adventure requires, but accompanied on his journey by the cheerleaders of the college football team—he should be so lucky!

We've defined our first and fundamental principle in treatment: it must be goal oriented, directed toward the achievement of an objective, removing the barriers that inhibit normal enjoyment of life. The second principle is: all treatment is patient oriented, that is to say, the treatment is programmed for each patient as an individual. Treatments are not directed solely at individual symptoms. Symptoms come attached to people and it is people we treat.

In recent decades the term "holistic" has come into use, much popularized by those without benefit of medical training who believe their methods are superior to those of the trained physician and by those who have had medical training but like to proclaim, "I thank thee Lord, I am not as other men." The word, however, is derived from the ancient Greek and we know from their writings dating back at least to Hippocrates that considering the patient "as a whole," not as a bearer of a collection of separate symptoms, was their method at that epoch, and it remains our method now. For this reason, there is no such thing in our rehabilitation program as "one size fits all." Or to use the vernacular, "We ain't cookie cutters."

Setting Up a Treatment Program

Who controls the treatment? Who organizes it? Who monitors it?

The word "paternalistic" in the dictionary means no more than acting like a father, and there must have been a time when fathers were believed to be well disposed to their children, or "Our Father" wouldn't have become an expression of religious acceptance. Today, however, "paternalistic" seems to have become a derogatory expression, yet somehow "maternalistic" has escaped opprobrium. A physician who dictates to his patient how the treatment plan will be conducted is going to be called "paternalistic." One who explains to her patients the reasons for her plan of action, explains the whys and wherefores, might just as well be called maternalistic, but she will certainly be more successful. I'm not sure whether the nurse in my office enjoyed the "Yes, Mother," when she explained my instructions to the patients, but she did have their respect and their cooperation.

The patient, immersed in a climate of confusion and uncertainty, should be involved through education about fibromyalgia, through the necessary adjustments in her life, the all-encompassing therapies designed for her personal range of symptoms designed to reduce the overall impact of the illness that burdens her life. Such a program will involve the judicial use of pharmacological and nonpharmacological interventions and must be monitored to determine its benefits or its failings. The patient must be fully aware that it will take time and that her treatment program will require regular follow-up (Russell 2004).

There needs to be a conductor of the orchestra, and that role is not one the patient should try to fill herself. In large part this program is designed to ensure the patient is fully informed about her condition, has full opportunity to discuss her concerns and to discuss the recommendations made to her. But recommendations should come from a knowledgeable person, and there should be a single person monitoring the patient's progress and one to whom she can turn for advice and support.

There are two unsatisfactory scenarios on the opposite side of the coin. One is a scenario where the patient goes from specialist to specialist, with no intercommunication, each making his own decision, each going his own way. The other unsatisfactory scenario is the patient selecting her own therapists, going from clinic to clinic, going from one type of treatment to another, always seeking that one advertised cure she reads about in the magazines or sees advertised in the newspapers, which somehow just never works for her.

I draw analogies. If I have trouble with my vehicle, I take it to a mechanic; in the same way, I take my tax problems to an accountant and my legal problems to a lawyer. Through a process over the years, not altogether without its misadventures, I am now fortunate in having the help of excellent experts in all these fields, and I trust them completely. I would not like to draw too tight an analogy with the patient who directs her own treatment program, but the legal profession does have an expression to the effect that "the lawyer who represents himself has a fool for a client."

The Conductor of the Orchestra

So if the conductor of the orchestra—and there will be an orchestra—is not going to be the patient, then who should it be? In Canada and most of Europe, the prevailing system is for each patient to have her own primary care physician, who ideally year after year will be the person who knows her, understands her, supports her, and assists her in finding specialized consultant advice when appropriate. In other countries where the patient has direct walk-in access to a specialist, she may have precluded the possibility of obtaining a primary care general physician, and this role might be played by a general internist, or possibly a specialist rheumatologist.

Whatever the designation, be it specialist or nonspecialist, there are certain fundamental requirements for the role of the "conductor." She must first of all "believe" in fibromyalgia. Not everyone does, and you won't make much progress with a doctor who doesn't: "Comments such as 'it's all in your mind' or 'I can't find anything wrong with you,' only add to the patient's frustration. The first crucial element in the treatment of pain, fatigue, and other diverse symptomatology in patients with fibromyalgia is empathetic listening and acknowledgment that the patient is indeed experiencing pain, that is, to validate the patient's illness" (Winfield 2007).

Making a correct diagnosis is crucial, and patients need to know a name exists for the mysterious symptoms they have been experiencing. They must be told in a straightforward manner that at present no outright cure exists, but with proper rehabilitation methods, they can be helped to regain control of their life and will achieve significant improvement (Gilliland 2007).

The Meaning of Words

To ensure there is no confusion, in modern medical usage, "to provide therapy" and "to treat" are essentially the same terms. Whereas "therapy" at one time meant "to wait upon," and "to treat" meant "to deal with," they are used now interchangeably.

The Philosophy of the Treatment Program Is Directed at the Whole Person

We reemphasize that our treatment, our therapy program, is of a person, not a disease, not a set of symptoms, but a person. I don't favor the word "holistic," which falsely implies something new and different. It's not new. It's not different. It's no more than common sense, and it's been the basis of the best practice of medicine for more than four thousand years (Keral Ayurvedic). Perhaps the word can more readily be understood in simple English if one were to put the W we irrationally use in English in front of the Greek stem *holos*, then it's seen that the word means no more than "whole," and there is nothing new or mysterious about it—Aristotle used it in his axiom, "The whole is more than the sum of the parts," and Socrates' axiom, "The part can never be well unless the whole is well." The message here is, beware the therapist who'd have you believe his "holistic" approach is new—they understood the concept in India long before Hippocrates was on the scene!

Attention needs also to be directed to your family, to your social and work background, the milieu from which you have come, in which you still exist and to which you will return after your initial period of treatment is completed. Are there problems with family members, finances, work, and so on that need attention? The close family relations and if indicated, the close work relations, need to be included in the overall treatment concepts. Treatment will continue for a long time and will perforce involve those with whom you are in contact.

Attention to Specific Issues

The concept of an "overlapping syndrome," postulated by Yunus as a "dysregulation spectrum syndrome," will be attended to later, but many patients with fibromyalgia have symptoms and signs of other concomitant (separate but also present) conditions. Just as having a head cold doesn't prevent you from also having appendicitis, so having fibromyalgia doesn't preclude having other conditions such as rheumatoid arthritis, irritable bowel syndrome, or bursitis. These other problems should have been recognized at the time the history was taken and in the physical examination.

Each concomitant condition will need attention on an individualized basis—individual to the patient and individual to the condition. For concomitant regional chronic pain syndromes, for instance, disorders of the jaw joint, or irritable bladder syndrome or low back pain, referral will be arranged if indicated to experienced consulting specialists who favor nonsurgical treatments.

The General Program

The general program is multifaceted, one that all patients will embark upon, and consists of a blend of active and passive treatments directed at the specific symptoms that characterize fibromyalgia, namely, the widespread pain, the fatigue, and the issues of sleep.

First, the program is directed to lifestyle. You will learn to order your life to match your capabilities, to realize your full capabilities, and when possible, to live within your capabilities every day, in order to avoid periods of inactivity that result from bursts of superactivity. These will be taught by psychologic and behavioral approaches to reduce distress, promote self-effectiveness and self-management by methods such as relaxation training, and activity pacing.

There is a developed program of medication, pursued along the traditional lines of "as little as possible; as much as necessary." The various therapists and physicians who will work with you are all familiar with the problems facing the patient with fibromyalgia, and all "believe" in the condition. They also believe improvement is possible, but they know from experience the extent of improvement rests less on the therapists' efforts than on the patient's. Here is one place where you will find reward for the efforts you make.

There is no single combination of all these forms of therapy that works best for everybody; there isn't a "one size fits all," but there are common features in the approach to therapy and once these have been started they will be tailored on an individualized basis. The emphasis is on minimizing your symptoms and improving your general health.

You've been told about the research we plan to use as our guide. The European League Against Rheumatism (EULAR) guidelines for treatment are derived from the opinions of eleven member countries, a review of one hundred forty-six published studies, from which were selected thirty-nine pharmacological and fifty-nine nonpharmacological reports. Despite the extent of the material available for review, and although they issued some general guidelines from their study, it is clear they did not find "the one best way to go" (Carville 2007).

Their guidelines emphasize the need to tailor the treatment to the person, to understand thoroughly the person's psychosocial background, and to use a multidisciplinary approach in the treatment program:

- Evidence of most benefit was from use of medication to achieve pain relief by antidepressants, tramadol, and pregabalin.
- Lesser benefit was obtained from use of a heated pool with or without exercise.
- Less enthusiasm expressed for exercises including aerobic and strength training, other forms of physiotherapy, relaxation, and psychological support.
- Slight enthusiasm only for cognitive behavioral therapy, but the material available for decision was not satisfactory.
- Definitely opposed to corticosteroids and strong opioids.

ADJUSTMENT OF BACKGROUND PSYCHOSOCIAL ISSUES

He was not without his critics, but it's not given to many of us to leave a legacy in the common speech such as Norman Vincent Peale has done with *The Power of Positive Thinking*, nor to keep new editions of a book flowing twenty years after the author's death (Peale 2007). It is the power to think positively that must be evoked by the treatment team, and the patient must see herself as the little engine who goes from "I think I can" to "I knew I could."

Many cases of fibromyalgia can be traced to their origins from a stressful experience. The role of stress and its effect on the neuroendocrine system will be discussed in another chapter. But for now, we accept that living with fibromyalgia is difficult and that some very positive thinking has to go into improving the situation.

Let's get some terms sorted out. Are you a fibromyalgic? No, you are a *person* burdened with a problem, known for lack of a better term as fibromyalgia. But you are a *person!* You are identified as a person, not as a bearer of a medical condition. The foundation of control in jail or the army is to turn you into a number, marked with a sentence and a uniform. Remember

Charles Dickens' "One hundred and five, North Tower"? Don't ever let them treat you as "Bed three, fibromyalgia." In medicine, you must remain a *person* who is burdened with a condition.

Are you disabled? What does that word mean? Various definitions range through insurance contracts, legalese and medical, sociological and moral judgments. Essentially, disabled people cannot function as they would wish and they may need some form of help with their lives. Didn't we all at one time? Were we born able to care for ourselves? Of course not. It's a question of timing and degree. We all need some help from others, at different phases of our lives. Even at our optimum state we're only *TAB*—temporarily able-bodied—that span of life between first and second childhoods.

The remaining issue you must apply to yourself. Will you accept help? Will you work with your therapists? That is the early task in the rehabilitation process designed to assist you to remove the barriers that prevent optimization of your abilities.

Role of a Fibromyalgia Program

There is no cookie-cutter model for rehabilitation. Each person willing to accept help, will relate as an individual to the other persons providing it. "Multidisciplinary" is a popular buzzword that means different things at different times in different places. Too often it means, "We've got a dozen consultants on staff, and you don't get out of here until they've all added their accounts to your insurance bill." Ideally it means you see only the consultants who have some useful advice for the "conductor of the orchestra," and you only see as many different types of therapists as will bring you real benefit. And all tests are kept to a minimum, performing only those reasonably necessary to exclude the likelihood of conditions other than fibromyalgia.

There is insufficient evidence to create an unquestionably perfect model for treatment, but the one proposed does have more support than any other (Karjalainen 2000; Sim 2002; Gilliland 2007; Carville 2007).

Specialized in cognitive behavioral therapy (CBT), therapists will work with you under the direction of the consultant psychologist. Although the EULAR study was uncertain of the place for CBT, more recent studies have shown value in persons whose lives were dominated by pain, exactly the issue in fibromyalgia (Escobar 2007).

Bio-Psycho-Social

That sounds like a word that covers the waterfront. Engel found it necessary to reinvent the wheel to remind us what the Greek physicians knew: mind and body are one, and what the French philosophers manage to distort. There must have been a Greek equivalent for "May the gods preserve us from philosophers!" The very obvious concept is that mind and body work together within the person who is also affected by the society in which she lives. The lesson to the doctor and patient who believed everything could be fixed by a pill was clear enough— it ain't gonna happen.

And that is the foundation of our fibromyalgia program. Attention is given to your place in society, your physical needs, and your mental needs.

To establish your place in society is not a question of whether you wear a diamond tiara or torn jeans, but of what support you have. An issue that's critical to any person in distress, and it is fully accepted that chronic pain is an issue of stress and distress. To be socially supported is to know there's someone who cares about you, that you haven't been abandoned, that you have emotional support. If it becomes apparent you are lacking in support, or your social ambience is downright negative, the psychologist and social worker will assist to reverse this. You may need advice on how to set about building a network of true friends, as contrasted with sympathizers. Family counseling may be indicated.

The therapist will discuss with you what you have in what she calls "instrumental support." Do you have practical help with the house and the kids? What about your finances? Your insurance? Matters of that kind. She will inquire also into what she terms "informational support." To whom do you go when you want to find out about getting help? Your family doctor? Your pastor or priest? The Internet? Is your source of information appropriate? She is fully aware disinformation is rife.

The Role of the CBT Therapist

The therapist will work with you throughout the program. She will constantly stress to you that this is your program. She will help you set realistic step-by-step goals, the best kinds have numbers, like a two-mile walk, a ten-minute meditation.

She will constantly stress to you that the effort to improve toward your goal is your effort, that it isn't going to be achieved by any person or pill from the outside, that achievements are yours to make from the inside.

She will constantly stress to you her role will be to evoke your thoughts about your problems and to assist you to work toward solutions. She will deal with the here and now and will not be discussing with you how you came to here but rather will be helping you to determine where you are going to go from here. She will encourage you with your realistic goals to do homework toward meeting those goals and to keep a diary of your achievements or the thoughts that were blocking you from realizing those goals.

Throughout the program she will emphasize she is not going to tell you what you should think nor what you should feel, but will guide you in turning away from negative thoughts of failure and unworthiness toward the development of positive thoughts of achievement.

Physical and Occupational Therapy and the Home Environment

The program is directed toward function, keeping you or restoring you to an active place in your family and society. Every effort will be made by means of a number of methods to relieve pain, but the prime role of physical therapy in this program is the restoration of function. There are two aspects that will be addressed, the removal of barriers to performance and the improvement of performance.

Also a therapist in that she is concerned with improvement of function, this person is going to assess what you need to do at home and at work, what is making it difficult for you, how it can be improved. She may visit your home and your place of work, or an ergonomist might be commissioned to do this.

The occupational therapist or the kinesiologist or the ergonomist will help you go through your physical activities at home, with advice on rearranging tasks and manner of setting about them. We warn you, occupational therapists are in love with gadgets, so see what you can manage with the equipment you already possess before taking on a host of new tools.

Stress, Tobacco, Sleep, Fatigue, and Diet

It is to be hoped that the stressful situation associated with the onset of your fibromyalgia was a one-off occasion, never to be repeated. On the other hand, if life remains stressful for you, this needs to be exposed fully in discussions with your therapists. If your conductor deems appropriate, techniques for stress management will be taught by psychotherapists, and possibly interventions will be made by counselors at home or at work to relieve your stress burden.

Issues of importance at home and at work should have been uncovered in the initial history taking. If they were not, you must make your physicians and therapists aware of them. Don't ask them to go into the ring to fight your fibromyalgia with one hand tied behind their back!

Smoking is definitely out. Apart from general health issues for the smoker and those around her, there are particular issues of aggravation of the symptoms of fibromyalgia, including interference with sleep. Help will be given, as needed, but any insistence on continuing to smoke might be interpreted as an expression of disinterest in pursuing a rehabilitation program.

Sleep is in itself a period of active rehabilitation, not an empty gap, not a mere hiatus between periods of activity. Sleep hygiene is critical, removing all the nasty habits acquired that prevent a full period of critically restorative sleep, and these will be discussed.

Proper sleep is important; so is proper nutrition. Fatigue, discussed later, is an even greater problem to the patient burdened also with a chronic fatigue syndrome. An effort must be made to increase activities progressively, and sometimes a log or diary of the day's activities will help in this regard. "Pace yourself" is good advice, but the pacing occurs between activities, not instead of them.

There is neither good nor bad in natural foods. There is nothing you must eat. There is nothing in an ordinary diet that you must not eat. Discussed later, neither is there any supplement nor any "magic in a bottle" that will help you.

MEETING THE THERAPISTS

The Orchestra

A successful rehabilitation program involves a team of professionals and various modalities individualized for each patient. The team includes physicians; a medical psychologist; physical, massage, and other therapists; and possibly an exercise physiologist. These professionals have expertise in the treatment of your condition. We know from others' experience, the sports medicine attitude to therapy, the "no pain, no gain" variety, will surely worsen your symptoms and is to be avoided. We accept "one size does not fit all," and we accept "one tailor does not dress all."

The Physical Therapist and the Purpose of Physical Therapy

This is the hands-on aspect of the treatment program. The field in which the therapist works is known generally in British areas as "physiotherapy" and in American areas as "physical therapy." There is no difference in the work, only the words. Often the term is abbreviated to "PT," and that must not be confused with "physical training."

The therapist, in most instances, has received four years of specialized training after the preliminary bachelor's degree and is highly informed and skilled in her own area of work. Some therapists work in hospitals and clinics under the overall supervision of a medical specialist, usually a physiatrist; some work in independent practice and direct their own clinics.

Ideally, the therapist is part of the orchestra and plays in harmony with the rest of the performers. A general program of therapy has already been initiated, all players having input to the relevant areas of its design; your therapist will modify this program to match individual needs as you progress in your own tailored program under the therapists' direct observation.

As of now, we do not have a cure for fibromyalgia, a fundamental statement that bears frequent repetition. What we do have is a number of approaches designed to alleviate the negative effects of fibromyalgia. Inherent in these approaches is the need for the patient to take charge of her own recovery, not to conduct the orchestra herself, but to accept responsibility for her own efforts on the path to recovery. And that defines the difference in meaning between the frequently used expressions of "active" and "passive" therapy.

Active therapy is done by the patient, for the patient, under the guidance of the therapist, and is the fundamental of the program (Jones 2002; Gowans 2004; Mannerkorpi 2005). Passive therapy is done by the therapist, to the patient; the patient receives the action and does not perform it. Undoubtedly there is a place for passive aspects of therapy, but they are adjuvants. They are add-ons. They are not the core of the program. The core is what you, the patient, will do for yourself. Graduated exercise is an essential part of optimum treatment for patients with fibromyalgia, but overly strenuous physical exercise before reconditioning is established will be avoided.

The Therapists' Assessment

Physicians talk of physical examinations and physical therapists talk of assessments. Either way, it's the same thing. At your first meeting with the therapist, you will find her in possession of your file, and she knows all about your problems; after all, she's a key member of the orchestra!

Once the pleasantries have been exchanged, and once she's explained that the object of the exercise is your improvement in function, she'll set about doing her own examination. In general, this will be directed at the difficulties you are experiencing, your baseline competence to exercise, and your level of fitness.

She will repeat the examination for back and joint movements, for flexibility, and for muscle tenderness or trigger points. She will examine your posture and your way of walking and discuss with you the proposed program and ensure there are no particular reasons inhibiting your participation. She will also discuss with you the need for regular and organized rest—rest must be just as organized as activity. She will discuss with you your sleeping habits and suggest any needed improvements in what is termed "sleep hygiene." Perhaps not the first day, but at an early stage the therapist will determine your ability to exercise, your breathing capacity and your pain and fatigue tolerance.

When she goes on to treatment, she will concentrate the beginning of the session on joint and soft-tissue mobilization to decrease spasm, there will be a stretching program, body mechanics training, breathing and stress reduction training, sleep hygiene training, individualized strengthening, functional activity, and self-management home treatments, and she will teach any necessary trigger point release methods.

ACTIVE PHYSICAL THERAPY—JANE FONDA VERSUS HULK HOGAN

Because many patients with chronic pain fear activity will make their pain and fatigue worse, they gradually become physically and emotionally out of condition; thus, aerobic and flexibility exercises are an essential component of the rehabilitation program.

If you're young and a jock, you'll have grown up with the word "aerobic." But since you're probably neither of those, we'll explain the word—and that's where Jane and the Hulk come in. Aerobic means no more than exercising your muscles within the boundaries of the amount of oxygen available to feed them, typically the type of light exercise with suitable warming up and stretching that Jane Fonda popularized. You might not get to look like her, you might not get to be as fit as her, but that's the direction for you to go.

Anaerobic is exercising the muscles beyond the boundaries of their available oxygen supply, to all intents and purposes it means weight lifting, heavy weight lifting, and although you might admire the Hulk, and you might have an ambition to be chosen as a firewoman's calendar girl, that's quite a ways down the road.

Graded exercise by low-impact aerobics, walking, water aerobics, stationary bicycle, dancing, and so on, will all start gently and then progress gradually to endurance and strength training. Encouragement and positive reinforcement can improve compliance. Obesity and poor posture will be addressed and progress tailored to each of you, both your ability and your willingness to cooperate with the program. We intend to avoid the experience of other clinics where drop-out rates as high as 47 percent have been reported (Richards 2002).

Exercise, however, was long ago recognized to have therapeutic benefits. In a study in which patients were randomized to receive twenty weeks of high-intensity exercise or were restricted to flexibility training, greater improvements in fitness, global assessment ratings, and tender point pain thresholds were obtained in the high-intensity exercise group than in the flexibility group. Subsequent clinical trials have confirmed the benefits of aerobic exercise and muscle strengthening on mood and physical functioning (McCain 1988). The benefits of exercise for patients with fibromyalgia include improvement in subjective and objective measures of pain and in an overall sense of well-being (Winfield 2007).

You will begin with gentle warm-up, flexibility exercises and progress to stretching all the major muscle groups. Low-impact aerobic exercise is necessary at least three times weekly, and will always start at low levels of exercise and progress slowly. The goal is to exercise safely without increased pain. The target exercise regimen is four to five times a week for at least twenty to thirty minutes each time; this may take months to achieve, but you will be encouraged to exercise at the highest level possible without worsening your symptoms.

As goals are met and symptoms change, your rehabilitation prescription will be modified. A number of trials of multidisciplinary treatment and exercise combined with education, cognitive behavioral therapy, or both have shown the patients had improvements on a six-minute walk, with significant decreases in pain. One trial of multidisciplinary rehabilitation showed continuing improvement in health-related outcomes in a nonclinical, community-based setting at fifteen-month follow-up.

Aquatic Therapy and Adjunctive Passive Therapy

Aquatic exercise may be the safest and gentlest aerobic conditioning exercise available for fibromyalgia. It not only enables aerobic conditioning but also flexibility, strengthening, and stretching exercises. When your body is supported by warm water, these are well tolerated and are especially helpful (Jentoft 2001; Altan 2003; Cedraschi, Desmeules, and Rapiti 2004; Gusi, Thomas-Carus, and Hakkinen 2006; Assis, Silva, and Barros 2006; Gilliland 2007). The remarkable features of the Dead Sea have been helpful when used (Buskila 2001) but clearly are not available to everyone.

The EULAR study supported the benefits to be obtained from exercising in a heated pool, some reports showed benefit in function, others in pain relief.

Massage is beneficial in patients with fibromyalgia, however, excessive dependence on administration of treatments by another person may block your own efforts to achieve your own methods of pain control. Heat, massage, and other treatments are sometimes useful. Diffuse and regional pain is eased by use of a sauna, hot baths and showers, hot mud, and massage. Trigger point injections, acupuncture, chiropractic manipulation, electrotherapy, therapeutic heat and myofascial release are usually appreciated by patients but they're passive methods of questionable long-term benefit.

OTHER FORMS OF TREATMENT

When I stroke my cat she purrs. She likes it and I like it. We both feel good. When I stroke my mare, she seems to like it, though mares don't purr. Clearly she likes it when she's brushed down, and she seems even more to like a good hand rubbing. I like doing that, too. I expect the whole thing has something to do with neurochemistry; pleasurable experiences must show up somewhere in the brain. The day will come when a mare can be put in an MRI and her brain scanned with chemical markers to show us in which part of her head she enjoys this experience. After all they've demonstrated the neurochemistry of the mating mole (Young 2004), of the young human while suffering the distressing condition the French are pleased to call *folie d'amour* (Carey 2005), the effects of an orgasm in an MRI (Holstege 2003), so we should be able to determine what happens in the brain when a person is enjoying a good massage.

But there is an intellectual hold-up. If fibromyalgia is a pain disorder due to an aberration in the central nervous system, and not to any tangible or visible peripheral problem, how can treatment to the surface of the body be expected to alleviate the pain of fibromyalgia?

History of Massage

The origin of the practice of massage predates recorded history, various methods have been used in medicine throughout the world for several thousand years. According to Major (1954), massage is mentioned in the earliest of known Chinese medical works and was already in a high state of development when recognized in the T'ang dynasty (619–906 AD) as a distinct branch of the healing arts.

Equally old, back into prehistory, is the practice of massage in the Indian Subcontinent, under the heading of Ayurvedic medicine; the numerous complicated forms of massage with oils and herbs are still popular and are still offered as therapeutic (Hentschel 2004; KAHC 2007). Massage continued on into Greek medical practice as a basic form of treatment.

The Web site of the National Center for Complementary and Alternative Medicine (NCCAM), a branch of the US Government National Institutes of Health, describes some aspects of massage. The term "Swedish" massage is used to define techniques developed by Per Henrik Ling of Sweden, and "Western" massage, effectively the same, to designate techniques used in the American continent.

The origin of the word in a way describes the earliest concepts of technique. Our word "massage" is derived from the French word *masser,* meaning "to rub," which, in turn, is derived from the Arabic word meaning to apply pressure to muscles and/or the Latin *massa,* a lump of dough that had to be kneaded. What used to be known in England as "medical rubbing" became "massage" in an 1818 encyclopedia (Skinner). In India it was called *chàmpnà* with the same meaning of kneading; this was corrupted in British India to "shampoo," which word was used to describe massage from the barber and later brought to Britain where for a time the same meaning applied (Yule 1994).

Massage: Acceptance, Definition, Techniques, and Theory

According to NCCAM, a survey in 2002 of thirty-one thousand persons in the United States revealed 9 percent had at some time received a professional massage and 5 percent had received massage within the previous twelve months. In the United States, approximately two to four billion dollars is spent each year for visits to massage therapists, which accounted for approximately 26 percent of the $11.7 billion spent on nontraditional healthcare in the 1990s (Wieting 2007).

Massage is manipulation of the soft tissues of the subject's body with a part of the therapist's body (hands, elbows, feet, etc.) or with some form of machine; however, massage primarily consists of hand movements. It has been reported as used by as many as 75 percent of persons with fibromyalgia (Pioro-Boisset 1996).

Over eighty differing forms of massage are described (NCCAM). The variable factors in the treatment include rhythm, rate, pressure, direction, and duration. Most massage methods involve a friction-reducing medium, so the hands of the practitioner move along the patient's skin with minimal friction. Powders or oils are often used. Massage strokes should be regular and cyclic.

In some approaches the rate is several times per second while in others it's much slower. The amount of pressure depends on the technique and the desired results. Light pressure may produce relaxation and relative sedation and may decrease spasm. Intervention at a deeper tissue level may require heavier pressure. Treatment of edema and stretching of tissues requires intermediate amounts of pressure. Direction of massage often is toward the heart, theoretically to provide better movement of fluids toward the central circulation.

When muscles are treated, motions generally are kept parallel to the muscle fibers. If the goal is to reduce adhesions, shearing forces are circular or at least include cross-fiber components.

Massage can have mechanical, neurological, psychological, and reflexive effects. Massage can be used to reduce pain or adhesions, promote sedation, mobilize fluids, increase muscular relaxation, and facilitate vasodilation (Wieting 2007). It may stimulate the release of endorphins, the body's own opium, and increase serotonin levels (Ironson 1996), and it is found to lower blood pressure. Although no consensus exists on the complete physiology of massage, the treatment is generally accepted as more than just the interaction of mechanical forces and human anatomy. Touch has a long history of being a natural, essential component of healing and health maintenance.

Massage may be used as a primary therapeutic intervention or in conjunction with other forms of therapy. It generally increases feelings of relaxation and well-being in patients. Whether this is from placebo effect or the result of some previously undiscovered reflex is not fully understood. Practitioners often incorporate a variety of psychophysical techniques.

A trial of massage therapy at a major US cancer center sought to examine massage therapy outcome in a large group of patients. Over three years, 1,290 patients were treated with regular light touch, or by foot massage, based on the request of the patient. The patients filled out symptom cards before and after an average twenty-minute massage session. Symptoms were reduced by approximately 50 percent. Anxiety, nausea, depression, and pain demonstrated the greatest improvement in symptoms (Wieting 2007), however, the long-term efficacy of massage has not been validated (Haraldsson 2006).

There is some evidence in regard to the effect of massage on neurotransmitters (more on these later). Field tested the benefit of massage on depressed adolescent mothers comparing massage with relaxation therapy; both groups showed reduction of anxiety. Only the massage therapy group showed measurable decrease in pulse rates and in cortisol levels in saliva and urine (cortisol gives a measurement of emotional stress).

Field also examined the effects of massage given by "significant others" to eighty-four depressed women in the second trimester of their pregnancies; he found lowered levels of anxiety and depression, higher dopamine and serotonin levels, and lower cortisol and norepinephrine levels; there were suggestions the offspring had also benefited.

What Place Does Massage Have in the Treatment of Fibromyalgia?

By all accounts, not much, as suggested by Alnigenis's study, and although emotionally satisfying to the recipient, as a one-on-one activity, it is very demanding of therapists' time (Chen), perhaps in itself the reason for the perceived benefit. It was not considered as a form of treatment in the EULAR study (Carville 2007).

Rosomoff describes heat and massage as minor adjuncts to other treatments for painful conditions. Staud (2007) refers to the pleasures of receiving a massage but warns that although pains may be eased, massage does not cure fibromyalgia. Blotman considers massage, as does Rosomoff, a preliminary to active physiotherapy but notes it may relieve the depression aspects accompanying fibromyalgia (Brattberg 1999; Alnigenis 2001).

Of the twenty-five hundred respondents in Bennett and associates' survey, 43 percent had received "massage/reflexology" with a perceived average benefit of just over six on the zero-to-ten Visual Analog Scale, putting massage/reflexology at the same level of benefit as pool therapy, substantially ahead of physical therapy at four and a half, and comparing favorably with the optimum physical activity, which was "resting," and rated at just over a six.

Heat

If heat was used for comfort before prehistory, we cannot know; one likes to think of a cave woman applying heated stones to her daughter's sore back after the men made her carry more than her fair share of the woolly mammoth they'd just downed. But it is known as a recognized therapeutic modality from as far back as we have records. By applying a heated substance to the surface of the body, there is a level of relaxation of the muscles, release of emotional tension, and an engorgement of superficial blood vessels. Surface heating causes these reactions but does not penetrate deeply and is therefore relatively safe.

Modern clinic technology is likely to employ hot packs, basically water, or heated paraffin wax; such heat does not penetrate the body's tissues more than a couple of centimeters, although the patient's sensation is that it enters much further. And then, of course, there is the opposite school that believes the application of cold packs creates a better effect. Electrical equipment generating ultrasound waves or short-wave diathermy penetrates further and is therefore more dangerous in use.

But does a sense of comfort translate to therapeutic benefit? One could reasonably suppose that when there are so many different methods of accomplishing the same objective, changing the temperature of the tissues is known technically as thermotherapy, the benefit derived might be slight. There does seem to be help in aiding mobilization of inflamed joints as in rheumatoid arthritis, but that is not an issue in fibromyalgia, and the Cochrane review conducted by Robinson did not suggest any verifiable benefit of thermotherapy, other than improving the range of joint motion in the treatment of rheumatoid arthritis.

An argument could well be made that if it makes the patient feel better, then why not use it? This might be supportable for home devices, but not at the expenditure of the therapists' time. Not all patients with fibromyalgia find heat of help, and when incorrectly used there are real dangers (Offenbacher and Stucki 2000).

Spa

Very popular for centuries in Europe, many spas have now turned to more profitable enterprises such as casinos, but Bath in the west of England, famous since Roman times, is now a respected center for research into rheumatism, and the Dead Sea in Israel continues as a therapeutic center. Buskila (2001) reported those who stayed at the Dead Sea resort and did not receive treatment were as much benefited as those who actually took the sulfur baths.

Treatments in the various spas offer mud packs, and a variety of minerals including the smelly sulfur; what they all have in common is a set of strange devices and personal attention at great expense, which must generate the benefits conferred by the placebo effect (discussed elsewhere) if no other.

Ultrasound

Sound is absorbed in the tissues and its energy converted to heat. Although there is supposedly also some mystical benefit in getting the tissues to vibrate with the frequency of the sound waves, this has yet to be explained. The energy penetration is deeper than surface heating, and ultrasound is convenient in that it can be applied to a small area such as an inflamed shoulder bursa; however, numerous studies have failed to prove it has any real value (Robertson 2001).

Transcutaneous Electrical Nerve Stimulation (TENS)

The therapeutic use of one form or another of electrical discharge antedates recorded history. In more recent times, Mesmer, of hypnotism fame, used extensively and with great personal benefit what he called "animal magnetism." Marie Antoinette insisted he stay in Paris to continue his "healing"; he escaped the revolution, Marie did not (Major 1945). Benjamin Franklin had an enthusiasm for therapeutic electricity as well as lightning conductors (Garrison 1929). An epidemic of young ladies' hysterical paralysis, associated with collapsing at inopportune moments, was successfully treated by electrotherapy in the latter half of the eighteenth century; Shorter (1992) has unearthed twenty-three publications describing its benefits.

There must be something appealing about electricity, for we're still doing the same thing. One of our current machines is called Transcutaneous Electrical Nerve Stimulation, or TENS for short, and is very widely used for control of both acute and chronic pain. Shorter found twenty-three reports for the eighteenth century, when they were blissfully unaware of words like "control studies." We now have literally hundreds of reports on TENS describing customer satisfaction, but not with scientific controls that prove it to have any more efficacy than placebo in reducing pain or even as helpful as Mesmer's highly successful animal magnetism.

A variety of newer transcutaneous or percutaneous electrical stimulation modalities has emerged recently. Interferential current therapy (IFC) is based on summation of two alternating current signals of slightly different frequency. IFC therapy can deliver higher currents than TENS. (If a little electricity is good, then more must be better. Stands to reason, don't it?)

Percutaneous electrical nerve stimulation (PENS) combines the advantages of both electroacupuncture and TENS. Rather than using surface electrodes,

PENS uses acupuncture-like needle probes as electrodes, placed at dermatomal levels corresponding to local pathology. The main advantage of PENS over TENS is that it bypasses the local skin resistance and delivers electrical stimuli at the precisely desired level in close proximity to the nerve endings located in soft tissue, muscle, or periosteum (Kaye and Branstater 2007). It's hard not to think of Mary Shelley, whose convincing living proof showed if only enough electricity is applied, the dead can be restored to life.

Although reports in the United States question the use of TENS in pregnancy, a BBC report states the most common indication for its use in the United Kingdom is by women in labor, applied to the spine and not the uterus (Macnair 2006).

Acupuncture

This is a highly contentious subject, so the author, having decided that one contentious issue per book is sufficient, relies on the government's description (NCCAM). Acupuncture is based on the concept that disease results from imbalance in the opposing forces of yin and yang (which is pretty much the foundation of all mysticism, religions, and bodice-ripping novels—the forces of purity opposed by the forces of evil). It is the stimulation of specific points on the body by a variety of techniques, including the insertion of thin metal needles through the skin. Complications have resulted from inadequate sterilization of needles and from improper delivery of treatments. When not delivered properly, acupuncture can cause serious adverse effects, including infections and punctured organs.

The 1997 National Institutes of Health Consensus Statement on Acupuncture found that, overall, results were hard to interpret because of problems with the size and design of the studies. In the years since the Consensus Statement was issued, the National Center for Complementary and Alternative Medicine (NCCAM) has funded extensive research to advance scientific understanding of acupuncture (the author is unaware of any further scientific support for this form of widely practiced treatment).

The Power of Auto-Suggestion and the Significance of Consumer Satisfaction

For seven hundred dollars you can buy a special electrically powered foot bath that claims to remove toxins from the body and improve health. The customers are very satisfied. And there is proof. As the subject sits with his or her feet in the bath, a rust-colored scum forms; the accumulated toxins are being released from the body. What is really happening is a simple process known as electrolysis. When the power is turned on, a small current flows through the water between a pair of electrodes built into the bath. One of the electrodes is made of iron; the iron is converted to rust. This is what is passed off as the toxins coming out of the body (Schwarcz 2008).

What Should We Learn from Franz Anton Mesmer?

Mesmer trained in theology and law and then in medicine at Vienna, the best medical school in Europe, where he graduated in 1766 and became a member of their teaching faculty. He believed there were invisible forces flowing through the body, an idea consistent with philosophers' thoughts at the time and not dissimilar from today's acupuncturists' ideas of yin and yang. He believed the flow could be controlled by the person's own "animal magnetism."

He moved progressively in his practice from using magnets, to electrodes, to séances in which groups sat around a tub of dilute acid, each person holding a protruding iron bar. From this, to accommodate a larger group, he moved on to "magnetizing" a tree with dangling ropes, one to a customer. Holding the rope induced a convulsion and a cure of whatever ailed them. It appears that the controlled experiment did not inhibit Mesmer's success, but Falconer in the city of Bath showed wooden paddles that could not possibly conduct any electricity worked just as well (Shorter 1992).

A school of therapists developed around Mesmer. Hundreds of books were written extolling the value of his treatments and he received royal patronage to continue his works from which hundreds of persons received cures of their overwhelming and distressing physical conditions.

What should we learn? That there's one born every minute? We all know that. That you can fool all of the people some of the time? No argument, we know that too. That people can be cured of their inexplicable problems by bizarre and scientifically unsound treatments? We have yet to learn that lesson.

MEDICATION

Medications (the pills and syrups you take) can help reduce the pain of your fibromyalgia and improve your sleep, but you should always combine the medication approach to your treatment with nonpharmacologic therapy, especially management of stress, aerobic exercise, in some persons psychotherapy, and ensure that any underlying depression will be thoroughly managed.

In their extensive survey, Bennett and associates' respondents rated "rest" as the most effective method of managing their symptoms; second in benefit came heat, and they placed medications for pain control in third place. Medications should be used with a program of proper diet, lifestyle changes, and mind work and body work; we react differently to each medication, and there is no cookbook recipe for fibromyalgia syndrome (Starlanyl 2006). There is no single right way to prescribe medicines for fibromyalgia, and more than one strategy may work for different people and for different physicians who will teach their patients basic goals in the use of medication. The most important of these is to understand there is no one magic pill that will get rid of all fibromyalgia symptoms. Prescribed medicines are, however, an important part of the treatment of fibromyalgia.

Many studies have been published that illustrate how numerous prescribed medicines can benefit those with fibromyalgia, but at the time of this writing there are only three specifically FDA-approved medications for the treatment of fibromyalgia—Lyrica (pregabalin), Cymbalta (duloxetine), and Savella (milnacipran). Physicians are able to prescribe other medicines "off-label" for fibromyalgia because of these evidence-based studies.

The medications prescribed—or bought over the counter with your physician's knowledge—will not relieve all of your pain but should relieve some of your symptoms. Pain relief, improved sleep, more energy, and better mood are examples of goals that prescription medicines can help you reach. Prescribed medicines can provide great benefits to many, so it's worthwhile to work together with your physician to try to find a successful medicine regimen. You must act responsibly in the use of analgesics and narcotics to take the edge off the pain, and you should educate yourself about what you can expect from medication. Always use the lowest effective dose of medicine and wean yourself from it as soon as possible. If you find the prescribed medication is simply not working, then rationally it should be discontinued, but your physician should be involved in this decision (Pellegrino 2007).

Another way to evaluate the effectiveness of any medication is to examine whether the patient chose to continue her treatment. Nonadherence to prescribed medications is reported to be common in fibromyalgia patients, but whether this is a result of lack of benefit, side effects, cost, or psychosocial factors is not known (Bennett 2007).

Patients with fibromyalgia have difficulty in tolerating regular doses of most medications and supplements. They are sensitive to medications, and adverse effects are common. People with fibromyalgia tend to be more sensitive to medications and often experience side effects such as nausea, drowsiness, or lightheadedness; lower doses of medicines than the usual should be considered. To avoid these problems, always start with the lowest dose available or perhaps one half to one quarter of the lowest usually recommended dose.

Your pharmacist and your physician will be aware that several medications should be avoided or used carefully, and to ensure you avoid complications and confusion, always have with you written instructions on scheduling and dosage. It is your responsibility to ensure that you understand these. As emphasized already, you should consult your pharmacist or your physician before starting any over-the-counter (OTC) medications or taking any supplements in order to avoid potentially harmful drug interactions.

Complaints of significant sleep problems are almost universal among patients suffering from pain. Improving sleep, quality and quantity, in patients with painful disorders may break the vicious circle and thereby enhance your overall health and quality of life (Onen 2005). But it must not be forgotten that the treatment of pain and sleep disorders cannot rely on a pharmacological approach alone. Other therapeutic modalities such as CBT (Smith 2007) should be tried first, or in association with drug therapy (Beaulieu 2007).

Central nervous system (CNS) agents, antidepressants, muscle relaxants, or anticonvulsants are the most successful pharmacotherapies. These medications affect serotonin, substance P, norepinephrine, and other neurochemicals that have a broad range of activities in the brain and spinal cord, including modulation of pain sensation and tolerance, which are described elsewhere in this book.

The Relief of Pain—The Words We Use

Analgesic. Any agent, applied or ingested, used with the intention of relieving pain.

Narcotic. Derived from the classical Greek, "narcotic" means a condition of being numb. As words, analgesic and narcotic are thousands of years old; as medicines, they were known to Hippocrates and Galen.

Opium. Also derived from classical Greek, "opium" is quite specifically "poppy juice," obtained from slitting the seed capsules—an action frequently seen on current television documentaries in relation to the fields of Afghanistan, and can be traced back to the Sumerians, in the land now known as Iraq, at least as long ago as 3400 BCE. They knew their product as the "joy plant." Morphine is a direct derivative from opium and is the standard against which other analgesic medications are compared. There has been some confusion in its name. It was originally developed by a Frenchman in 1803, then by a German who named his rediscovery "morphium" in 1805, in honor of Morpheus, the god of dreams, but it did not become well known until 1817. In England it was called morphia, in France morphine (Skinner 1961). Both names remain in common use, but morphine is probably the better accepted term. Heroin is a chemically altered form of morphine. Originally marketed as a child's cough medicine (Askwith 1998), it is in fact both more potent and more addictive than the morphia it was designed to replace. (Parents loved the way it quieted their children who went to sleep with a happy smile.)

Opiate. A term used to describe the many naturally occurring narcotic substances that collectively compose the whole of opium. Morphine is the strongest of these in terms of pain relief. Another medication, directly derived from opium and of major medical significance, is codeine. There are nearly thirty chemicals designated as opiates, but most are now of little importance in medical usage.

Opioid. The word is clearly a variation of "opium," the "oid" tacked onto the end implies the substance is "like" opium, but does not mean that it's chemically the same, nor does it imply a common origin; it just means an opioid behaves or functions like opium in bringing relief of pain as a result of acting like morphine, binding to specialized points found in the nervous system and gastrointestinal tract, known as "opioid receptors" (more about these later in the book).

- *Natural forms of opioid* are the opiates, for example, morphine and codeine.
- *Semisynthetic forms of opioids* are those derived by chemical manipulation from the natural opiates; examples are heroin, hydromorphone, hydrocodone, oxycodone.
- *Totally synthetic forms of opioids* are methadone, pethidine, propoxyphene, fentanyl, tramadol.
- *"Endogenous" forms of opioids* are those the body produces by its own internal chemical mechanisms known variously as endorphins, endomorphins, enkephalins, dynorphins.

Anti-inflammatories. Every medical student was taught the classical signs of inflammation, possibly the only Latin she now remembers: *calor, rubror, tumor, dolor*; or in the English: heat, redness, swelling, and pain. Medical conditions associated with inflammation have "itis" tacked on to the end of the word, such as tonsillitis, appendicitis, arthritis. We used to talk of "fibrositis," but since one of the few things everyone agrees about—there is no inflammation—the name of the condition was changed to fibromyalgia, dropping the "itis." All part of our tendency as doctors to confuse ourselves and the rest of the world into thinking changing the name implies progress. Does the patient in pain really care whether the doctors use an "itis"?

Salicylate. Derived from the bark of willow trees, salicylate was an early home-remedy form of this chemical, later altered by Bayer to be acetylsalicylic acid and sold as aspirin (Jeffreys 2004). It has anti-inflammatory properties of no value in fibromyalgia where there is no inflammation, but it also has analgesic properties and when used in fibromyalgia its purpose is as an analgesic. Acetaminophen is in the same grouping. Other anti-inflammatory medications have been developed. The most startling was cortisone. As pure anti-inflammatory medications they have no place in the treatment of fibromyalgia. Not infrequently rheumatoid arthritis or other connective tissue disorders, however, are found in the patient who also has fibromyalgia (known as a concomitant or comorbid condition) and in such circumstances a true anti-inflammatory medication may be required for the treatment of the rheumatoid arthritis.

Steroids. A huge chemical family, including among many other chemicals, the male and female sex hormones, cholesterol, and cortisone. In speaking of using "steroids" to control joint pain, it's usually derivatives of cortisone (prednisone, prednisolone) that are meant. These are used to control inflammation in arthritis. There is no inflammation in fibromyalgia. They are not used for the treatment of fibromyalgia but may, as described, be employed in the treatment of concomitant inflammatory conditions.

NSAIDs. A class of drugs remarkably defined by what they're not. Nonsteroidal anti-inflammatory drugs were a response to the need for a medication that had the ability to reduce inflammation but did not have the unfortunate side effects found with the continued use of cortisone and its derivatives. Aspirin is the most obvious of these, but since it was in use long before the term NSAID came into common parlance, aspirin is not usually spoken of as a member of the group. Apart from anti-inflammatory properties, this group has analgesic properties, and perhaps that is their most common indication when they're prescribed in the treatment of fibromyalgia. There are many variants, among which are ibuprofen and diclofenac; literally billions of NSAID tablets and capsules are sold every year. A variant, known as the COX-2 inhibitor, has been criticized for reported side effects. Some forms have been withdrawn from the market.

Anticonvulsants. It's going to seem strange to the patient that medications used to prevent seizures, known also as convulsions, are used to alleviate pain in fibromyalgia. It seems just as strange to physicians. Perhaps more strange, *Lyrica,* a member of this group, is the first medication to be approved by the Food and Drug Administration of the US Government (FDA) for treatment of fibromyalgia. Of course, that doesn't mean they disapprove of the use of the others; the FDA doesn't go for black and white, "approved" or "disapproved." Prior to approval two studies were conducted on 1,800 patients and the results "support approval for use in treating fibromyalgia" (FDA News 2007).

Antidepressants. A group of medications, such as amitriptyline, are used primarily in the treatment of depression, but they are often prescribed for relief of pain in fibromyalgia. A controlled study conducted on patients with fibromyalgia confirmed their benefit in relieving pain, stiffness, fatigue, and difficulties with sleep (Mease 2005).

SSRIs and SNRIs. When translated from initials to doctor-speak, Selective Serotonin Reuptake Inhibitors and Serotonin Norepinephrine Reuptake

Inhibitors are forms of widely used antidepressant medication. Both serotonin and norepinephrine are involved in the transmission of signals in the pain pathways of the central nervous system (Mease 2005; Dadabhoy 2006; Arnold 2006; Sumpton 2007) discussed in another part of this book. At the end of 2007, FDA approval was sought for specific use in fibromyalgia of milnacipran, a medication in this group, which was believed to have shown value in the requisite trials (RTT News 2007). If approval is granted it will be the second specifically given in pharmacological treatment of fibromyalgia.

Dopamine agonists. Medication currently approved by the FDA for treatment of Parkinson's disease is also employed in the treatment of fibromyalgia (Sumpton 2007).

Guaifenesin. Much is written, books even, all based on a rather bizarre and totally unproven theory regarding a commonly used element of OTC cough medicines. What has been proven, by acceptable scientific methods, is that guaifenesin has no value in the treatment of fibromyalgia. Results of the only known randomized clinical trial showed guaifenesin had no significant effects on pain, or any other symptoms, over twelve months in patients diagnosed with fibromyalgia (Bennett 1996).

Some might argue that if it does no harm, then why not use it? The reason against that specious argument is the same as ordering bottles of pink water and lies in the probable loss of the patient's confidence in all medications if one so highly publicized does not work, and the possible abandonment of a modestly effective medication for a totally ineffective one. We don't absolutely know what causes fibromyalgia, but we do know it certainly is not due to "an excess of phosphates," as the guaifenesin enthusiasts would have you believe (Wallace 2003).

Over the counter. Habitually abbreviated OTC, these are the medications a pharmacist may sell to you without the law requiring a prescription from a physician. The group is not defined by its actions, only by the absence of legal ordinance. Legal control varies from state to state, from country to country. What is legal and usual in one country is forbidden in another. Medications that may be sold OTC in the United States may be unavailable in Canada. The decision to allow medication to be sold without prescription may be based in part on the strength of the tablet; for instance, although codeine is an opiate, the tablet sold OTC contains a very safe amount of the drug, often combined with another medication, such as acetaminophen. There are other less logical reasons, some based on "grandfathering."

Individual medications and their pluses and minuses are considered in detail in another chapter. It is useful here to examine what Bennett and associates found in their 2007 survey. Respondents rated in order of merit the most effective management modalities as rest, heat, pain medications, antidepressants, and hypnotics. The questionnaire listed two hundred and fifty-three medications and asked, "Which of the following medications do you currently use, or have tried in the past to relieve symptoms due to fibromyalgia and were they helpful?" His table is modified here to show the pain medications used and the benefit found by the patient:

Pharmaceutical name	Drug category	Common trade name	% ever used	% used now	% considered helpful
Acetaminophen	Analgesic	Tylenol	94	35	36
Ibuprofen	NSAID	Motrin, Advil	87	36	51
Naproxen	NSAID	Naprosyn, Aleve	66	13	39
Celecoxib	NSAID (Cox-2)	Celebrex	48	6	40
Rofecoxib (Cox-2)	NSAID (Cox-2)	Vioxx	48	0	39
Codeine compound	Opiate (mild)	Tylenol #2, 3, 4	47	4	55
Tramadol	Opioid, synthetic	Ultram	46	13	44
Hydrocodone compound	Opioid, semisynthetic	Vicodin	44	18	75
Propoxyphene	Opioid, synthetic	Darvocet	44	8	54
Oxycodone compound	Opioid, semisynthetic	Percocet	32	7	67
Tramadol compound	Opioid, synthetic	Ultracet	27	7	49
Gabapentin	anticonvulsant	Neurontin	33	36	46
Fluoxetine	antidepressant	Prozac	39	8	42
Paroxetine	antidepressant	Paxil	36	4	32

This survey was conducted before the approval of Lyrica, but Neurontin (gabapentin) was an earlier form of a similar medication.

According to Bennett (2007),

> Interestingly, there is a discrepancy between the most commonly used and the most effective medications. This discrepancy may be associated with the heavy use of over-the-counter drugs, which are generally cheaper than prescription drugs. There may also be a reluctance of physicians to provide ongoing prescriptions of opioids and benzodiazepines. The perceived effectiveness of hydrocodone preparations is of some interest as this medication has never been formally tested in fibromyalgia patients.

The most commonly used medications were acetaminophen, ibuprofen, naproxen, cyclobenzaprine, amitriptyline, and aspirin. The medications perceived to be the most effective were: hydrocodone preparations, alprazolam, oxycodone preparations, zolpidem, cyclobenzaprine, and clonazepam. Nonadherence to prescribed medications is reported to be common in fibromyalgia patients (Sewitch 2004), but whether this is a result of lack of efficacy, side effects, cost, or psychosocial factors is not known.

The COX-2 group of NSAIDs has either been taken off the market or are under scrutiny involving the discrepancy between "use now" and "consider helpful." Where the numbers in these two columns are close together may indicate they can be bought easily and cheaply without a prescription (OTC), as with acetaminophen and NSAIDs. Hydrocodone compound, a strong opioid, was considered the most effective (75 percent), but only 18 percent of respondents were still using it—was this due to reluctance to take it or reluctance to prescribe it?

On the Use of Morphia

Among my favorite axioms: *The easy and obvious solution is nearly always the wrong solution.*

Not infrequently one reads: if a physician will give morphia to a patient with pain from cancer, he ought to be willing to order it for a patient whose pain is just as severe, but in her case it's caused by fibromyalgia. That would seem to be an entirely logical argument. The fallacies are: not all pain is the same; not all pain pathways are the same; not all pains respond to the same medication.

"Are opioids effective for chronic pain?" was rhetorically asked by Field (1997) and answered with, "This question has been argued for decades with hardly a shred of clinical evidence to either support or reject the hypothesis. . . . It is not known whether they retain their effectiveness when used chronically. It might be the case, that opioids play a causative rather than a curative role in chronic pain." Somatic and visceral pain is susceptible to relief from morphia; fibromyalgia is not in that group, explaining why most investigators recommend using narcotics sparingly (Gilliland 2007).

The College of Physicians and Surgeons of Ontario organized a task force to consider what should be the approved use of narcotics in the treatment of pain caused by conditions other than cancer (designated as "nonmalignant" pain, and unfortunately sometimes called "benign" pain). Literature was reviewed up to 2005, it included forty-one randomized trials on over six thousand patients who were experiencing pain from a number of conditions including fibromyalgia. Their conclusion was, "There is now strong consistent evidence that opioids relieve chronic neuropathic and nociceptive pains and improve function in placebo-controlled trials with patients who suffer chronic non-cancer pain" (CPSO; Mailis-Gagnon 2005). A further Canadian origin meta-analysis confirmed this opinion, but tramadol was the only opioid used in the two fibromyalgia studies, comprising nearly four hundred patients (Furlan 2006). The value of tramadol, which has only 10 percent the potency of morphine, in treating fibromyalgia was confirmed (Bennett 2003).

The argument that morphia and other narcotics should only be given to those in the most extreme pain or to those at death's door is no longer supported. The general view held in the profession is that it should be given whenever it is reasonably indicated by the severity of the pain and whenever it works to relieve that pain, observing appropriate precautions, just as one would with any other form of treatment. But there is no point giving a narcotic, or continuing to give it, if it fails to work.

Apart from scientific explanations, there are simple explanations from experience: not everyone has found opioids of benefit in relieving the pain of fibromyalgia. Gardner-Nix, a specialist in pain control, records her difficulty in bringing pain reported at a level of eight (the maximum is ten) down even to a five, but could lower perceived pain disability by "mindfulness-based chronic pain management," otherwise known as meditation. Rheumatologists Russell and Aaron (2003) agreed narcotics are appropriate for painful osteoarthritis of the hip, where palliative care is the goal, or for short-term problems, such as postherpetic neuralgia. But they reported on a large number of patients, perhaps the largest diagnostic group in their practice, who had chronic musculoskeletal pain with no clear-cut structural basis. These medically unexplained symptoms included fibromyalgia. In their experienced opinion, the introduction of narcotics might provide transient pain relief, but there was no convincing evidence they would restore function, get patients back to work, or indeed have any long-term benefit whatsoever. The patients themselves typically described opioids as merely "taking the edge off the pain." To barriers to prescribing opioids, they wished to add the lack of evidence of any long-term beneficial impact, in particular improvement of function or restoration of a more normal lifestyle.

Opioids, hypnotics, anxiolytics, and certain skeletal muscle relaxants must be used with caution because of the potential for abuse. An occasional patient with severe allodynia may require tramadol or opioid analgesics in order to improve quality of life and to restore function. The physician should expect several weeks or months spent adjusting the dosage after initiating opioid therapy. Monitoring of patients receiving opioid medications requires frequent reevaluation for efficacy, improvement in daily functioning, and adverse effects during initiation, dose alteration, and maintenance therapy. The patient should sign a narcotics contract that specifies one prescribing physician, one dispensing pharmacy, and acceptance of no early prescription of opioids if medication runs out early or is lost or stolen (Winfield 2007).

Physicians who regularly prescribe narcotic medications put themselves at some legal risk and become targets for drug seekers (Rosenberg 2007; Henry 2007). Pellegrino (2007) reports in his substantial experience that opioids (codeine, hydrocodone, oxycodone, morphine, fentanyl) do not alter the fibromyalgia, but they can help take the edge off pain by blocking the central pain pathways. Narcotic medications, however, have potential for adverse side effects including drowsiness, difficulty with concentrating, and addiction, so they should be used carefully. As a pain specialist, he will frequently prescribe analgesics, including narcotics, for patients experiencing severe pain but requires the patient to sign a written agreement when using scheduled medicines for pain.

The view from France is: "Pure opiates are badly tolerated and ineffectual; as a rule they have no place in the treatment of a chronic condition like fibromyalgia" (Blotman 2006).

The European League Against Rheumatism (EULAR) recommended tramadol for pain, weaker analgesics as needed, but did not recommend the stronger opioids (Carville 2007).

On the Use of Muscle Relaxants

There is a huge market for a group of medications known as muscle relaxants. Of course, there are muscle paralyzers: the South American Indians use curare on their arrows; in Texas and other states they use succinylcholine to paralyze execution victims before killing them. Our anesthesiologists use both. But that's not the kind of muscle relaxant used in office practice.

The medications prescribed for the fibromyalgia patient are in their chemical structure akin to the tricyclic antidepressant amitriptyline and work in a similar manner. The patient may be made drowsy and unsafe to drive or to use machinery. In fibromyalgia, taken in the evening, this may help her to sleep and may make her more comfortable, but since there is not in fibromyalgia an issue of "muscle spasm" as there might be in a back sprain, there is therefore no more indication for a medication that relieves muscle spasm than there is for one to relieve inflammation—neither condition exists.

In many years of practice, I never ordered this medication, and I've always told my patients (many of whom expected to have it ordered for them) that these were "mind relaxers" but not muscle relaxers.

Nevertheless, they are ordered in large quantities for patients with fibromyalgia, who may not know the side effects of taking them. A review of five groups of fibromyalgia patients treated with muscle relaxants did show a sensation of general improvement (perhaps due to improved sleep) but no alteration in daytime fatigue, nor was there any reduction in tender points (Tofferl 2004).

Other Views on Muscle Relaxants

The Mayo Clinic (2007) suggests that taking the medication cyclobenzaprine (Flexeril) at bedtime may help treat muscle pain and spasms. Muscle relaxants are generally limited to short-term use. According to Pellegrino (2007), muscle relaxants can decrease pain in people with fibromyalgia. The most common side effect is drowsiness; muscle relaxants do not really decrease muscle spasms or truly "relax" muscles. Rather, the medicine appears to help by a central neurological mechanism that reduces muscle pain. If drowsiness is a side effect, this medicine should only be taken in the evening so it doesn't interfere with driving or concentration. Flexeril is a popular medicine for evening use. Although it is a muscle relaxant, it is very similar to amitriptyline in structure and effect, hence the benefits reported.

The EULAR report did not consider the use of muscle relaxants, possibly an indication of their opinion of their value.

On the Use of Antidepressants in the Treatment of Pain

Fibromyalgia and every other chronic, painful condition is emotionally depressing. Fibromyalgia is not, however, directly caused by depression.

A group of medications widely used for the clinical condition of depression is helpful in easing some of the symptoms of fibromyalgia and in fact is commonly used in many conditions of chronic pain. As the patient, you must understand that when the physician, nurse, pharmacist, or whoever lets it slip that the medication ordered is an "antidepressive," you have not been told "it's all in your head," you've been told that a medication ordered for you has been extensively shown to help patients with fibromyalgia, in addition to helping those suffering from depression. To draw a crude analogy: a screwdriver is so-called because of its effect in driving screws; however, it's also the right tool to use to lever the lid off the paint can—not what it was designed to do, but if it does the job, why not use it?

How does an antidepressant help? There are chemicals involved in the transmission of messages in the central nervous system (the brain and spinal cord); such chemicals, notably those named serotonin and norepinephrine, are targets for these medicines (explained in more detail elsewhere). Over the years, it has been found at times that as our knowledge expands the first explanation of a mechanism of action is replaced by another. What matters to you the patient is: does it help you? And are the side effects you experience worth tolerating for the benefit obtained? There are substantial side effects, so that the advice to the prescribing physician has been "Start low; go slow," as she works with her patient to balance benefit against undesirable side effects, noticeably drowsiness.

The greatest benefit is usually improved sleep; there is less benefit obtained from relief of the symptoms of pain and morning stiffness (Arnold 2000; O'Malley 2000). The EULAR study found antidepressants to be effective in reducing pain and improving function in fibromyalgia and supported their use (Carville 2007).

The Relief of Anxiety

There are specifically defined psychological conditions known as "anxiety disorders." Everyone, no matter how phlegmatic, matter-of-fact, or casual seeming, has at some time experienced a degree of apprehension. "Apprehensive" is defined as viewing the future with anxiety, and "anxiety" is defined as an apprehensive uneasiness of mind, and so we go around in a circle. Most people will have little difficulty in separating them, if we think of apprehensive as mild and staying mild, but anxiety having the potential for building into something far worse.

A person suffering from chronic sleep disturbance and having difficulty concentrating is likely to be apprehensive that she might not be able to continue in this task. If her employer asks her to step into his office to discuss her performance review, she might be anxious about the family finances. These are very real social issues with very real emotional consequences, which contribute to pain, muscle tension, and irritability. They are best met with nonmedicinal approaches. If the level of anxiety mounts, a pharmaceutical adjunct might be appropriate but should not be the first line of therapy. If your physician thinks the anxiety has mounted to the level where it meets the defined criteria of a "disorder," the advice of a psychologist or psychiatrist might be appropriate. Although a psychologist might be appropriate, psychiatrists are licensed to prescribe medication when indicated, and psychologists are not.

Antidepressants might be prescribed, but the group of medications most commonly specifically used for anxiety are the benzodiazepines (street parlance: "benzos"). These are controlled drugs, with risk of dependence and other significant side effects. The latter must be understood, but properly used they have made life more tolerable for many distressed persons.

Sleep Medication and Hypnotics

Pharmacologic and nonpharmacologic treatment of poor sleep is crucial for improving the patient's overall sense of well-being. Complaints of significant sleep problems are almost universal among patients suffering from pain. Improving sleep quantity and quality in patients with painful disorders may break the vicious circle and thereby enhance patients' overall health and quality of life (Onen 2005). Sleep disorders are characterized by a circular interrelationship with chronic pain—pain may lead to disordered sleep, which may lead to an increase in pain perception and so on, round and round (Lavigne 2007).

Beaulieu (2007) discussed the problems of the interconnected difficulty with sleep while experiencing pain and proposed an algorithm for tackling this problem. He emphasized adequate management of sleep disturbances should involve comprehensive assessment of the symptoms as well as education about sleep hygiene, and only if necessary the use of pharmacologic agents. Many of the drugs that are used to regulate sleep and wakefulness are thought to act directly on the wake and sleep systems. The complex relationship between sleep and pain is a delicate problem when it comes to determining the most appropriate treatment for a given patient.

Beaulieu's algorithm for sleep and pain interactions:

Step 1. Comprehensive Evaluation. Evaluate symptomatology to determine presence or absence of a primary sleep disorder. Consult a sleep specialist to eliminate the possibility of sleep apnea, insomnia, periodic limb movements, and so on.

Step 2. Review of Sleep Hygiene. Total time of sleep (six to nine hours, depending on the subject); sleep environment (calm less than 35dB, comfortable bed, room ventilation, etc); wake/sleep cycle (nap less than twenty minutes); lifestyle (coffee, smoking, diet, alcohol, exercise).

Step 3. Pharmacological Intervention.

- Short-term therapy: analgesics, acetaminophen, NSAIDs, either alone or combined with a myorelaxant in the evening.
- Mild cases: myorelaxant or sedative and analgesics; low-dose cyclobenzaprine; clonazepam; acetaminophen and NSAIDs; sleep enhancer; triazolam (not in the elderly); temazepam; zaleplon (ideal for night awakenings); zopiclone, eszopliclone; zolpidem.
- Severe or persistent cases: low-dose amitriptyline in the evening; trazodone; nefazodone; gabapentin, pregabalin; codeine, morphine; herbal remedies.

Dopamine Agonists, Topical Applications, and Other Medications in the Treatment of Fibromyalgia

A group of medications (e.g., pramipexole, sinemet) employed in the treatment of Parkinson's disease have been found helpful by some workers in treating restless leg syndrome. Topical anesthesia with lidocaine (5 percent Lidoderm patch) can be helpful in postherpetic neuralgia, but it remains to be shown if it would be of value in fibromyalgia (Scudds 1995). Capsaicin, from red peppers, is a traditional constituent in Chinese medicines, the possibility of benefit as a local application in fibromyalgia has yet to be established although it is extensively used in other conditions as a counter-irritant (Chen 2005). Beta-blockers and/or increased fluid and sodium/potassium intake may benefit a subset of patients with orthostatic hypotension, palpitation, and vasomotor instability. Growth hormone and cytokine therapies are still experimental (Winfield 2007). Trials have not supported the use of thyroid hormones, melatonin, calcitonin, or dehydro-epiandrosterone in the treatment of fibromyalgia (Gilliland 2007).

PLACEBO AND NOCEBO

Placebo remains the foundation of the "bedside manner." Who wants to see a grumpy, uncaring doctor? How could he help? Who wants to be told, "There's no medicine for that"? So the kindly doctor sends you off with a prescription for an antibiotic to treat your virus infection or suggests you increase your vitamin intake when you complain of fatigue.

They don't call it a placebo, but how is that different from snake oil, sugar pills, and bottles of pink water laced with a little alcohol? Drug companies to this day remain conscious of the importance of the color of their pills (James 2007). How else could the sellers of pills for fibromyalgia stay in business? The screeds of advertisements for sure cures? If they're so sure, why does fibromyalgia still exist?

Placebos are supposed to be inert substances, incapable of altering the body, the reason they are used in controlled trials to determine whether that new drug confers any real benefit.

But we talk of the "placebo effect." How can an inert substance have an effect? Bit like military intelligence—an oxymoron?

For a long time in drug trials, it's been known that as much as a third of any benefit in the trial of a new drug might be due to this placebo effect, since the persons given only the placebo, and not the new drug, were also improved (Beecher 1955). This was variously attributed to suggestibility, the power of persuasion, or some inner mechanism of unknown spiritual powers. With more recent studies, we find placebos really can be shown to have an effect, and that effect can be demonstrated and measured with biochemical techniques.

Placebos don't work on the tangible. They don't make bones heal faster, but there are "objective measurements," such as blood pressure, that may be altered. Pain may be reduced. A good nurse "talks down" an anxious patient in pain; a lesser nurse gives more morphia. Women in childbirth may be troubled less by pain if they deliver in a supportive ambience. We've kept the mind and the body separated for too long; it's taken hundreds of years to undo the damage caused by philosophers like Descartes! If Pavlov's dogs could be made to salivate at the sound of a bell, nonphilosophers would've known there was something going on between the dog's ears and his salivary glands. The professional torturer knows the thought of pain is as frightening as the pain itself.

Common to the benefits achieved by the placebo effect is the work of the autonomic nervous system and the hypothalamic-pituitary-adrenal axis (HPA) discussed in more detail in another chapter. Chemicals, rationally called neurotransmitters because they transmit messages in the nerve system, are liberated as a response to pain. These can be measured. The body produces its own pain-relieving substances called endorphins. These can be measured. The action of endorphins at specialized pain receptor sites in the brain can be imaged by positron emission tomography (PET scan) and by functional magnetic resonance imaging (fMRI). It has been shown that under sham conditions, the same pain-suppressing mechanism can be activated by the "placebo effect" (Wager 2004). Perhaps not of much practical use, but these techniques will even permit the subject to determine whether her favorite cola drink has been taken or whether it's the "other brand."

The Nocebo Effect

Every good story for children of all ages has a hero and a villain, a good guy and a bad guy, a good fairy and a bad witch. And so it is with our brain. The bad witch, the villain, they all pronounce, "Nocebo—I will harm!"

The placebo effect is the body's mechanism to heal itself. There are other mechanisms that unite bones and heal wounds; the body's own opium, which we call endorphins, diminishes the effect of the pain-causing chemicals produced in the inflammatory response to injury. Creating a negative response to the possibility of benefit from treatment is the reverse of the good bedside manner. A rude or seemingly indifferent doctor sends his patients away angry and frustrated; not only will they fail to have the positive results of the placebo effect, they are liable to suffer the negative effects of a nocebo. They not only fail to improve with the medicine he ordered, they become definitely worse.

Everyone knows the story of the priest who gave last rites to the wrong person, who obligingly died forthwith. True? Who knows? There is evidence that when a patient is convinced he will suffer side effects from taking a drug, then very likely he will. Experienced surgeons have learned not to operate on the patient who fears he will die under the anesthetic—too often he does!

Wager and his group demonstrated a pain-suppressing mechanism came into play when a sham painful experience was induced. Researchers in Turin have shown a neurotransmitter is released when the subject fears he will suffer a painful experience, and sure enough, he does have pain; but if a blocking agent is used to prevent the action of the neurotransmitter, the anticipated pain does not occur (Colloca 2007).

And So?

We depend on physical signs, what we see, feel, or hear, to make a diagnosis. We listen to symptoms that give us clues, but we need signs to support them. Before Roentgen and the x-ray, we had a pretty good idea about most pathologies; we could always open up the live patient on the operating table, or failing that, on the autopsy slab.

But pain we couldn't see. We all learned as students about the hysterical women who'd been cured of their overwhelming pain by sham surgery (Shorter 1992), but we didn't question whether they really had pain and whether an unexpected mechanism had come into play to cure it. Now we are closer to being able to make a picture of pain, imaging pain. We know more about the mechanisms that carry the messages from the abused area to the brain, where the messages are interpreted. We still have a long way to go. Rome was built brick by brick.

NUTRITION

A basic premise is that nutrient needs should be met primarily through consuming foods, pretty much what we've always done, even before Eve bit into that troublesome apple. But it is reported patients with fibromyalgia are influenced heavily by information promoting complementary and alternative approaches to treatment, so we discuss here principles of sound general nutrition, and what if anything is appropriate to take in the way of vitamin and other supplements, to maintain *mens sana in corpore sano*—a healthy mind in a healthy body.

Poor diet will surely burden the symptoms of fibromyalgia, whereas some nutritional changes might lessen them. Most patients with fibromyalgia consume enormous amounts of carbohydrate-rich foods, which may contribute to their symptoms. You must forgo junk foods, all those processed snack foods, replete with large amounts of delicious sugar and salt!

The nutritionist will help you to choose menus that are nutritionally balanced yet satisfying. She will help you to set reasonable and attainable goals in your dietary changes and your optimum weight. She will show you how to keep a food journal so you will be able to see what changes you have made and what benefits you've received, and what adjustments you still need to make. You must wean yourself from coffee, slowly so you don't get an increase in fatigue and pain, nor the headaches, anxiety, and sleep disturbance that persons who are giving up coffee will sometimes experience. Meals with fresh vegetables, fish, and fiber are preferable; you will learn green, leafy, and yellow vegetables are preferred by nutrition experts because of their low carbohydrate content.

Key Recommendations of the US Guidelines

The US Government Department of Health and Human Services has made readily available on the Internet "Dietary Guidelines for Americans," which provides science-based advice to promote health and to reduce risk for major chronic diseases. Appropriate amounts of physical activity, combined with a diet that does not provide excess calories, should enhance the health of most individuals.

Use a two-thousand-calorie level as a reference. Recommended calorie intake will differ for individuals based on age, gender, and activity level. At each calorie level, individuals who eat nutrient-dense foods may be able to meet their recommended nutrient intake without consuming their full calorie allotment. Consume a variety of nutrient-dense foods and beverages within and among the basic food groups while choosing foods that limit the intake of saturated and trans fats, cholesterol, added sugars, salt, and alcohol.

To maintain body weight in a healthy range, balance calories from foods and beverages with calories you use up. To prevent gradual weight gain over time, make small decreases in food and beverage calories and increase your physical activity. For those who need to lose weight, aim for a slow, steady weight loss by decreasing calorie intake while maintaining an adequate nutrient intake and increasing physical activity.

Engage in regular physical activity and reduce your sedentary activities to promote health, psychological well-being, and a healthy body weight. Achieve physical fitness by including cardiovascular conditioning, stretching exercises for flexibility, and resistance exercises for muscle strength and endurance.

Two cups of fruit and two and a half cups of vegetables per day are recommended. Choose a variety of fruits and vegetables each day. In particular, select from all five vegetable subgroups (dark green, orange, legumes, starchy vegetables) several times a week. Choose fiber-rich fruits, vegetables, and whole grains often. Eat three or more ounce-equivalents of whole grain products per day, with the rest of the recommended grains coming from enriched or whole grain products. Drink three cups per day of fat-free or low-fat milk or equivalent milk products. Less than 10 percent of your calories should come from saturated fatty acids, and less than 300 mgs/day of cholesterol, and keep trans fatty acid consumption as low as possible.

Keep total fat intake between 20 to 35 percent of calories, with most fats coming from sources of polyunsaturated and monounsaturated fatty acids, such as fish, nuts, and vegetable oils. Make choices that are lean, low fat, or fat free when selecting meat, poultry, dry beans, milk or milk products.

Choose and prepare foods and beverages with little added sugars or caloric sweeteners and with little salt (less than one teaspoonful a day). At the same time, consume potassium-rich foods, such as fruits and vegetables.

Dietary Supplements

While sometimes necessary, supplements cannot replace a healthful diet.

A dietary supplement (also known as a food supplement) is intended to supply nutrients (vitamins, minerals, fatty acids, or amino acids) that are missing or not consumed in sufficient quantity in a person's diet.

Some important definitions under the US Dietary Supplement Health and Education Act of 1994 (DSHEA):

A **dietary supplement** is defined as a product that is intended to supplement the diet and contains one or more of the following dietary ingredients: vitamin; mineral; herb or other botanical (excluding tobacco); amino acid; a **dietary substance** is for use by people to supplement the diet by increasing the total dietary intake, or a concentrate, metabolite, constituent, extract, or combination of any of the above. It must be: intended for ingestion in pill, capsule, tablet, powder or liquid form; not represented for use as a conventional food or as the sole item of a meal or diet; and labeled as a "dietary supplement."

It's important to understand that the Food and Drug Administration regulates dietary supplements as foods, not as drugs.

Unlike the pharmaceutical companies, manufacturers of supplements are not required to prove the safety or effectiveness of their products; the FDA can take action only after a dietary supplement has been proven harmful. *In addition, the purity and quality of individual brands of dietary supplements are unregulated.*

Confusion about the implications of DSHEA was shown in an October 2002 nationwide Harris poll when 59 percent of respondents were found to believe supplements had to be approved by a government agency before they could be marketed; 68 percent believed supplements had to list potential side effects on their labels; and 55 percent believed supplement labels could not make claims of safety without scientific evidence. All of these beliefs are incorrect.

The claims made about a dietary supplement are key to its classification. If a dietary supplement claims to cure, mitigate, or treat a disease, it would be considered to be an unauthorized new drug and in violation of the applicable regulations and statutes. The FDA must be notified of these claims within thirty days of their first use, and there is a requirement that these claims be substantiated.

Vitamin Supplementation, Free Radicals, and Antioxidants

Unnecessary vitamin intake may actually be harmful to your health. A study published in the *Journal of the American Medical Association* found regular supplementation with vitamin E, beta-carotene, and vitamin A increased mortality by 4, 7, and 16 percent, respectively. The same study also suggested that vitamin C and selenium had no effect, one way or the other, on longevity (Bjelakovic 2007).

"Free radicals," just one of the current buzz phrases, is used by salesmen to induce us to buy their products, coupled inevitably with "antioxidants." Ask what they mean, ask what they do, and you won't get much more than an increase in pressure to buy lots of them. Free radicals are the demons circling the earth, and antioxidants are the magic charms you must buy to ward them off.

What are free radicals? Why are they damaging to the human body? And how do vitamins C and E and other antioxidant nutrients help protect the body against free radical damage? Why should you eat fruits and vegetables? How can they benefit your health? A free radical is a hungry fellow, looking to stabilize his life and not too worried about whom he harms as long as he gets what he wants. Sound familiar? Happens at all levels! The hungry fellow in this instance is an atom. Atoms have rings of electrons layered around them. At times the outer layer finds itself short of an electron, and this electron-deficient atom is the so-called free radical. It's a usual part of normal cellular metabolism, but it's more frequent in abnormal circumstances such as inflammation. The electron-deficient atom seeks to satisfy its needs by stealing an electron from a neighbor, who is then obliged to take one from his neighbor, and off goes the chain. Normal when controlled, but destructive to the cell when out of control.

The controlling factors, or one of them, is the so-called antioxidant effect of vitamins C and E. They neutralize free radicals by generously giving one of their own electrons, ending the electron-stealing reaction. The antioxidant nutrients themselves don't become free radicals by losing an electron; they're stable in either form. They act as scavengers, helping prevent cell and tissue damage that might otherwise lead to disease. Vitamin C is the most abundant water-soluble antioxidant in the body and acts primarily in cellular fluid; vitamin E is the most abundant fat-soluble antioxidant in the body and one of the most efficient chain-breaking antioxidants available. Although the antioxidants help to protect the body from free-radical damage, more is not always better.

Vitamins in General

The body is a highly efficient chemical factory; it manufactures most of the chemicals it needs for its normal function by taking the foodstuffs ingested, breaking them down to smaller components, then reassembling these components into the new chemicals it wants. It's extraordinarily clever at doing this, but not quite clever enough. There are some components of proteins that the human body cannot manufacture and must obtain by eating them; hence, they're called the "essential" amino acids. There are chemicals that, although not converted into other structures, are essential in the transformation or maintenance of those structures. What we've learned about these came originally from studying the diseases that occurred when these essential chemicals were missing, called deficiency diseases, the best known of which is scurvy, with lemon juice as the best-known cure.

It cannot be overemphasized that a normal diet, one that follows all the routines of a normal life, contains all the vitamins needed, and taking more vitamins than are required conveys no additional benefit.

There is a serious misconception that if a small amount of a vitamin is good, then a large amount must be even better. To make a not altogether apt analogy, it's a bit like needing a pinch of salt to bring out flavor, but adding more than a pinch has no benefit and may even be harmful. Or to try another analogy, if your car will easily do one hundred miles an hour, which is as fast as you ever wish to drive, why would you surrender your good sense to the salesman who'll tell you this "new and improved" model will easily do two hundred fifty?

Abuse of Vitamins

Despite the known lack of medical value, more than one hundred million Americans regularly use nonprescribed vitamins. In the United States, consumer spending on vitamins and minerals has doubled in the last six years, reaching $6.5 billion annually. What fantastic power of salesmanship! Excessive use of vitamins is not merely wasteful of money; it leads people to believe that this magic is all they need to stay healthy and so they evade proper nutritional responsibility. Can we blame the epidemic of obesity on that misconception?

Excessive quantities of vitamins can be toxic, particularly to young children who get into their parents' unsecured medicine cupboard, and it's the iron-containing vitamin pills that are the most toxic to infants and small children. Overall, 57,801 exposures to different types of vitamins were reported to poison control centers across the United States in 2003, accounting for sixty-three major adverse outcomes and four deaths. Of the total exposures, 45,352 occurred in children younger than six years (Rosenbloom 2007).

Vitamin A

Summary for fibromyalgia:

- Normal diets contain sufficient vitamin A.
- Vitamin A may be deficient if chronic diarrhea is present; advice on the need for supplements should be sought if also suffering from irritable bowel disease.
- There is no benefit to be gained from taking more than the standard suggested amount of vitamin A.
- There is substantial possibility of harm from significantly exceeding the usual quantity of vitamin A, in particular osteoporosis with threat of hip fracture. Liver damage, neurologic injury, and fetal injury are also possibilities.

Role of vitamin A. The vitamin is an important participant in vision, bone growth, reproduction, fetal cell differentiation in which a cell becomes either part of the brain, muscle, lungs, blood, or other specialized tissue. It helps to regulate the immune system, which helps against infections by making white blood cells, which in turn destroy harmful bacteria and viruses. The vitamin promotes healthy surface linings of the eyes and the respiratory, urinary, and intestinal tracts. When those linings break down, it becomes easier for bacteria to enter the body and cause infection.

Sources of vitamin A. Vitamin A in foods that come from animals is called "preformed" vitamin A. When derived from colorful fruits and vegetables it's called, "provitamin A carotenoid." Preformed vitamin A is absorbed in the form of retinol, one of the most active forms of vitamin A. Sources include liver, whole milk, and some fortified food products. Provitamin A can be made into retinol in the body. Vitamin A in foods that come from animals is well absorbed and used efficiently by the body. Vitamin A in foods that come from plants is not absorbed as well as the animal sources of vitamin.

Most fat-free milk and dried nonfat milk solids that are sold in the United States and Canada are fortified with vitamin A to replace the amount lost when the fat is removed during processing. Fortified foods such as fortified breakfast cereals also supply vitamin A.

Who May Need Extra Vitamin A to Prevent a Deficiency?

Vitamin A deficiency is common in developing countries: as many as half a million malnourished children in the developing world become blind each year from a deficiency of vitamin A. In the United States, vitamin A deficiency is rare and is most often associated with extreme self-imposed dietary restrictions or excessive alcohol intake. Fat malabsorption can result in diarrhea and prevent normal absorption of vitamin A. Over time this may result in vitamin A deficiency. Healthy adults usually have a reserve of vitamin A stored in their livers and should not be at risk of deficiency during periods of temporary or short-term fat malabsorption. Strict vegetarians who eat neither eggs nor dairy foods need provitamin A carotenoids to meet their need for vitamin A, and should eat daily a minimum of five servings of dark green leafy vegetables and orange and yellow fruits.

Excessive Intake of Vitamin A

Toxic symptoms of hypervitaminosis A can arise after consuming very large amounts of preformed vitamin A over a short period of time. Signs of acute toxicity include nausea and vomiting, headache, dizziness, blurred vision, and muscular uncoordination. Although hypervitaminosis A can occur when large amounts of liver are regularly consumed (don't eat polar bear liver), most cases result from taking excessive amounts in supplements. It's not too uncommon to see a very young child with orange-tinted skin as a result of being fed too much mashed carrot. The US Government Institute of Medicine (IOM) has established Tolerable Upper Intake Levels (ULs) for vitamin A that apply to healthy populations. The UL was established to help prevent the risk of vitamin A toxicity, which increases at intakes greater than the UL.

Osteoporosis is a serious health problem besetting the elderly, women sooner than men, whites sooner than blacks. Women who consumed three times the recommended daily intake of vitamin A had an increased risk of experiencing a hip fracture (Melhus 1998; Feskanich 2002; Michaelsson 2003). Other adverse effects of hypervitaminosis A are fetal birth defects, liver abnormalities, and central nervous system disorders.

Vitamin B Complex

Summary for fibromyalgia: A normal diet contains adequate vitamin B complex. Only in exceptional circumstances might you require particular supplements, such as B_{12} for older persons and persons with gastrointestinal problems, and folic acid for those at risk of becoming pregnant.

Vitamin B was the original. The word "vitamin" is a contracted form of "vitamine," itself a contracted form of the original term coined by Casimir Funk, the Polish doctor working in England who called his product "vital amine," incorrectly believing it to be an amino acid (Carpenter 2000).

The B vitamins. Eight water-soluble substances that play important roles in cell metabolism were once thought to be a single vitamin, referred to as vitamin B. Later research showed they are chemically distinct vitamins although often coexisting in the same foods. Collectively, all eight B vitamins are generally referred to as a vitamin B "complex." Individual B vitamin elements are identified by specific number, for example, B_1, B_2, B_3, and less often by name.

Actions. The B vitamins have been shown to support and increase the rate of metabolism; maintain healthy skin and muscle tone; enhance immune and nervous system function; promote cell growth and division, including the red blood cells that help prevent anemia; combat the causes of stress, depression, and cardiovascular disease.

Sources. Potatoes, bananas, lentils, chili peppers, liver, turkey, and tuna. Nutritional yeast (or brewer's yeast) and molasses are especially good sources of vitamin B. Due to its high content of brewer's yeast, beer is also a good source. All B vitamins are water soluble, and are dispersed throughout the body. Most of the B vitamins must be replenished daily, since any excess is excreted in the urine; however, a six-year cobalamin (B_{12}) store can be found in the liver.

Deficiency States of Vitamins B

- Vitamin B_1 (thiamine): Deficiency causes beriberi, rarely seen in the United States (Carpenter 2000). Symptoms of this disease of the nervous system include weight loss, emotional disturbances, impaired sensory perception, weakness and pain in the limbs, periods of irregular heartbeat, and swelling of bodily tissues. Heart failure and death may occur in advanced cases. It was common in military prisoners held by the Japanese during World War II. Chronic thiamine deficiency can cause Korsakoff's syndrome, an irreversible psychosis characterized by amnesia and confabulation (found in the United States in chronic alcoholics).
- Vitamin B_2 (riboflavin): Deficiency symptoms may include cracks in the lips, high sensitivity to sunlight, inflammation of the tongue (found in the United States in chronic alcoholics).
- Vitamin B_3 (niacin, includes nicotinic acid and nicotinamide): Deficiency causes pellagra. Symptoms include aggression, dermatitis, insomnia,

weakness, mental confusion, and diarrhea leading to dementia and death (now rare in the United States).

- Vitamin B_5 (pantothenic acid): Deficiency may uncommonly result in paresthesia.
- Vitamin B_6 (pyridoxine).
- Vitamin B_7, also vitamin H (biotin).
- Vitamin B_8 (myo-inositol) is no longer classified as a vitamin because it is synthesized by the human body.
- Vitamin B_9 (folic acid): Deficiency results in a macrocytic anemia. Deficiency in pregnant women can lead to distressing spinal defects in the child. Recommended daily supplementary intake is an exception to the rule that a normal diet is all that's necessary, in that this supplement is highly recommended during pregnancy, or even if at risk of exposure to an unintended pregnancy, which in the view of some means any woman between menarche and menopause. If there is to be a birth defect, it happens in the very earliest stages of embryonic development, before the woman even knows she's pregnant.
- Vitamin B_{12} (cobalamin): Deficiency is most likely to occur among elderly people as absorption through the gut declines with age, or in persons with some gastrointestinal problems. It results in macrocytic anemia, peripheral neuropathy, memory loss, other cognitive deficits, and the "pernicious anemia," which in extreme cases results in paralysis.

Vitamin C

Summary for fibromyalgia: A normal diet with appropriate fruit and leafy vegetables should provide quite sufficient quantities of vitamin C.

Role. What humans and guinea pigs have in common is an inability to make their own vitamin C; most other animals do not have that inefficiency in metabolism. You don't very often see a dog eating lemons. Vitamin C is an essential nutrient for humans and is required for a range of metabolic reactions. In humans, vitamin C is a highly effective antioxidant with an important role in the formation of collagen, the framework of the body. Its actions allow the collagen molecule to assume its triple helix structure, thus vitamin C is essential to the development and maintenance of scar tissue, blood vessels, cartilage, bone, and all collagen-containing tissues. It also has a critical role essential for the transport of fatty acids into mitochondria for the generation of the energy chemical, adenosine triphosphate (ATP), in the synthesis of norepinephrine from dopamine, and in innumerable other biochemical activities in whose absence the body's chemical factory would grind to a halt.

Daily requirements. There is continuing debate over the best dose schedule of vitamin C for maintaining optimal health. The North American Dietary Reference Intake recommends ninety milligrams per day and no more than two thousand milligrams per day. It's generally agreed a balanced diet without supplement contains enough vitamin C to prevent scurvy in an average healthy adult, while those who are pregnant, smoke tobacco, or are under stress may require slightly more. High doses (thousands of milligrams) may result in diarrhea. Proponents of alternative medicine claim the onset of diarrhea to be an indication of where the body's true vitamin C requirement lies—stuff yourself with vitamin C until you're forced to go to the toilet!

Effects of deficiency. It is widely known as the vitamin whose deficiency causes scurvy in humans. The human body can store only a limited amount of vitamin C, which is soon depleted. Without this vitamin, the already formed collagen is too unstable to meet its function. Sailors used to report their healed scars would break down. Gums became spongy; there was bleeding from all mucous membranes. In advanced scurvy, there are open, suppurating wounds; loss of teeth; and eventually death.

Sources. Rose hips are a particularly rich source, and children in Europe were sent out during the war to collect them. The richest natural sources are fruits and vegetables. While plants are generally a good source of vitamin C, the amount in foods of plant origin depends on the length of time since it was picked, the storage conditions, and the method of preparation. Vitamin C is also present in some cuts of meat, especially liver, and least present in the muscle. Since muscle provides the majority of meat consumed in the Western human diet, animal products are not a reliable source of the vitamin. Vitamin C is present in mother's milk and, in lower amounts, in raw cow's milk, but pasteurized milk contains only trace amounts and is not usually supplemented. (Check the package for the listed contents.)

Food preparation. Fresh-cut fruit does not lose significant nutrients when stored in the refrigerator for a few days. Despite popular opinion, boiling water at 100°C is not hot enough to cause any significant destruction of the vitamin, which decomposes only at 190°C and above. However, pressure cooking, roasting, frying, and grilling food is more likely to reach this temperature. Longer cooking times also add to the destructive effect, as will the use of copper food vessels.

Historical. While the earliest known documented case of scurvy was described by Hippocrates around the year 400 BCE, the need to include fresh plant food or raw animal flesh in the diet to prevent disease was known from more ancient times. Early peoples incorporated this knowledge into their medicinal lore; spruce needles were used in temperate zones in infusions, and the leaves from species of drought-resistant trees were used in desert areas.

In 1536, the French explorer Jacques Cartier, traveling the St. Lawrence River, was helped by the indigenous knowledge that pine tree needles could save his men who were dying from scurvy.

In what might be the first modern scientific controlled experiment, James Lind, a ship's surgeon in the British Royal Navy, in May 1747 provided some crew members with fresh citrus fruit and others with various of the bizarre scurvy preventatives the admiralty insisted should be used. The results conclusively showed citrus fruits prevented the disease. Lind published his work in 1753 in his *Treatise on the Scurvy*. Although Lind indubitably proved his point, and although he later was in charge of the enormous naval hospital at Haslar, he didn't force the issue against his superiors who were reluctant to accept his findings, and many sailors and soldiers continued to die from scurvy (Brown 2004).

Adverse effects. While being harmless in usual quantities, as with all substances to which the human body is exposed, vitamin C can cause harm under certain conditions. Relatively large doses of vitamin C may cause indigestion, particularly when taken on an empty stomach. When taken in large doses, vitamin C causes diarrhea.

Controversy. There is a strong movement advocating large doses of vitamin C led by scientists and doctors such as the two-time Nobel Prize laureate Linus Pauling. If one were to believe their argument, and if we all took as much vitamin C as they suggest, there would be very little disease in the world and probably a lot less death. Proponents such as Pauling consider that if it is given "in the right form, with the proper technique, in frequent enough doses, in high enough doses, along with certain additional agents and for a long enough period of time," it can prevent and, in many cases, cure, a wide range of common and lethal diseases, ranging from the common cold to heart disease, and we would all live forever. "You just have lots of ideas and throw away the bad ones," Pauling said. "You aren't going to have good ideas, unless you have *lots* of ideas and some principle of selection." Pauling died in 1994, leaving his "principle of selection" open to question.

Vitamin D

Summary for fibromyalgia: A normal diet should be sufficient for most persons; older persons pregnant and/or lactating mothers might be recommended to take supplements.

Chemistry. Vitamin D, like vitamin B, is a group of substances, the two major forms of which are vitamin D2 (ergocalciferol) and vitamin D3 (cholecalciferol) produced in the skin exposed to sunlight, specifically ultraviolet B radiation. A critical determinant of vitamin D3 production in the skin is melanin, which acts as a light filter in the skin. Individuals with higher skin melanin content require more time in sunlight to produce the same amount of vitamin D as individuals with lower melanin content. Once vitamin D is produced in the skin or consumed in food, it is converted in the liver and kidneys to form the physiologically active form of vitamin D.

Actions. Calcium and phosphorus: vitamin D regulates levels in the blood by promoting their absorption from food in the intestines and reabsorption of calcium in the kidneys, and by its action on the parathyroid gland. Bone formation and mineralization: vitamin D is essential in the process of development and maintenance of the skeleton. Immune system: vitamin D promotes and strengthens its effects.

Deficiency. Vitamin D deficiency is caused by inadequate dietary intake, inadequate sunlight exposure, or both. Specific medical problems may interfere with absorption, or conversion of the vitamin into its active state. Deficiency results in impaired bone mineralization; the collagen framework of bone is present, but it's not reinforced with the crystals of bone mineral. Rickets is a childhood disease characterized by restricted growth and deformity of the softened long bones; osteomalacia, an adult form of failure to mineralize the collagen framework of bone, is characterized by bone fragility and muscle weakness. Prior to the fortification of milk products with vitamin D, rickets was a major public health problem. In the United States, milk has been fortified with vitamin D since the 1930s, leading to a dramatic decline in the number of rickets cases. Prior to the Second World War, cities in England were covered by a pall of smoke, and 30 percent of the children suffered rickets. Rickets was supposed to be a thing of the past but is now reported at the 1 percent level in certain at-risk minority groups in England, principally due to failure to take the available supplements (BBC 2007).

Groups at greater risk of deficiency. Vitamin D requirements increase with age, due to diminished ability of the skin to create the vitamin. There may be need for increased vitamin D supplements in older persons. Obese individuals may have lower levels of the circulating form of vitamin D, and are at higher risk of deficiency. Patients with chronic liver disease or intestinal malabsorption disorders may also require larger doses of vitamin D. The use of sunscreen with a sun protection factor of eight inhibits more than 95 percent of vitamin D production in the skin. To avoid vitamin D deficiency, dermatologists recommend supplementation along with sunscreen use. Conversely, in the winter, diminished hours of sunlight have led the Canadian Cancer Society to recommend adult Canadians to consider taking 1,000 IU of vitamin D during the fall and winter months.

Sources. Season, geographic latitude, time of day, cloud cover, smog, and sunscreen affect ultraviolet-ray exposure and vitamin D synthesis in the skin, and it is important for individuals with limited sun exposure to include good sources of vitamin D in their diet. Very few foods are naturally rich in vitamin D, and most vitamin D intake is in the form of fortified products including milk, soy milk, and cereal grains, which are often fortified with vitamin D. In some countries, foods such as milk, yogurt, margarine, oil spreads, breakfast cereal, pastries, and bread are fortified with vitamin D to minimize the risk of deficiency. In the United States and Canada, for example, fortified milk typically provides 100 IU per glass, or one quarter of the estimated adequate intake for adults over the age of fifty. Natural sources of vitamin D include fatty fish, such as salmon, catfish, mackerel, sardines, tuna, eel, and cod liver oil. (I recall seeing Newfoundland fishermen drinking cans of cod liver oil as they worked on the "fish flakes.") Vitamin D is also to be found naturally in mushrooms, eggs, and yeast, but fortified foods represent the major dietary sources of vitamin D, as very few foods naturally contain significant amounts.

Daily requirements. The US Dietary Reference Intake for Adequate Intake (AI) of Vitamin D for infants, children, and men and women aged 19–50 is 200 IU/day. Adequate intake increases to 400 IU/day for men and women aged 51–70 and to 600 IU/day past age 70.

Overdose. The symptoms of vitamin D toxicity are a result of an elevated level of calcium in the blood caused by increased intestinal calcium absorption. Gastrointestinal symptoms of vitamin D toxicity can develop, including anorexia, nausea, and vomiting. At very high levels, vitamin D will promote the resorption of bone. Exposure to sunlight for extended periods of time does not cause vitamin D toxicity. Within twenty minutes of ultraviolet exposure in light-skinned individuals, the concentration of vitamin D precursors produced in the skin reaches an equilibrium, and any further vitamin D that is produced is degraded. Normal food and pill vitamin D concentration levels are too low to be toxic in adults; most historical cases of vitamin D overdose have occurred due to manufacturing and industrial accidents, and toxicity usually occurs only if excessive doses in prescription forms have been taken. All known cases of vitamin D toxicity with raised serum calcium levels have involved intake of or over one hundred times the recommended daily intake. In the United States, overdose exposure of vitamin D was reported by 284 individuals in 2004, leading to one death.

Vitamin E

Summary for fibromyalgia: A normal diet contains sufficient vitamin E; supplements should not be needed for persons with fibromyalgia alone; if there are concomitant bowel problems, this might need to be reviewed.

What is vitamin E? During feeding experiments with rats, Evans concluded in 1922 that apart from vitamins B and C, an unknown vitamin had to exist.

Although every other nutrient was present, the rats were not fertile. This condition could be changed by additional feeding with wheat germ. It took until 1936 when the substance was isolated from wheat germ, and its structure was determined in 1938. It was given the name "tocopherol" from the Greek words meaning "to carry a pregnancy," with the ending "-ol" signifying its status as a chemical alcohol. Natural vitamin E exists in eight different forms. Each has a slightly different biological activity. Various derivatives with vitamin activity may correctly be referred to as vitamin E. All are antioxidants.

Role. Numerous claims are made that vitamin E does more than help infertile male rats. None of these claims have been satisfactorily proven.

- In the eye: adding vitamin E appeared to help protect the retina from glaucomatous damage; diminished tendency to cataracts reported with regular use of vitamin E supplements; age-related macular degeneration; possibly protective effect in combination with other antioxidants, like zinc and vitamin C.
- Alzheimer's disease: in combination with vitamin C, the onset reduced between 64 and 78 percent.
- Parkinson's disease: moderate to high intake of vitamin E found to lower the risk.
- Cancer: by protecting against the damaging effects of free radicals, by enhancing immune function, vitamin E may contribute to the prevention of chronic diseases such as cancer.
- Heart disease: a widely held belief that vitamin E may help prevent or delay coronary heart disease was not supported by large controlled studies; in fact, vitamin E supplements may increase the risk for heart failure.

Contrary to the expectations of those who believe the vitamin will preserve health, a review of all randomized controlled trials in the scientific literature by the Cochrane Collaboration found an increase in mortality of those using vitamin E, estimated at four hundred per ten thousand persons (Bjelakovic, Nikolova, and Gluud 2007).

The influence of a group of enthusiasts can be very strong. The Shute Clinic in southwest Ontario had a regional influence akin to that of the Mayo Clinic in Minnesota; their enthusiasm for applying vitamin E to a wide group of conditions left its mark.

Deficiency. Vitamin E deficiency is usually characterized by neurological problems due to poor nerve conduction. Individuals who cannot absorb fat may require a vitamin E supplement because some dietary fat is needed for the absorption of vitamin E from the gastrointestinal tract. Anyone with malabsorptive problems should discuss the need for supplemental vitamin E with their physician.

Sources. The IOM states that most North American adults get enough vitamin E from their normal diets to meet current recommendations. In foods, the most abundant sources of vitamin E are vegetable oils such as palm oil, sunflower, corn, soybean, and olive oil. Nuts, sunflower seeds, seabuckthorn berries, kiwi fruit, and wheat germ are also good sources. Other sources of vitamin E are whole grains, fish, peanut butter, and green leafy vegetables. Fortified breakfast cereals are also an important source of vitamin E in the United States.

Excess. "Megadoses" of vitamin E are not recommended by many government agencies, due to a possible increased risk of bleeding.

NONTRADITIONAL TECHNIQUES AND SUPPLEMENTS

Perhaps we were in fact getting to a point where we were separating the mind from the body and perhaps we needed to be jerked back to what Hippocrates knew, not to mention the practitioners of the art of medicine in China and India in even earlier periods. Too often employed to justify the myriad supposedly traditional forms of medical care for which there is no scientific or rational basis, holism has become a euphemism for nonscientific.

I have difficulties with the idea that the principles of medical practice in China a thousand years ago are any more appropriate to medical practice in the Western world today, than are the principles of medical practice in western Europe a thousand years ago—snakes' tongues, lizards' tails and all. Hippocrates would laugh his head off!

Physical Alternatives in Treatment

Cervical collars. There are three kinds of neck braces:

1. Fixed, supported from the torso, with a cup under the chin, another at the base of the skull, worn by tetraplegics whose head would otherwise droop to the chest. The cervical spinal cord is no longer at risk—it's already been destroyed.
2. Rigid, made of leather or plastic, often with extensions over the chest and back, applied with the intention of severely restricting movement of a spine considered "at risk" after an injury or surgery, when there is serious question of damage to the spinal cord if the weight of the head is not supported. Often known in the trade as a "Philadelphia" collar. The kind used by paramedics is a ring, closed by Velcro and easily applied to move in safety a potentially injured person. It's not comfortable—comfort

wasn't the reason it was applied—and the emergency room physician is urged to give priority to its removal.

3. Soft, made from stockinette stuffed with cotton batten, or scarves, or proprietary foam rubber bought at the drug store. Essentially no more than a "Hey! Look at me! I've hurt my neck!" statement, since it does absolutely nothing to support the weight of the head or to restrict movement at the neck. There's a type of patient who cannot be separated from her neck collar, but she usually wears it loosely so as not to impede ease of movement.

Belts. Men doing heavy work have traditionally worn wide leather belts. These do have some purpose. Think of bending forward to pick up a heavier-than-usual weight. You hold your breath. What's actually happening is the air in the abdomen acts as a balloon beneath the spine, supporting it. You hold your breath to stop the diaphragm from moving. To be vulgar, sometimes air is expelled from the anus with the effort. Heavy loads cannot be lifted by a person with a paralyzed or severely weakened abdomen. The belt helps to reinforce the balloon of the abdomen. Abdominal strengthening exercises and reducing a bloated belly would be part of the treatment. The usual soft belt, however, worn loosely on the outside of the clothing, is also no more than a "Hey! Look at me!" device, and serves no treatment or functional purpose.

Magnets. The current Food and Drug Administration (FDA 2007) statement is, "Magnets marketed with medical claims are considered to be medical devices because they are promoted to treat a medical condition or to affect the structure or function of the body. The law requires that manufacturers of medical devices, including magnets intended for medical use, obtain marketing clearance for their products before they may offer them for sale. This helps protect the public health by ensuring that new medical devices are shown to be either safe and effective or substantially equivalent to other devices already legally marketed in this country.

To date, the FDA has not cleared for marketing any magnets promoted for medical use. Because these devices do not have marketing clearance, they are in violation of the law and are subject to regulatory action. "Action is taken on a case by case basis depending on the significance of the medical claims being made. Significant claims that are likely to trigger regulatory action include, but are not limited to, treatment of cancer, HIV, AIDS, asthma, arthritis, and rheumatism."

An anonymous editorial in the *British Medical Journal* (2006) states a billion dollars a year are spent on magnet therapy; publicity has been gained by "notables" participating in the advertising to promote the product. Studies on fibromyalgia claimed benefits for the participants but were considered invalid in their design (Colbert 1999; Alfano 2001). Barrett (2002) describes several of the reasons magnet therapy has not been approved, the unsatisfactory nature of the research, and the litigation undertaken by FDA against unreasonable and unsubstantiated claims. Read the section again on Mesmer; initially he had his patients swallow an iron solution then placed magnets on the body to stimulate the flow of fluids, but even Mesmer gave up on the use of magnets.

Oral Supplements

Excellent information is available from the Web site of the NIH, Office of Dietary Supplements, National Institutes of Health, US Government. In normal health there is no indication to take any of the widely advertised supplements.

Calcium

Calcium plays a vital role in our anatomy, physiology, and biochemistry. Its obvious role is in the bone mineral, its less obvious role is in the passage of nerve signals, muscle activity, and cell function. Calcium's function in muscle contraction was found as early as 1882 by Ringer and led the way for further investigations to reveal its role as a chemical messenger about a century later. Vitamin D assists its absorption from the gut; the hormones secreted by the parathyroid gland regulate the resorption of calcium from bone where it is "stored."

Deficiency. Very tightly regulated by a balancing act controlled by hormones and vitamins, the serum level of calcium is one of the least variable in the biological system. Bone is used as a reservoir, and bone suffers at the expense of the needs of the rest of the body, so in deficiency states rickets and osteomalacia result. Birds use their bones as a reservoir for the egg's shell. A form of muscle spasm may occur in the type of severe deficiency that follows inadvertent surgical removal of the parathyroid glands.

Excess. If the parathyroid gland is overactive, the normally tightly regulated calcium blood level rises above its normal level.

Magnesium

Magnesium is an essential element in biological systems and is found in every cell in every organism. It is involved in virtually every metabolic pathway, and much of nucleic acid biochemistry requires magnesium, in particular all reactions that require release of energy from adenosine triphosphate (ATP). In the process of nerve conduction, magnesium acts in balance with calcium.

Deficiency. May result in muscle spasms, anxiety disorders, migraines, and osteoporosis, and may occur as a drug side effect or with chronic alcoholism and diuretics.

Excess. Oral magnesium poisoning in adults with normal renal function is very rare; diarrhea may occur. There are some medical conditions where the therapeutic use of magnesium is critical, for example, eclampsia and with an unusual form of cardiac irregularity.

Zinc

Zinc is an essential element, necessary for sustaining all life; it is now considered a neurotransmitter and is an activator of certain enzymes.

Food sources. Found in most animal proteins, beans, nuts, almonds, whole grains, pumpkin seeds, and sunflower seeds.

Deficiency. Results from inadequate intake of zinc, or inadequate absorption of zinc into the body: hair loss, skin lesions, diarrhea, and wasting of body tissues occur. Severe deficiency during pregnancy may impede fetal brain development.

Excess. Swallowing a US one-cent piece (98 percent zinc) can cause damage to the stomach lining due to the high solubility of the zinc ion in the acidic stomach. Zinc toxicity, mostly in the form of the ingestion of US pennies minted after 1982, is commonly fatal in dogs, where it causes a severe hemolytic anemia.

Essential Fatty Acids

Because of its high fuel value, fat is an important component of diet. As a form of energy storage in the body, fat has more than twice the value of protein or carbohydrate. Some terms used when describing fatty acids are confusing to those not grounded in biochemistry. "Saturated" fatty acids are structured without a double bond; "unsaturated" fatty acids have one or more double bonds. Animals fed a diet of vegetable oil (unsaturated fatty acids) have soft fat relative to ruminants (e.g., cows) in whose stomachs micro-organisms convert unsaturated fatty acids to the saturated form, and thence a firmer body fat (known in the stockyard as "finishing").

What Are "Essential" Fatty Acids?

Like the essential amino acids, "essential" fatty acids are those the human body specifically cannot manufacture for itself and must obtain from ingested foodstuffs. "Indispensable" is sometimes used as an alternative word and is easier to understand.

In simple terminology these foodstuffs are known as linoleic, linolenic, and arachidonic acids. More recently introduced is "omega," the last letter in the Greek alphabet (ω), written like a rounded lowercase letter w. The far end of the fatty acid chain is designated omega. Then the actual participant in chemical reactions is counted along the chain back from omega, designated with a minus sign and numeral, so linolenic acid becomes "omega minus three," or ω-3, and linolenic acid is ω-6. You'll find this at extra cost in the supermarket on the shelf selling milk.

What Do They Do? Will Supplements of EFA Help Me?

Most of our knowledge of nutrition comes from studies on the rat—we owe a lot to rats! It was found that these fatty acids were "essential" to the rat's growth in the absence of any other fat. It is agreed the human cannot manufacture them, but the effects of not ingesting them are rather less clear. We know the EFAs are active in forming other structures, but the need to take supplements or the benefits to be obtained remain uncertain despite extensive experiments and fervid claims of benefit they'll inhibit the effects of aging, dementia, and various neuro-cognitive problems (AHRQ 2005).

This has given rise to an industry that not only will sell you the EFAs ω-3 and ω-6 but also offers ω-9, which your body is quite capable of making for itself. A quick tour through Google produces some exhilarating opportunities to purchase "wild deep sea north pole salmon oil" with its "high content of omega three." And, if you love your dog and cat, you'll buy the same for them!

Evening Primrose Oil

Evening primrose (NCCAM 2006) is a plant native to North America but also grows in Europe and parts of the Southern hemisphere. Its pretty yellow flowers bloom in the evening.

Use. Evening primrose oil contains gamma-linolenic acid (GLA), an essential fatty acid, as described above; the oil is extracted from the seeds and put into capsules. Since the 1930s the oil has been used for eczema, more recently for other conditions involving inflammation, such as rheumatoid arthritis, and for conditions affecting women's health, such as breast pain associated with the menstrual cycle, menopausal symptoms, and premenstrual syndrome. It is used during pregnancy in attempts to shorten the duration of labor and is also advocated for cancer and diabetes.

What the science says. Evening primrose oil may have modest benefits for eczema, and it may be useful for rheumatoid arthritis and breast pain. However, study results are mixed, and most studies have been small and not well designed. There is not enough evidence to support the use of evening primrose oil for other health conditions.

Side effects and cautions. Evening primrose oil is well tolerated by most people, mild side effects include gastrointestinal upset and headache; it appears to be safe for use during pregnancy, but scientific information is limited.

Lecithins

Relationship to fibromyalgia. There are many advertisements and blog-style reports suggesting the use of lecithins in fibromyalgia. No particular benefit is known except as a supplement for those on severely restricted diets. No therapeutic value.

What is it? Lecithin is the name for a group of chemicals widely distributed throughout the cells of the body, and particularly important in the metabolism of fat. They are mostly a mixture of glycolipids, triglycerides, and phospholipids. Lecithin is the major component of a phosphatide fraction, which may be isolated from egg yolk (in Greek, *lekithos*) and soy beans. Lecithin is commercially available in high purity as a food supplement and for medical uses. Lecithin is an integral part of cell membranes and can be totally metabolized, so it is virtually nontoxic to humans; it's especially used by vegetarians as an alternative to meat. Lecithin is approved by the US Food and Drug Administration for human consumption with the status "Generally Recognized As Safe."

Value as additive. A Cochrane review (2007) of twelve trials did not find any benefit for cognitive impairment in Alzheimer's or Parkinson's diseases; a "dramatic result" was obtained in favor of use of lecithin for subjective memory problems—they presumed this was "spurious."

NADH

Relationship to fibromyalgia. No deficiency status is known. No benefit is known from taking it as a supplement or additive.

What is it? Nicotinamide adenine dinucleotide, abbreviated NADH, is found in all living cells. It plays key roles in metabolism, as an oxidizing agent, and in cell signaling. Due to the importance of these varied functions in metabolism, NADH is a target for the additives industry.

Methylsulfonylmethane (MSM)

Relationship to fibromyalgia. It's heavily advertised on Google and elsewhere. No clear evidence of need as a supplement or benefit as a therapeutic agent.

What is it? MSM is promoted as a natural source of sulfur by the supplement and health food industry, suggesting that people are deficient in sulfur intake. However, protein in the diet is an abundant source of sulfur, which is contained in the amino acids methionine and cysteine. Clinical research on the medical use of the chemical is limited to a few pilot studies that have suggested beneficial effects. US retail sales of MSM as a single ingredient in dietary supplements amounted to $115 million in 2003 despite the biochemical effects being poorly understood. Some researchers have suggested that MSM has anti-inflammatory values (Morton and Siegel 1986; Murav'ev et al. 1991; Childs 1994). MSM is the primary metabolite of DMSO in humans. Any health effects of dimethyl sulfoxide (DMSO) may be mediated, at least in part, by MSM (Williams, Burstein, and Layne 1966; Kocsis, Harkaway, and Snyder 1975). Jacob, of the Oregon Health and Science University, reports using MSM to treat over eighteen thousand patients with a variety of ailments (Jacob 2003).

Evidence from clinical trials. Clinical evidence for the usefulness of MSM is limited. Pilot studies of MSM have suggested some benefits, particularly for treatment of osteoarthritis. In 1978, the FDA approved dimethyl sulfoxide (DMSO) for instillation into the bladder as a treatment for interstitial cystitis (see later in book). Since DMSO is metabolized to MSM by the body, it is possible that MSM is the active ingredient in DMSO treatments (Childs 1994). Although not well studied, MSM has been used clinically to treat conditions such as snoring, scleroderma, fibromyalgia, systemic lupus erythematosus, repetitive stress injuries, and osteoarthritis (Jacob 2003).

Glucosamine Sulphate

Relationship to fibromyalgia. Many advertisements advocating benefits on Google and elsewhere. Questionable evidence of benefit in osteoarthritis. No evidence of benefit in fibromyalgia.

Does it help? In a study published in the *New England Journal of Medicine*, the popular dietary supplement combination of glucosamine plus chondroitin sulfate did not provide significant relief from osteoarthritis pain among all participants. However, a smaller subgroup of study participants with moderate-to-severe pain showed significant relief with the combined supplements. This led the National Institutes of Health to fund a large, multicenter clinical trial studying reported pain in osteoarthritis of the knee, comparing groups treated with chondroitin sulfate, glucosamine, and the combination, as well as both placebo and Celecoxib (NSAID). The results of this six-month trial found patients taking glucosamine, chondroitin sulfate, or a combination of the two had no statistically significant improvement in their symptoms compared to patients taking a placebo (Clegg 2006).

Glutamine

Relationship to fibromyalgia. Multiple advertisements advocating use. No evidence of need or benefit except in severe states of malnutrition.

What is it? Glutamine is the most abundant naturally occurring, non-essential amino acid in the human body, where it's found in the blood and stored in the skeletal muscles. It's widely available through both plant and animal sources.

What does it do? Glutamine is necessary for DNA synthesis, plays a major role in protein synthesis, is needed in the metabolism of cells lining the inside of the small intestine, is a source of fuel for the brain. It has been shown to be useful in treatment of serious illnesses, injury, trauma, burns, cancer. It's thought intestinal intake of glutamine is higher than that for other amino acids, and it's the best option when attempting to alleviate conditions of undernourishment relating to the gastrointestinal tract—not an issue in fibromyalgia, nor even in irritable bowel syndrome.

WHAT'S KNOWN ABOUT THE RESULTS OF TREATMENT?

No treatment program will work if the patient doesn't follow it (Dobkin 2006). The pills left in the bathroom cupboard will not help you sleep. A mental attitude of confidence has to be projected by the medical team and reciprocated by the patient. "This doesn't usually work but why not try it?" will do no good. "This is the latest thing and is bound to help you," will be just as bad, and in the long run more damaging, when it's found to be ineffective. Ineffective treatment deters the patient from continuing with the modestly effective one she was previously trying.

The patient must understand the purpose of what is proposed, must be willing to pursue the exercises, and must be emotionally supported in her activities (Dobkin 2005, 2006). The patient has in all likelihood not been prone to taking regular exercise, therefore a special incentive must be built into her program to make it as interesting as possible.

Measuring Outcomes

Because so much of the range of symptoms in fibromyalgia is subjective, to gain an objective comparison measurement is difficult (Mease 2005; Rooks 2007). If one wishes to know whether the treatment has served its purpose, it's essential to define the symptoms at regular intervals and to make comparative measurements over a period of time. Measured and recorded levels of physical and emotional function are important for chronic pain intervention studies.

Among the available measuring techniques are:

* Visual analog scale (VAS), which can be applied to the symptoms of pain, fatigue, and sleep (Burckhardt 1991)
* McGill Pain Questionnaire (Melzack 1987)
* Pain and sleep diaries (Williams 2004; Gendreau 2005)
* Beck Depression Inventory (Beck 1974)
* Beck Anxiety Inventory (Beck 1988)
* Fibromyalgia Impact Questionnaire (Burckhardt 1991; Bennett 2005)
* Short Form 36 Health Survey (Ware 1994)
* Leisure Time Physical Activity Instrument (Mannerkorpi 2005)
* Physical Activity at Home and Work Instrument (Mannerkorpi 2005)

A 30 percent improvement in any one symptom variable is required before the treatment can be considered to have met clinical efficacy (Rooks 2007).

Treatment Results

Bennett and associates' (1997) frank but gloomy statement that treatment modalities for fibromyalgia seldom lead to long-term relief is not wholly supported by later studies. The resistance of fibromyalgia symptoms to contemporary treatments was described by Wolfe (1997). Five hundred and thirty fibromyalgia patients were followed in six US tertiary referral centers over seven years. There was no significant improvement in pain, functional disability, fatigue, sleep disturbance, or psychological status. Half the patients were dissatisfied with their health, and 59 percent rated their health as only fair or poor. It was found fibromyalgia patients used an average of nearly as many as three different fibromyalgia-related drugs in every six-month period.

Despite this dismal picture, in Bennett's later view there is evidence that fibromyalgia patients can be helped (but not cured) by a multidisciplinary approach that emphasizes education, cognitive behavioral therapy, therapeutic treatment of pain, participation in a stretching and aerobic exercise program, prompt treatment of psychological problems, and attention to the associated syndromes (Goldenberg 1994, Clark 1994, Martin 1996, Wigers 1996, Goldenberg 1996).

The Oregon Health Sciences University Fibromyalgia Treatment Group has employed a multidisciplinary treatment method using a team of interested health professionals comprising nurse practitioners, clinical psychologists, exercise physiologists, mental healthcare workers, and social workers (Bennett 1996). In this way, groups from ten to thirty patients can be seen in designated sessions several times a month. Patients are usually appreciative of meeting others who share similar problems and the interaction in group therapy assists in cognitive behavioral modifications. Such groups can be encouraged to develop a sense of camaraderie in solving mutual problems. This form of therapy has proved beneficial in a six-month program, with continuing improvement up to two years after leaving the program (Bennett 1996). Another group has published similar encouraging results (Turk 1998).

A Cochrane review examined the benefits of exercise in fibromyalgia. Their material comprised thirty-four studies of forty-seven interventions on twelve hundred patients. It was concluded there was "gold"-level evidence that supervised aerobic exercise training has beneficial effects on physical capacity and fibromyalgia symptoms, and strength training may also have benefits (Busch 2007).

Rooks (2007) recruited two hundred and seven women taking medication for fibromyalgia between 2002 and 2004. For sixteen weeks, the women were randomly assigned to one of four groups: fifty-one performed aerobic and flexibility exercises only; fifty-one also did strength training; fifty received a self-help course on managing fibromyalgia; and fifty-five participated in all the exercises and the education course. The exercise groups met twice weekly, gradually increasing the length and intensity of their workouts, with instructions to perform a third day of exercise on their own. A total of one hundred and thirty-five women completed the study and underwent a six-month follow-up assessment. As measured by two self-assessment questionnaires and one performance test, women who participated in all forms of exercise improved their physical function, an effect that was larger in the combined education and exercise group. "Social function, mental health, fatigue, depression and self-efficacy also improved. The beneficial effect on physical function of exercise alone and in combination with education persisted at six months" (when the study terminated).

Results of Use of Medication

The value of tricyclic antidepressant (amitriptyline) use reported from nine placebo-controlled trials showed only a meager benefit in less than half of the participants (Arnold 2000). A controlled study of pregabalin (Lyrica) showed some of the participants sustained greater than 50 percent relief of pain over a six-month period (Crofford 2005). Tramadol is reported to allow improvement in quality of life by relief of pain and improvement in physical and work activities (Bennett 2007). More recently, the manufacturers of milnacipran reported to the FDA the results of a trial study in one and a half thousand patients with fibromyalgia and have asked for approval for use in that condition (RTT News 2007).

CHAPTER FIVE

PROGRAM PROGRESSES

WHAT IS PAIN?

Everyone has experienced pain. Everyone knows how to use the word, but do we all use it the same way? Do we all mean the same thing? When politicians and generals lachrymosely spout, "We share your pain," what does that mean?

The respected International Association for the Study of Pain (IASP) published its definitions (Merskey 1994), the prime one being the meaning of the word "pain," not in fact easy to define and not a definition that met universal approval. IASP concluded pain is: "An unpleasant sensory and emotional experience associated with actual or potential tissue damage, or described in terms of such damage."

The IASP experts note pain is always subjective. Each individual learns the application of the word through her own experience. Many people will report pain when there has been no tissue damage or any likely pathophysiological cause; usually this happens for psychological reasons. (Where does this leave fibromyalgia?) If one accepts this subjective report, there is usually no way to distinguish their experience from pain resulting from tissue damage. If they regard their experience as pain and if they report it in the same way as pain caused by tissue damage, it should be accepted as pain.

A fundamental rule in the practice of medicine: the patient has as much pain as she says she has.

The IASP classification concerns itself largely with the various characters of pain, giving definitions that everyone could use, putting clinicians and researchers on effectively a level verbal playing field. Some definitions are:

Allodynia: Pain due to a stimulus which does not normally provoke pain. [The original provocation is normally nonpainful, but the later response is painful, for example, sunburn. Allodynia involves a change in the quality of a sensation, whether tactile, thermal, any other sort.]

Analgesia: Absence of pain despite a stimulation which would normally be painful.

Causalgia: Sustained burning pain.

Central Pain: Pain initiated or caused by a primary lesion or dysfunction in the central nervous system.

Dysesthesia: An unpleasant abnormal sensation, whether spontaneous or evoked.

Hyperalgesia: An increased response to a stimulus which is normally painful [but not as painful as the response suggests].

Hypoalgesia: Diminished pain in response to a normally painful stimulus.

Hyperesthesia: Increased sensitivity to stimulation, excluding the special senses [such as hearing, seeing, etc.].

Neuralgia: Pain in the distribution of a nerve.

Neuritis: Inflammation of a nerve.

Neuropathic Pain: Pain initiated or caused by a primary lesion or dysfunction in the nervous system. Peripheral neuropathic pain occurs when the lesion or dysfunction affects the peripheral nervous system. Central pain is the term used when the lesion or dysfunction affects the central nervous system.

Neuropathy: A disturbance of function or pathological change in a nerve.

Nociceptor: A receptor [for example, at a nerve ending] sensitive to a noxious stimulus or to a stimulus which would become noxious if prolonged.

Pain Threshold: The least experience of pain which a subject can recognize.

Pain Tolerance Level: The greatest level of pain which a subject is prepared to tolerate.

Paresthesia: An abnormal sensation, whether spontaneous or evoked.

Pain may also be classified by the region involved, which is the usual in clinical practice. A patient who presents herself at the emergency department triage desk is written up by the nurse as "chest pain," "abdominal pain," and so forth. After the doctor comes to her conclusion about the patient, the pain is narrowed down to an organ or a disease process, such as "gallbladder stone," "coronary thrombosis," and so on. Between these steps the doctor will likely ask about time sequences. Not only "When did this attack start?" but "When did you first have this pain in this place?" Thus a time component as well as the component of location is introduced.

Then there is the very important "character of the pain" component. "Crushing chest pain" is a coronary thrombosis until you prove otherwise; "bolt of lightning down my leg" is sciatica. "All over, all the time" may be fibromyalgia.

Other issues in classification are the cause of the pain, typically falling into the groupings of traumatic, infectious, neoplastic, degenerative, and those due to the most troubled organ in the body—the brain (Sessle 2007).

Bearing these issues in mind, there is yet one more classification of pain based on the mechanism: somatic (from the general frame of the body, skin, muscle bone, etc.), visceral (from the inner organs, heart, stomach, gut, etc.), and nociceptive and neuropathic (Woolf 1999; Woda 2005).

Why Do We Have Acute Pain?

The ability to feel pain must be there to protect us from putting our hands on a hot stove, from walking barefoot on sharp pebbles, from inhaling ammonia. But what would happen if we were unable to sense pain?

A condition called "tabes dorsalis" used to be common (and fortunately now is rare), due usually to tertiary syphilis that diminished the sensation of pain and position. Hence there was no feeling of pain when the joints were distorted and a form of severe arthritis ensued. A knee would be markedly swollen, the bone ends chewed up, but the patient wasn't particularly bothered by this because he felt no pain. Not uncommon these days is a similar condition of diminished joint sensation due to diabetes. Usually it's the foot that's affected; the joints dislocate and the arch collapses.

Common in tropical countries where leprosy is still found is a different type of joint destruction due also to the loss of feeling ensuing from nerve destruction in the lepromatous process. A very rare condition is congenital indifference to pain, where the child ends up, if not protected, with multiple wrecked joints.

So, yes, we're fortunate to have a sense of acute pain as a protective mechanism. It gets an A plus. But this is *teleological* thinking. We presume the mechanism of pain exists because it's convenient to the preservation of our lives and limbs to have such a mechanism in place, and we are happily confident that's why it exists.

Why Do We Have Chronic Pain?

There's a need to distinguish between conditions where pain persists unremittingly, for instance, rheumatoid arthritis or osteoarthritis, and conditions where the pain recurs over a prolonged period, for instance, gallbladder disease. If they've lasted for more than an arbitrary time frame of three or six months, both types are called chronic. Both undoubtedly are pains.

Is that pain useful? Probably. It tells us something is wrong. It tells us that certain activities or certain foods are damaging to the body and should be avoided. So accepting we have a pain mechanism that protects us by telling us something is wrong—this just squeezes past the post with a C minus.

What about the Inexplicable Pain?

Staats (1996) states, "Pain is pain." As an expert in the field, Staats intends to provoke. But there is a third kind of pain clearly defined by G. J. Bennett (1997):

> When peripheral somatosensory nerves are damaged by disease or trauma, a small percentage of cases develop positive symptoms, almost always various kinds of pain. Such pains are said to be neuropathic because they are believed to be due to a dysfunctional nervous system. Neuropathic pain ranges from mild and dysesthetic to excruciating torture. The conditions are usually chronic (months to years) and very often fail to respond to any current therapies.

Bennett (1997) lists the commonest conditions associated with this form of pain, but he did not mention fibromyalgia: diabetic neuropathy, postherpetic neuralgia, cancer, spinal cord injury, multiple sclerosis, reflex sympathetic dystrophy (for which the term "causalgia" was coined), phantom limb pain, poststroke central pain, HIV associated, tic douloureux, low back pain, and a wide variety of peripheral nerve disorders.

What conceivable use does this kind of pain provide? It certainly deserves an F minus, which raises the question, is the perception of pain just something with which we happen to be endowed? Just something that is at times useful and at other times harmful, but not truly related to utility?

SOMATOFORM PAIN DISORDERS

Psychosomatic illness is one in which physical symptoms, produced by the action of the unconscious mind, are defined by the individual as evidence of organic disease, and for which medical help is sought. Their problems qualify as genuine diseases. There is nothing imaginary or simulated about the patient's perception of illness. Although the symptoms may be psychogenic, the pain or the grinding fatigue is very real. Just like the conscious mind, the unconscious is influenced by the surrounding culture, which has models of what it considers to be legitimate and illegitimate symptoms; there is great pressure on the unconscious mind to produce only legitimate symptoms (Shorter 1992).

The *Diagnostic and Statistical Manual of Mental Disorders, Fourth Edition, Text Revision* (DSM-IV-TR) is the codex created for, and used by, those members of the healing professions who deal with conditions of the mind. It classifies these conditions and details their features quite specifically to avoid confusion—rather similar to the American College of Rheumatology's 1990 decision that it needed to stipulate exactly which features should be considered to justify the diagnosis of fibromyalgia. The DSM views are generally accepted in the medical profession but, like everything in that inexact science, are open to dispute.

Fibromyalgia is characterized by an intense unwillingness to accept a diagnosis that is not based on a physical status. For fibromyalgia to be classed under "rheumatic diseases" is quite acceptable, even though no joint is involved. To be classed under "emotional disorders" is totally unacceptable to the patient. Blotman (2006) quotes his patients saying, *"Docteur, ne me dîtes pas que je somatise!"* ("Doctor, don't tell me I'm a psychosomatic!")

Common Features of Somatoform Disorders

The common feature in a grouping of conditions known collectively as "somatoform disorders" is defined in DSM as, "Physical symptoms that suggest a general medical condition and are not fully explained by a general medical condition, by the direct effects of a substance, or by another mental disorder. The symptoms must cause clinically significant distress or impairment in social, occupational, or other areas of functioning."

Pain Disorder

Among the seven disorders included in this somatoform disorder grouping is pain disorder, for which, according to the DSM-IV-TR, the criteria necessary to support a diagnosis are:

1. Pain which causes clinically significant distress in one or more anatomical sites is the predominant focus of the clinical presentation.
2. Psychological factors are judged to have an important role in the onset, severity, exacerbation, or maintenance of the pain which is not intentionally produced and is not better accounted for by a mood, anxiety, or psychotic disorder and does not meet the criteria for dyspareunia.

Somatization Disorder

Another of the seven subcategories of somatoform disorder is "somatization disorder," for which the (condensed) criteria necessary to support such a diagnosis include a history of many physical complaints that started before age thirty. In addition, the sufferer must have four pain symptoms related to at least four different sites of functions, two gastrointestinal symptoms other than pain, one sexual symptom other than pain, and one pseudoneurological symptom other than pain. A general medical condition does not account for these symptoms, nor are they intentionally produced.

Undifferentiated Somatoform Disorder

Various articles have pointed out how frequently the primary care physician is confronted with a physical complaint for which she cannot with any degree of comfort make a diagnosis. Estimates are given that 25 to 75 percent of the primary care physicians' time is spent dealing with essentially psychosocial problems masked by somatic complaints, taking up half her office hours; somatization has been described as the fourth-commonest problem in primary practice. Because many patients did not fit the criteria for the disorders described above, new categories appeared in journal articles, with titles such as "subsyndromal somatization disorder" and "multisomatoform disorder." These are now covered by the DSM-IV "undifferentiated," described as a "residual category" for presentations not meeting the full criteria outlined for other disorders. "Undifferentiated" criteria are a physical complaint of six or more months that cannot be fully explained by any known condition, and the complaints and impairment are grossly in excess of what the history, examination, and lab findings would indicate.

Somatoform Disorder Not Otherwise Specified

This is a kind of "holding" category where the symptoms are of less than six months' duration.

Unless one insists that fibromyalgia is a "general medical condition" that fully explains all of the patient's symptoms, it would not be difficult to read them as fitting the categories of a pain disorder. If the patient also suffers from some of the other problems of the "overlapping syndrome" (described in later chapters), such as irritable bowel disease, chronic pelvic pain, and temporomandibular joint disorder, it is not difficult to see why some clinicians think the condition is consistent with the terms describing a somatization disorder.

Psychogenic and psychiatric therapies are recommended for patients who have no demonstrable underlying medical disorder, but patients with somatization disorder are extremely resistant to these treatments (Venuturupalli 2005).

In Russell's view (2004), a patient cannot be diagnosed as having both fibromyalgia and the somatization disorder; the diagnosis must either be one or the other.

MEASURING PAIN

One illogical aspect of medical practice is the general lack of measurement of pain. In most instances, the patient seeks care because she has pain. Her range of movement will be recorded in degrees, her white count in numbers, the date the pain started will be there, but her degree of pain is not scaled, nor as a rule is the effect of the pain on her life. Sometimes a verbatim account, such as "pain described as horrible," is recorded, but at the next visit, there probably will be no record of the pain beyond "says feels a little better today, prescription renewed."

The difficulty lies in pain being the patient's subjective concern, not something the physician sees, hears, or feels. How then should she measure a subjective complaint?

The answer is predicated on the fundamental of medical practice: a patient has as much pain as she says she has. So the scale of recording must be based on what the patient says she has. This may either be reduced to numbers—scientists love numbers—or it can be recorded in words. The difficulty with the latter system is, do you use the doctor's words or the patient's? And then how do you put numbers to words so it can be entered into the computer?

Wherever there's an issue in medicine, a specialty will be created. Just as polling the people as they leave the voting station has developed into a less-than-perfect science, so we have experts ready to devise innumerable ways of measuring subjective sensations and concerns. The physician employing their methods must know the benefits, limitations, and potential misdirections. You, the patient, subjected to them, must know what benefit they might bring to you, and you must understand the need for thoughtful and accurate answers.

What Should Be Measured?

Pain is technically described as a multidimensional experience. When the dimensions are separated, your pain can be analyzed at a minimum into categories of its severity (intensity), the suffering it causes (known as affect), and its effect on your life. All of these are variable factors, altering from hour to hour, week to week. For this reason, the records must be developed so they can be tracked over a period of time, and the time intervals should remain constant.

Visual Analog Scale (VAS)

Without discussing whether the words are appropriate, we'll explain that this is a commonly used simple device to ask the patient to record the *severity* of her pain. In its simplest form, it is a line with "no pain" at one end and "the greatest pain imaginable" or similar wording at the other end. You are then invited to put your mark somewhere between the extremes. The person recording your result will convert into numerals the point where the mark is placed, usually between zero and ten; some scales come with these marks already printed, and you are asked to choose a number. The pain may be "at the moment" or the "average for the week" or whatever seems appropriate to the physician caring for you or his research assistant who set up the system. The system has the advantage of simplicity and reproducibility; it is computer friendly; and it has all the features that lead an experienced physician to distrust it because simplicity usually leads to impressive numbers with little practical value.

The average patient does not think of her pain in terms of numbers. She doesn't come into the office and say, "My pain is six." She says, "My pain is horrible." When the patient gets brainwashed to the point of saying, "Yesterday I was a six. Today I'm an eight," the physician should know his system is working against, not for, the patient's interests.

Computers do numbers. People should do words.

Verbal Rating Scale (VRS)

People do words. But the physician must ensure she knows to which subjective issue you are applying your word. Is it "horrible" because it never lets up, "horrible" in its severity, or "horrible" in the effect it's having on your life?

These are all separate issues, and each may need to be addressed separately from a treatment point of view. Each needs to be followed over time, months stretching into years, to determine the effect of the treatment and/or the need to alter it.

Fortunately, the geniuses who apply their minds to analyzing issues of this kind have devised rating scales for any and all subjective issues. Unfortunately, there are a lot of geniuses out there, each of whom is intent on making a name for himself, and your doctor has to choose which of the hundreds of available scales she's going to use. They can be applied to "as of this minute," "average through the day," or "worst of the week," and so forth.

Some commonly used scales are:

- *SF-36 Bodily Pain Scale.* Choice of words offered to describe severity of pain, varying from "none" through "moderate" to "very severe."
- *McGill Pain Questionnaire (MPQ).* Choice of words offered to describe the nature of the suffering (affect), varying from "mild" through "distressing" to "excruciating." The full MPQ is a list of one hundred and two adjectives describing sensory, affective, and evaluative aspects of pain. The MPQ is generally considered to be too long and too dependent on language skills. For this reason, a Short Form McGill Pain Questionnaire (SFMPQ) was devised, which is reduced to only fifteen adjectives and generally simplified. Its acceptability is signaled in having been the questionnaire used in the Lyrica (pregabalin) study.
- *Behavioral Rating Scale.* Choice of phrases offered to describe the effect of the pain on your life, varying from "can easily be ignored," through "interferes with all tasks," to "have to stay in bed."
- *Pain Diagrams.* These are often used in pain clinics. For the patient with fibromyalgia, pain is not usually restricted to one point and tends to vary in location and in severity, so this is not of much help. Sometimes the violence of shading is indicative of the patient's emotional attitude.
- *Faces and "Ouch."* These are pictures of persons' faces indicating varying degrees of distress. They were devised for children but can be used for persons unable to communicate by numbers or words, by virtue of illiteracy, language barrier, age, and such.
- *Analgesic Consumption.* A record of analgesics taken can be entered into the computer and a graph of some kind made from it. It is not thought to be a good indicator of the pain experienced or of the effects of the pain.
- *Specific to Fibromyalgia—Tender Point Assessment.* The assessment should include not only the ACR-designated eighteen points but also a selection of control points, which can be expected not to be tender, although they are reported as unreliable and positive in 60 percent of fibromyalgia patients (Wolfe 1998). Attention has been given to increase or decrease in the number of tender points (TePs); although attempts have been made to measure intensity of pain with a designated "myalgic score" to evaluate benefits of trial medications, this has not proved satisfactory.
- *Fibromyalgia Impact Questionnaire.* Designed specifically for fibromyalgia, this is a mix of two VAS-type questionnaires. One component, scaled in boxes from one to ten (without visible numbers), asks "severity" questions in regard to pain, ability to work, fatigue, stiffness, anxiety, and depression. The other component asks specific functional type "were you able to?" questions, such as household activities, walking,

and so on, with a numeric scale ranging from "always" to "never."

- *Arthritis Impact Measurement Scales (AIMS).* Many persons with fibromyalgia are treated in arthritis (rheumatology) clinics, where this scale is commonly used. The form has six item subscales for depression and for anxiety, both issues of importance in the person suffering chronic pain but not considered to be the cause of the problem.
- *Sleep and Fatigue Assessment.* There is a twelve-point multidimensional assessment of sleep (Medical Outcomes Study [MOS] Sleep Scale) and the even more complex Sleep Assessment Questionnaire (SAQ), which only those of you most severely troubled by insomnia will be asked to complete. Simple VAS scales are to be used, indicating on an unnumbered line your current level of fatigue, how well you slept, and how refreshed you felt when you woke.

WHAT IS SLEEP?

The more simple a question, the more fundamental we know it to be, the more difficult it is to provide a satisfying answer. So to this simple question there is an equally simple answer. We truly don't know why we sleep.

What we do know is a little bit like the old "Everyone does it, the birds and the bees, they do it," for all birds and mammals, and some insects, have periods of sleep (Peever 2007).

Do We Need to Sleep?

Since all animals do it, it's hard to believe sleep has no purpose in life. Possibly it's a mechanism for conserving energy expenditure. Sleep appears critical to our survival. Extended periods of sleep deprivation have led to subject death; mammals (Rechtschaffen et al. 1983), fruit flies (Shaw 2002), and rats deprived of sleep will die as surely and as rapidly as if deprived of food (Peever 2007).

How Much Sleep Is "Normal"?

Large animals sleep for shorter periods than small animals; a fruit fly sleeps longer than an elephant (Zepelin 2005). The larger the animal, the slower the rate of metabolism; thus the "normal" length of sleep appears to be related directly to metabolic rate.

Our lives revolve around the natural periods between one rising of the sun and the next, a twenty-four-hour period, or put another way, "about a day." The only excuse for stating the obvious is the need to introduce a less obvious but widely used term, "circadian rhythm," an expression coined by Franz Halberg, who joined the Latin words *circa* and *dies*, to indicate "about a day." An understanding of this rhythm is essential to the understanding of normal and disordered sleep.

All living creatures follow their circadian rhythm—people, animals, plants, fungi, even the photosynthesizing cyanobacteria, which have been around for billions of years. For all, the circadian rhythm is built in. The "about a day" rhythm continues when all external evidence of change (external stimuli) has been removed; for instance, when a person or a plant is kept in total isolation and in total darkness in a deep cave. The "clock" can, however, be reset when we move from one time zone to another.

What Is Sleep?

The average person spends almost a third of his or her life sleeping. Someone who lives for seventy-five years will have spent twenty-five of them asleep.

Sleep is not a mere passive and inactive state that follows waking; rather, it's a carefully controlled and highly orchestrated series of states that occur in a cyclical fashion each night. Sleep is generally defined by behavioral quiescence that is accompanied by closed eyes, recumbent posture, limited muscular activity, and a reduced responsiveness to sensory stimuli; however, sleep differs from coma in that it can be readily and quickly reversed (Peever 2007). Sleep onset is associated with decrease in skeletal muscle activity, heart rate and breathing frequency, body temperature, and blood pressure.

Sleep is not a state of a massive system shutdown but quite to the contrary. During sleep, the brain is active, constantly communicating with the body. Many neurohormones, antibodies, and other molecules are synthesized during sleep; therefore, when sleep is disrupted, biochemical abnormalities can occur, leading to multisystem disturbances (Gilliland 2007).

The Study of Sleep

Nathaniel Kleitman, known as "the father of modern sleep research," died in 1999 with his mental faculties intact at the fine old age of 104 years. His classic 1963 text cites over four thousand references on the subject of sleep. He was not alone in having studied brain waves during sleep; Loomis and his associates were publishing papers in this field in the mid-1930s. Together with Eugene Aserinsky, Kleitman, however, brought the phases of sleep to the world's attention.

Prior to 1953, the general understanding of sleep was rather like the electric lightbulb—switch off until next needed. Aserinsky's revelation is a fine example of Pasteur's axiom, "Chance favors only the prepared mind." Living in the poverty that typified graduate students of the period, Aserinsky used his eight-year-old son as a model for studying continuous brain wave tracings. He taped electrodes to the child's scalp and adjacent to the eyes. While his son slept in the next room, Aserinsky found as he sat monitoring his machine, instead of the anticipated quiet brain wave emission, there were sudden bursts of activity. Up to this time, brain wave tracings with the electroencephalogram had been brief, about twenty minutes maximum; on this occasion, the tracing was prolonged. Thinking his son Armond had woken, Aserinsky went to him, but on checking, the child was still asleep. Aserinsky reported his startling discovery to his supervisor, Nathaniel Kleitman, who required the experiment to be repeated on Kleitman's own daughter. (Aserinsky supposed this to be a wish to eliminate the possibility of trickery as an explanation for the unanticipated discovery.) From this time, it was known that jerking eye movements, predominantly horizontal, are found occurring in bouts during normal sleep. Aserinsky at first contemplated the use of the term "jerk" but wisely chose "rapid" to precede "eye movements," hence REM (Brown 2003).

Sleep Architecture—The Meaning of REM

One cannot begin to comprehend the abnormal without a full understanding of the normal, a truism that applies to sleep as much as anything else.

Kleitman and Aserinsky, later joined by Dement, showed there are two separate and distinct states within sleep, which they divided into periods of non–rapid eye movement (non-REM or NREM) and rapid eye movement (REM). Some persons have found it confusing to characterize a period of sleep by a negative, by what is *not* happening. What else is defined by what it isn't? Call a zebra "not a donkey"?

Over the years, further information has been progressively acquired; each period of sleep is further characterized by distinct behavioral, neurochemical, physiologic, and electrophysiological attributes. The two main parts, designated respectively as NREM and REM, alternate cyclically throughout the night, starting always with NREM sleep. NREM accounts for three-quarters of the total time we sleep and is itself divided into four stages by those who study the field, the REM stage making the fifth in each cycle of approximately ninety minutes' duration.

These stages are characterized by changes in frequency and voltage of the brain waves (the higher voltage gives a taller wave, also called the amplitude), which are named by their features. The wave form on the EEG is, like the wave form on the heart's equivalent, the ECG, an adding up of all the electricity caught at the point of application of the electrode. As in the heart, different electrode placements around the head pick up different wave forms. These wave forms were named (Greek letters, of course) by their characterizing frequency and size (amplitude) long before sleep studies came along. The same names for the characteristic wave forms are used in sleep studies. Alpha rhythm typifies the awake patient, at rest with his eyes closed, and has a periodicity of 8–12 Hz. (Not going to explain that—it's a measure of frequency—just focus on the number!) Theta rhythms come in at 4–7 Hz and delta rhythms at 1–3 Hz. Interestingly, in books written before sleep studies were being made, the delta rhythm is described as "never seen in the normal EEG."

The first stage, lasting from one to ten minutes, constitutes *light sleep*. There is slow movement of the eyeballs and slight general muscular activity. We can easily be woken from this stage, may even deny we'd been to sleep, "just closed my eyes," or may remember fragmented images we've "seen." Sometimes there are sudden muscle contractions called *hypnic myoclonia*, a sensation of being about to fall, similar to the sudden movements made when "startled." The EEG shows theta rhythm at 4–7Hz.

The second stage lasts from ten to twenty-five minutes. Eye movements stop, brain waves are slower, but there are occasional clumps of rapid bursts, *sleep spindles*. In the third stage, extremely slow waves of higher amplitude, *delta waves,* begin to appear, with occasional smaller, faster waves. After a few minutes, Stage 3 moves into Stage 4, in which the waves are at their highest and slowest.

Stages 3 and 4 represent *deep sleep*, also called slow wave sleep. During deep sleep, there is neither eye movement nor any general muscle activity. If forced to waken from deep sleep, the person might be fully alert. Children's bed-wetting and sleep walking occur during this phase.

Stage 4 of NREM is followed by REM, lasting in the first cycle for about five minutes. The brain waves in Stage 5, REM sleep, are rapid, of low-amplitude (low-voltage) *theta activity*. Multiple differences in body activity during REM include:

- breathing is likely to become rapid, shallow, and perhaps irregular
- the heart rate increases, blood pressure rises
- the eyeballs jerk rapidly in various directions, mostly horizontal
- the muscles of the limbs are temporarily paralyzed
- there is penile erection or clitoral engorgement

It's common to wake for a short time at the end of an REM phase. During REM, the summed activity of the brain's neurons is quite similar to that during waking hours; for this reason, the phenomenon is often called *paradoxical sleep*, meaning there are no dominating brain waves during REM sleep.

As the sleep period continues, the approximately ninety-minute cycles have longer and longer Stage 5 REM components at the expense of reduced, deep sleep; Stages 3 and 4 and REM phases ultimately make up about a quarter of the total time of the four to six cycles of a night's sleep.

Age Changes

The relative proportion and duration of REM sleep varies considerably with age. A newborn baby is likely to be asleep for sixteen hours, to spend more than 80 percent of total sleep time in REM (Bliwise 2005), to have a sleep cycle of sixty minutes compared with the adult ninety minutes, and to pass rapidly from wakefulness into REM sleep. The high-voltage, slow pattern of late-stage NREM sleep is not found until six months of age. NREM sleep is 40 percent reduced by the age of twenty (Carskadon 2005). Whereas it is nearly impossible to rouse a young child from the "deep sleep" of stages 3 and 4, elderly persons are woken easily, and possibly a lowered arousal threshold explains their complaint of "restless sleep" (Boselli 1998; Bliwise 2005).

Sleep Studies

Polysomnography (PSG) is a technique employed to display sleep cycles and stages through the use of continuous recordings of brain waves (electroencephalograph, or EEG), electrical activity of muscles, eye movement (electrooculogram, or EOG), breathing rate, blood pressure, blood oxygen saturation, heart rhythm, and direct observation of the person during sleep. These studies are usually conducted in a sleep center and through the night, and electrodes are placed on the chin, scalp, and outer edge of the eyelids. Monitors are placed to record heart and breathing rates. Total body movements may be recorded by videocamera.

Neurotransmitters

There are special chemicals, neurotransmitters, that carry instructions to the cells of the nervous system, neurons. Among these are *serotonin* and *norepinephrine*, which keep our brain active while we are awake and control our sleeping or waking states.

A region known as the brain stem lies between the bulk of the brain, the visible outer wrinkled part, and the spinal cord and is concerned with the unconscious and most fundamental of the body's activities. The hypothalamus, lying at the floor of the brain, above the base of the skull and the pituitary gland, is a kind of switching station for signals to and from the brain. As far back as the 1920s, it was known from human experience that damage to the posterior hypothalamus resulted in persisting sleepiness, and damage to the anterior hypothalamus resulted in insomnia; one has to turn that around as a mirror image to understand the normal function of these zones in the undamaged state. Later studies in animals have confirmed the anterior hypothalamus is normally responsible for non-REM sleep, and if damaged, insomnia results. REM sleep, it was found, is controlled in a quite different part of the nearby brain (Saper 2005). Nerve signal transmission is by means of the densely packed nerve fibers in the region, but the message is ultimately carried through chemicals (discussed elsewhere) of which serotonin is one. The pharmacology of sleep control, and to some extent also pain control, is open to manipulation of these chemicals, which transmit the nerves' signals.

Sleep and Fibromyalgia

The American College of Rheumatology criteria for diagnosing fibromyalgia require a three-month minimum of widespread pain and provoked tenderness in at least eleven of eighteen designated points (Wolfe 1990); disturbance of sleep was not one of the defining criteria, but such is very commonly reported in patients suffering fibromyalgia, so commonly that it is generally considered a feature of the syndrome and is reported by up to 80 percent of those experiencing the condition (Dauvilliers 2001).

Of the eighty-one forms of sleep disorder recognized in the *International Classification of Sleep Disorders*, in fibromyalgia the most commonly reported are delayed onset of sleep, problems with sleep maintenance, and early-morning awakening. In interpreting their concerns, the patients describe their sleep as nonrestorative, superficial, and fragmented (Harding 1998; Dauvilliers 2001; Mease 2005), but it has been remarked that these complaints of unsatisfying sleep lead to daytime problems of "fatigue" rather than reports of sleepiness (Dauvilliers 2001; Moldovsky 2005).

The relationship between intensity of pain and the quality of sleep was sought with the help of fifty women maintaining a diary over thirty days (Affleck 1996). Poor sleepers had more pain the day following a poor night's sleep and had poor sleep after a painful day—a well-recognized circular relationship (Lavigne 2005). Interpretation is difficult in the face of other factors that might affect pain intensity; patients with fibromyalgia who also suffer a clinical depression find a worsening of mood on more painful days.

Sleep dysfunction is considered an integral feature of fibromyalgia. About 70 percent of patients recognize a connection with poor sleep and an increased pain, along with feeling unrefreshed, fatigued, and emotionally distressed. Several studies have linked abnormal sleep with these symptoms and have shown patients with fibromyalgia have disordered sleep architecture (Dauvilliers 2001). Also germane, sleep disturbances are found in other conditions, including psychiatric (Tsuno 2005).

This abnormality has been identified as a sleep anomaly of alpha-wave intrusion, or alpha-delta sleep, which occurs during NREM Stage 4 sleep. This intrusion into deep sleep causes the patient to awaken or to be aroused to a lighter level of sleep. It has some importance since "alpha-delta intrusion" is one of the buzzwords, like "Substance P," which is tossed around during discussions on fibromyalgia, most of the participants having little idea what they mean.

We've defined the characteristics of both the alpha and the delta waves—alpha is fast, delta is slow. The intrusion is in a period of about 20 percent of deep sleep, which should be represented by slow delta waves but shows instead the rapid alpha waves. Although Hauri and Hawkins described this in 1973 in psychiatric patients, it somehow became thought of as a diagnostic feature of fibromyalgia when Moldofsky demonstrated it two years later (1975). The same alpha-delta intrusion is found in various components of Yunus' Overlapping Syndrome, but it can also be found in healthy normal persons (Scheuler 1988), as well as those troubled with psychiatric problems. Deliberate interference with sleep at the delta-wave stage has been shown in normal persons to result in muscle fatigue, tenderness at the characteristic fibromyalgia points, and disorders of mood (Moldofsky 1976).

Some describe the altered sleep physiology and somatic symptoms as a non-restorative sleep syndrome. This dysfunction is believed to be linked to the numerous metabolic disturbances associated with fibromyalgia, including abnormal levels of neurotransmitters (serotonin, substance P) and neuroendocrine and immune substances (growth hormone, cortisol, interleukin-1). These metabolic imbalances are thought to be responsible for the increased symptoms associated with this sleep disorder of alpha-wave intrusion by impairing tissue repair and disturbing the immunoregulatory role of sleep.

Most alpha-wave intrusions occur during the first few hours of sleep, decreasing throughout the night to normal levels by early morning. This hypothesis has been well correlated with patients' frequent reporting that their best sleep is obtained in the early-morning hours just before arising.

Dauvilliers and Carlander (2007) review the multiple propositions to explain the relationship fibromyalgia bears to unsatisfying sleep; these include suggestions covering hormone, autonomic nervous system, and neurotransmitter dysfunctions. To date, no satisfactory explanation has been established.

Treatment of Sleep Disorders in Fibromyalgia

Poor sleep worsens and perpetuates symptoms, so aggressive treatment is indicated. Since most persons understand little about the nature of sleep, our patients are instructed on the basics of proper sleep hygiene. Hygiene (from the Greek *Hygieia*, daughter of Aesculapius and goddess of health) is a euphemism for what is in fact self-regulated discipline. Initiating and pursuing this education has been one of the most helpful of the program.

Smith and Haythornthwaite (2007) suggest:

1. Regular sleep-wake patterns must be established by rising at the same time each and every day, regardless of how well you've slept; limit daytime naps to less than thirty minutes; eat regular meals; avoid large meals within two hours of bedtime; use the bedroom only for sleep and sex, not as a refuge when in pain; establish a relaxing bedtime ritual.
2. Ensure adequate light exposure in the morning and into the evening; relax with a thirty-minute hot bath ninety minutes before going to bed; keep the clock face turned away, do not focus on how much you're awake in the night; keep the ambience dark, quiet, comfortable, and slightly cool.
3. Exercise regularly each day; avoid vigorous exercise immediately before bedtime.

Some further suggestions by Gilliland (2007) are:

1. Avoid caffeine and alcohol.
2. Restrict fluids in the evenings, if urinary frequency is a nighttime problem.
3. Only after proper education and instruction on sleep hygiene and dietary changes should consideration be given to medications to improve sleep.
4. Keep a sleep diary for two weeks before starting any new medications; it provides useful information for selection of medications. Include a list of medications taken during the two weeks, noting the time of going to bed, the approximate time falling asleep, the number of awakenings, the times of rising, a general description of how well rested you found yourself.

WHAT IS FATIGUE? WHAT IS TIREDNESS?

Chronic fatigue syndrome and fibromyalgia syndrome have clinical features in common. The major symptoms of each disorder are present in the other (Moldofsky 2005). The complaint of chronic fatigue and sleep disturbance results in the patient being sent to a sleep disorders specialist whose task is to determine whether there is a primary sleep disorder.

"Tired" is a troublesome complaint that is commonly used to describe an unpleasant ill-defined subjective experience that frequently brings people to their physicians.

This is one of the many words in the English language that means different things to different persons, and because there are large numbers of persons obliged to use English although that is not their mother tongue, confusion can easily arise. The medical worker must be sure she understands quite exactly what the patient means by "I'm tired" without putting answers in her mouth. The word "fatigue" is even worse, tending to be used almost in a pejorative sense, as in "donor fatigue."

1. Central fatigue—description given of mental exhaustion, impeding thinking. This may be a simple issue of lack of motivation and boredom. Or it may signal more significant problems such as degenerative brain disease, schizophrenia, major depressive disorder, or somatoform disorders.
2. Physical fatigue—resulting from physical effort. Sense of overall exhaustion; the possibility of significant disease processes, such as cancer and anemia, or the abuse of drugs must be ruled out.
3. Sleepiness—an urge to sleep although not fatigued. Whereas fatigue is eased by rest, only sleep relieves sleepiness.

Who Is Tired?

A quarter of the US adult population reports having experienced persisting fatigue (Price 1992). Internationally, an average of 8 percent of patients report fatigue persisting for more than one month, and smaller numbers, up to 1.5 percent, report fatigue of six months' duration (Kawakami 1998; Jason 1999).

Debilitating fatigue is reported by 76 percent to 81 percent of patients diagnosed with fibromyalgia (Wolfe 1990, 1996) and the poverty of the quality of their sleep is in proportion to the number of tender points elicited (Yunus 1991).

Diagnostic Characteristics of Tiredness of Fibromyalgia

When tiredness or fatigue is due to muscle weakness, these symptoms are relieved by rest and sleep. Tiredness associated with a major depressive disorder is worst on awakening and eases through the day. The patient with fibromyalgia reports both pain and fatigue on waking in the morning, with some improvement through the day, only to worsen toward evening (Moldofsky 2001).

Horne (2006) shows the Epworth Sleepiness Scale, which questions the likelihood of dozing off while:

- sitting and reading; watching TV
- sitting inactive in a public place (theater, meeting)
- passenger in car for one hour without break
- lying down in the afternoon to rest
- sitting and talking; sitting after lunch
- sitting in a car stopped at traffic

This type of scale does not seem to take into account the habit instilled in soldiers—never miss an opportunity to sleep, you never know when the next chance will come.

There is also the Beck Depression Inventory (Beck 1961), the Multidimensional Fatigue Inventory (Smets 1995), the Fatigue Severity Scale (Krupp 1989) and Chalder's scale (1993), none of which according to Moldofsky (2005) exclude simple sleepiness.

WHAT CAUSES FIBROMYALGIA?

Very few years ago, fibromyalgia review articles were likely to begin with the admonition, "The cause of fibromyalgia is not known."

Fibromyalgia is part of the spectrum of chronic pain. An improvement in our knowledge and our understanding of underlying neurologic pathways and the chemistry of chronic pain have increased our knowledge of the etiology and pathology of fibromyalgia. Which is far from saying that the mystery is solved, but there is sufficient evidence now to suggest there may be:

1. a predisposing state with one or more significant factors
2. a precipitating (triggering) factor
3. a progressive entrenchment of changes
4. an alteration in the structure and function of the central nervous system, which has resulted in a state of chronic widespread pain

Is It Nurture or Is It Nature?

No single cause for fibromyalgia has been accepted universally, though many theories have been proposed. Are these abnormalities the causes or are they the effects?

It's generally agreed most patients enjoyed a healthy active lifestyle prior to the onset of their fibromyalgia. Although stress in their lives may have been a risk factor, this is not fully proven. In fact there probably is no single predisposing, precipitating, or initiating cause common to all persons with the fibromyalgia syndrome. With some persons the onset of symptoms was gradual and no prodromal cause has been recognized (Russell 2003).

Predictability of Chronic Widespread Pain

There are various definitions, ranging from the inexact "all over" to the more exacting American College of Rheumatology definition requiring persisting pain in all four quarters of the body and in the axial spine. Not all patients with chronic widespread pain have fibromyalgia, but all patients with fibromyalgia, by definition, suffer chronic widespread pain. There is legitimate interest in determining whether this type of pain is predictable.

To determine whether psychological and physical indicators of the process of somatization could predict the development of new chronic widespread pain the arthritis research unit in central England undertook a survey of fifteen hundred subjects; a battery of questionnaires were completed, covering general health, somatic symptoms, fatigue, and illness attitude. These same persons were examined again a year later. Eight percent had developed chronic widespread pain; a strong relationship between certain baseline test scores and the subsequent risk of developing chronic widespread pain was shown, supporting the contention of predictability (McBeth 2001).

From the same unit a study was made of over three thousand persons who completed a battery of questionnaires examining psychosocial distress, health-seeking behavior, sleep problems, and traumatic life events. They were reexamined fifteen months later; it was found 10 percent had developed chronic widespread pain in the interval. On examining their data the researchers found degrees of predictability from the Somatic Symptoms checklist, the Illness Behavior Subscale, and the Sleep Problem Scale. High scores on all three scales put the subjects at twelve times the risk of developing chronic widespread pain as compared to those with low scores (Gupta 2007). In the same unit, it was also found that subjects initially free of chronic widespread pain are at risk of its development if they have a high tender point count, and they concluded a low pain threshold was likely a result of distress rather than the cause of its symptoms (Gupta 2007).

Between the years 1964 and 1966 more than two thousand entry-level university students in North Carolina were subjected to the MMPI screen (described elsewhere). Thirty years later a follow-up questionnaire was completed to determine who had developed chronic pain; a statistically significant relationship was shown between certain MMPI responses and the development of chronic pain, suggesting the possibility of identifying the population at risk at an early stage (Applegate 2005).

What Are the Suggested Predisposing Factors?

Abuse in childhood is always a popular theory brought forward to explain away the hard to understand problems that may confront adults. Several attempts have been made to link abuse to the onset of fibromyalgia (Goldberg 1999; Finestone 2000), but repeated studies have failed to find consistent evidence to support this theory (Russell 2003).

Retrospective studies comparing anonymous responses of healthy normal controls with patients diagnosed either with fibromyalgia or rheumatoid arthritis found 40 percent had had one stressful trauma prior to the age of eighteen, but there was no statistically significant difference between the two groups (Russell 1992). It has been suggested that fibromyalgia patients might have internalized more, but it was concluded "the evidence is just not there" to implicate childhood sexual abuse in the etiology of fibromyalgia (Hudson 1995).

Raphael (2001) conducted a prospective study of 676 adults who had been severely abused in childhood, compared with 520 controls; the interviewers were deliberately kept unaware of the group from which each person was derived. They found no differences in regard to pain or painful illnesses; there was a relationship between unexplained pain and depression in those *who had not been abused*, but no such relationship was found for those who had been abused.

In his self-reporting survey of two and a half thousand persons with fibromyalgia, Bennett (2007) obtained an 8.7 percent prevalence of childhood sexual abuse. He was aware of Alexander's study of the prevalence of sexual abuse in fibromyalgia, as high as 57 percent. Since the report in Bennett's survey was so much lower, he postulated there might be differences in "candidness" between an Internet-based survey population and a one-on-one, face-to-face interview.

Bennett's study found no association between fibromyalgia and sexual abuse, but did report a threefold increase over the national average of women who'd been raped. Thus, it was hypothesized that chronic stress, in the form of post-traumatic stress disorder, may mediate the relationship between rape and fibromyalgia (Ciccone 2005).

Some authors suggest that an inheritance factor may be involved, that the genetic predisposition manifests itself when the person reaches a critical age or sustains an external insult, such as trauma or illness (Gilliland 2007). This suggests that subjects destined to develop fibromyalgia are either genetically predisposed (nature) or have past life events or experiences that favor its later development (nurture).

There is evidence to support the concept that genetic factors play a role in the etiology of fibromyalgia. Buskila (1996) considered the global well-being, quality of life, and physical functioning were all suggestive of a genetic rather than an environmental basis for fibromyalgia. He reported a strong familial trend, showing an overall prevalence of 25 percent in first-line relatives with the fibromyalgia syndrome, distributed as 83 percent mothers; 50 percent sisters; 33 percent daughters; 15 percent sons; 0 percent fathers.

Yunus (1999) reported forty families with two first-degree relatives involved, distributed as: 74 percent siblings; 53 percent of children; 39 percent of parents had fibromyalgia.

Russell (2004) reported a survey of one hundred and twenty-four fibromyalgia patients: 20 percent indicated first cousins with like symptoms; 2.4 percent indicated two members in the family affected, but the diagnosis had not been confirmed by medical examination.

Russell (2004) also reported an ongoing search of the entire genome of one hundred and sixty families with two or more fibromyalgia members clearly suggestive of genetic implications, probably by an autosomal dominant mode of vertical transmission inheritance (Roizenblatt 1995; Buskila 1996; Yunus 1999).

The most probable mode of inheritance is polygenic. According to Olson (2004), early results of studies involving more than one hundred forty families may confirm that the genes associated with serotonin play a role in fibromyalgia (Russell 2004).

Hudson (2004) and Arnold (2004) pursue a concept there may be a genetic link between fourteen associated conditions, grouped together as affective spectrum disorder, in which they appear to include fibromyalgia. Although Buskila (1996) found members of fibromyalgia families had lower pain thresholds than matched healthy controls, Yunus (1999) found no differences between affected and unaffected persons in regard to anxiety or depression.

No racial predilection exists in fibromyalgia; researchers have reported the condition in all ethnic groups and cultures (Gilliland 2007), including desert Bedouin women (Doron 2004).

Why Women?

It is universally agreed that the sex distribution ratio of fibromyalgia patients is in the order of nine women to every man (Russell 2004; Gilliland 2007). Why should this be?

Various explanations are offered, most of which characterize women as a different species from men, incorporating issues such as female hormones, menstruation, higher levels of anxiety, increased prevalence of depression, poor coping strategies, and a postulated increased behavioral response to pain. As females they may have had adverse experiences during childhood and may have a psychologic vulnerability to stress. It is considered a background of a stressful, often frightening, environment and culture are important antecedents of fibromyalgia. Statistically sound research has supported some possibly associated or causative factors, such as higher levels of anxiety, increased prevalence of depression, poor coping strategies, increased behavioral response to pain, more willingness to take their complaints of pain to a doctor. No universally accepted explanation exists for this disproportion in adults; differences in fibromyalgia between prepuberty boys and girls are hardly recognized (Gilliland 2007).

But, it is reported, when a man does get fibromyalgia his symptoms may be worse than a woman's. Anyone who has run a medical office is fully aware of the willingness of many men to visit their physicians with trivial complaints, and it seems unrealistic to presume an unwillingness for a man to report pain can be an explanation—men are quite willing to report their minor back and knee pains.

Women it is said have more pain at all sites, use more analgesic medication, are more sensitive to pain stimuli, and have central pain modulatory systems influenced by phasic alterations in reproductive hormone levels. Even in rats, the female exhibits increased primary afferent input to the central nervous system and decreased activation of pain inhibitory systems. Stressful tasks are more likely to evoke changes in brain chemistry signifying pain, and psychologic responses in female compared to male rats (Winfield 2007). Women report unexplained somatoform symptoms 50 percent more often than men, which correlates with anxiety and depression; other data, however, do not support somatization as more common in females than males. It remains unclear if sex differences are genetic or learned (Winfield 2007).

Sociodemographic Factors

Fibromyalgia has been linked to several sociodemographic factors, compared to the norm:

- increased divorce rate (Hawley 1991; Wolfe 1995)
- failure to graduate from high school (Wolfe 1995)
- lower family incomes (Wolfe 1995)
- abnormally high body mass index, linking fibromyalgia to obesity (Wolfe 1995)
- disproportionate use of medical and surgical services (Wolfe 1995)

Bennett's (2007) survey showed a divorce rate of 17.4 percent; education level was not reported; they were "moderately overweight," having gained fifty pounds since age eighteen; 50 percent had a household income between twenty and eighty thousand dollars. (The author has no expertise in this field, and Bennett didn't offer comparative statistics, but those figures would seem to be pretty much the nation's average.)

What Are the Suggested Precipitating, Triggering Factors?

Bennett reported people with fibromyalgia often associate a specific event to the onset of their symptoms. Clearly, emotional stress (73 percent) is a major theme running through the great majority of them. His respondents replied to the question, "Have any of the following potential triggering events occurred around the same time that your fibromyalgia symptoms first became apparent?" Twenty-one percent of responders could not identify any precipitating (triggering) association. Of those who did indicate some triggering event and could identify a precipitating (triggering) association, 73 percent attributed their fibromyalgia to an emotional trauma or chronic stress. Of those who indicated some triggering event, these are subcategorized:

- 26.7% reported an acute illness
- 20.6% physical or emotional abuse as a child; 15.1% as an adult
- 16–17% reported for surgery, the same for motor vehicle collisions, and other injury
- 10% of the respondents related the onset of symptoms to menopause
- 9% of respondents cited childhood sexual abuse

Sometimes fibromyalgia is divided into primary (spontaneous) and secondary (known cause). Bennett's respondents seem only to be 21 percent without known cause. If one looks at that figure, it actually represents 21 percent no known cause remembered, or alternatively, not chosen to report. Does every woman abused in childhood, sexually or otherwise, remember it? Or choose to report it if she does? As already recorded, Alexander had a report of 57 percent childhood sexual abuse.

Symptom Intensity Scale

With the intention of determining whether fibromyalgia is a discrete disorder, and to investigate causal and noncausal factors, twenty-five thousand patients were evaluated on a self-reporting Symptom Intensity Scale that combined a count of pain in nineteen places in the body, which were not joints, and also measured fatigue. This provided information of general demographics, clinical symptoms, serious medical illnesses, hospitalizations, work, and death. High scores were found in those with varying forms of socioeconomic disadvantage and for all clinical variables, but there was no clinical basis by which fibromyalgia could be identified as a separate entity (Wolfe 2006).

Other Suggestions Made Regarding Triggering Factors

Almost all patients with fibromyalgia sleep poorly; a night of poor sleep is followed by a more painful day. Abnormal sleep affects the stress response system and contributes to negative mood and cognitive difficulties. Some researchers theorize that disturbed sleep patterns may be a cause rather than a symptom of fibromyalgia.

An injury or trauma, particularly in the upper spinal region, may trigger the development of fibromyalgia in some people. An injury may affect the central nervous system, which may trigger fibromyalgia (see "Secondary Fibromyalgia," below).

Chronic pain states may also develop during or after some infections (Simms 1990; Leventhal 1991; Sigal 1994; Barkhuizen 1996). Bennett (1997) describes experiments in rats demonstrating a neural pathway whereby proinflammatory cytokines can cause a hyperalgesic state, supporting a hypothesis that several discrete stimuli may initiate fibromyalgia via a common final pathway that generates a central pain state through the sensitization of second-order spinal neurons (anatomical structure explained in another chapter).

Sympathetic nervous system dysfunction occurs in people with fibromyalgia, particularly at night, which leads to fatigue, stiffness, dizziness and other signs and symptoms associated with the condition.

Deconditioning and decreased blood flow to muscles may contribute to decreased strength and fatigue. Differences in metabolism and abnormalities in the hormonal substance that influences the activity of nerves may play a role. The periosteum, ligaments, tendons, fascia, and muscles are sensitive to pain. The tender points in fibromyalgia are primarily where ligaments, tendons, and muscles attach to the bone. Ligaments are flexible but cannot stretch very far. Unlike muscles, ligaments have a poor blood supply, particularly at the point where they attach to the bone. Thus ligaments often do not heal completely and can remain in a "stretched-out" position. When weakened ligaments or tendons are stretched or the joints are moved too much, sensory nerves can become irritated or compressed, causing local and/or referred pain (Russell 2004). (The author has a lot of difficulty with this theory.)

SECONDARY FIBROMYALGIA

This is a highly contentious, medico-legally charged, issue. Russell (1973) believes there is consistency of evidence that physical trauma such as a motor vehicle accident or a fall can trigger fibromyalgia, and Russell gives extensive references and anecdotal reports to support this contention, such as 19% of 973 fibromyalgia patients attributed fibromyalgia symptoms to trauma (Lessard), and 23% of 127 patients attributed fibromyalgia to trauma (Greenfield 1992). In addition, 176 post-traumatic fibromyalgia patients (Waylonis 1994) reported a triggering trauma: 60.7% motor vehicle accidents, 12.5% work, 7.1% surgery, 5.4% sports, 14.3% other. Comparing the incidence of fibromyalgia after a motor vehicle accident, Weinberger (1977) found 1.7% for fractured leg bones and 21.6% for neck injuries. According to Buskila (1997), the incidence of fibromyalgia one year after automobile accidents causing whiplash was 22% and after leg fractures 1%. In patients where fibromyalgia was precipitated by trauma (Wolfe 1986), 40% had a neck injury, and 31%had a lower back injury.

Russell (1973) theorizes on how injuries to the cervical region may be more prone to cause chronic pain than are fractures of the leg. Yunus (1997) believes there is a compelling argument that trauma plays a role in some, but not all, cases of fibromyalgia. Bennett (1997) states most fibromyalgia patients causally relate an acute injury, repetitive work-related pain, athletic injuries, or another pain state to the onset of their fibromyalgia; he points out that although many persons with fibromyalgia attribute the onset of their problem to trauma, most persons who are injured do not develop fibromyalgia.

The opposite evidence is recounted by Winfield (2007), arguing sometimes from the same evidence: Patients who attribute their fibromyalgia to trauma are more disabled than those with primary fibromyalgia; they have more perceived disability, more self-reported pain, more life interference, and more affective distress than those with idiopathic onset. He views from the opposite point the study that showed patients with neck strain had increased rates of fibromyalgia compared to those with fractured legs (Buskila 1997), and adds there is no convincing evidence that minor trauma induces inflammation or permanent change in muscle or connective tissue. Examination of three current texts devoted to the subject of whiplash injury shows the potential for fibromyalgia is not even mentioned as a possible sequel to the injury (Ameis 1988; Foreman 1995; Gunzburg 1998).

There is no consensus in the medical community that trauma causes fibromyalgia. Fibromyalgia related to trauma appears chronic as well as severe (Greenfield 1988).

The Progressive Entrenchment of Changes

It's frequently reported that a patient may over a substantial period see as many as six doctors before being told her diagnosis is fibromyalgia. There is one widely circulated report of more than twenty-five doctors before fibromyalgia was diagnosed. Reports of this kind leave the impression that the symptoms were static, that is to say, the symptoms she presented to doctor number six were exactly the same as those she presented to doctor number one.

There are two reasons to make this improbable. The first, over a period of time symptoms change. Fibromyalgia is polysymptomatic, a semi-Greek way of saying there are a lot of them. If she had seen all six doctors, one after the other on the same day, that might be possible. If her mind was like a blank and empty slate, and remained that way, it might be possible; but since all animals including humans learn from experience, it's difficult to accept that patients don't learn anything from the questions the doctor poses. "Do you suffer from headache?" from doctor after doctor is liable to leave all but the most resistant minds with the concept, "Yes. But I've always supposed that was normal," and there goes another checkmark.

In Association with Other Conditions—Symptoms with Signs

Fibromyalgia is more common in those with other medical and musculoskeletal disorders, and the numbers accumulate with age.

It is found in rheumatology clinics in new patients from 12% (Wolfe and Cathey 1983) to 20% (Yunus 1981), in general medical clinics 5.7% (Campbell 1983), and in family practice 2.1% (Hartz and Kirchdoerfer 1987). Fibromyalgia is commonly found (Bennett 1997) as an accompaniment of rheumatoid arthritis (Urrows 1994), systemic lupus erythematosus (SLE) (Morand 1994; Middleton 1994; Bennett 1997), low back pain (Borenstein 1995), Sjögren's (Bonafed 1995; Vitali 1989), and osteoarthritis. In addition, 20–35% of patients with rheumatoid arthritis or SLE have concomitant fibromyalgia.

Psychiatric Associations

There is a significant increase in depression, an inverse association with health satisfaction and global health perception, and fibromyalgia can be conceived of as a general distress disorder (Wolfe 1993). Raphael (2004) and associated psychiatrists noted the synchronous (comorbid) findings of fibromyalgia and major depressive disorder. From a study of persons with depression, they concluded that (1) fibromyalgia is a depression spectrum disorder and (2) depression is a consequence of living with fibromyalgia.

A group of psychiatrists at Harvard (Hudson 2003) studying families concluded fibromyalgia was part of an affective spectrum disorder, in which, as well as fibromyalgia, they included a long list of conditions: major depressive disorder, attention deficit and hyperactivity syndrome, bulimia, cataplexy, dysthymic disorder, generalized anxiety disorder, irritable bowel syndrome, migraine, obsessive-compulsive disorder, panic disorder, post-traumatic stress disorder, premenstrual dysphoric disorder, and social phobia.

Psychiatrists in Chicago (Katz 1996) also proposed fibromyalgia should be considered to be part of an affective spectrum disorder after studying the families of sixty persons with fibromyalgia and establishing a prevalence of depression and alcoholism; they believed the depression was not simply reactive to the pain.

The Changed Mind

Winfield (2007) observes fibromyalgia is considered by many to be one of a series of essentially symptom-based conditions—symptoms but no signs:

- primarily associated with fatigue: chronic fatigue syndrome, fibromyalgia
- regional pain syndromes: myofascial pain syndrome, atypical chest pain, irritable bowel syndrome
- attributed to chemical, food, yeast sensitivity: at least twenty-one conditions
- associated with silicone breast implants: mostly fibromyalgia
- modern office buildings: sick building syndrome
- Persian Gulf War: mostly men

The hallmarks of fibromyalgia are chronic widespread pain, fatigue, conjoined with multiple other somatic symptoms, which have neurophysiologic and endocrinologic underpinnings. The suggestion is made that they derive primarily from psychologic issues that have led to chronic unrelieved stress and ensuing distress. Thus, to understand fibromyalgia requires a bio-psycho-social viewpoint such as proposed by Engel, who postulated outcomes in chronic illness are influenced by the interaction of biologic, psychologic, and sociologic factors.

The frequent comorbidity of fibromyalgia with mood disorders suggests a major role for the stress response and for neuroendocrine abnormalities (Gilliland 2007).

The Changed Body

Current thinking centers around a theory called "central sensitization." This theory states that people with fibromyalgia have a lower threshold for pain because of increased sensitivity in the brain and spinal cord to pain signals. Researchers believe repeated nerve stimulation causes the spinal cords and brains of people with fibromyalgia to change. This change, termed neuroplasticity, involves an abnormal increase in levels of certain chemicals in the spinal cord and brain that signal pain (neurotransmitters).

In addition, the brain's pain receptors, which receive signals from the neurotransmitters, develop a memory of the pain and become more sensitive, and may later overreact to pain signals. In this way, pressure on a spot on the body that wouldn't hurt someone without fibromyalgia can be very painful to someone who has the condition. But what initiates this process of central sensitization is not clearly known.

In Russell's view (2004), there are well-established physiological and biochemical abnormalities (Crofford 1994; Kang 1998; Russell 1998) that provide compelling evidence permitting identification of fibromyalgia as a biological and distinct clinical disorder involving many body systems (Russell 1999; Rau 2000).

IS WHIPLASH A CAUSE OF FIBROMYALGIA?

Since money is at stake, the issue of whether any one case of fibromyalgia can be attributed to an injury becomes highly contentious, and after the question of whether fibromyalgia is a "real" disease, its relation to trauma is the next most hotly debated issue. Reading the articles that address particular aspects of the subject does not allow the perspective given by years in practice. The author therefore takes the liberty of expressing undocumented views based on long experience in several branches of medical practice and from over four thousand tertiary examinations of injured persons for insurance and legal opinions.

Without any reference to motor vehicle accidents, it must be understood that very few people can accept "I don't know" as an answer. They ask their doctors, "Why did this happen to me?" They want the reason for their arthritis or their cancer or their child's birth defect explained, and "I don't know" doesn't satisfy them. They can generally get an easy, obvious, and totally erroneous explanation from somewhere in that all-embracing term "the healthcare field," the more superficial your knowledge the easier it is to conjure up glib explanations. The patient himself will commonly, and quite genuinely, believe an accident is the cause. If he has arthritis of his hip he will remember a fall at work. If he has brain cancer he will remember getting hit on the head when he was in the army thirty years ago. There's no disputing the certainty that all problems have a cause, and there's no point in arguing against, "Obvious, isn't it?" In particular, any doctor who wishes to disagree with the putative cause will find herself lined up against an angry patient, a tribe of relatives and supporters, a batch of assorted therapists, the legal profession, and the media. Why would any doctor expose herself to that?

Don't Confuse Me with Facts

Wallace (2003) has counted forty-seven different reported causes for fibromyalgia; the most frequent was trauma, either as a single event or as repetitive injury. He describes 2 to 5 percent of patients who, following several months of treatment after a whiplash injury, became worse rather than better, and their pains diffused into uninjured areas of the body: "Ultimately they are diagnosed with fibromyalgia." Wallace suggests this might have come about as a result of sleep disturbance or by "neuroplasticity" (implying neuropathic pain); he also observes that the likelihood of getting this diagnosis of fibromyalgia depends on the treating doctor (rheumatologists 65 percent more likely than orthopedists) and that the injury may in fact have drawn attention to a preexisting but undiagnosed fibromyalgic status.

Bennett and associates in their study (2007) of twenty-five hundred persons reported a panel of "Perceived triggering events of fibromyalgia onset." This is explicitly stated as "when symptoms first became apparent." Twenty-one percent of the responders could not identify such an event. Of those who could (presumably 79 percent), the totals given for the various triggers add up to 213 percent, so perhaps for some there was more than one event. Of these responders, 17 percent cited nonvehicle trauma, and 16 percent cited motor vehicle trauma as the triggering factor.

There are numerous retrospective references describing the patient diagnosed with fibromyalgia who anecdotally attributes her condition to trauma. To put studies of this kind in proportion, one would need to know how the fibromyalgia patient compares with the general population. When she is asked months or years later, "Was there an accident?" how would others who do not have fibromyalgia reply?

Al-Allaf and associates (2002) conducted a postal questionnaire and received responses from fifty-three fibromyalgia patients and an equivalent number of age- and sex-matched controls. Of the fibromyalgia group 39 percent remembered a significant physical trauma within six months prior to the onset of their condition. Pretty convincing evidence? Should satisfy any reasonable jury when put to them by a convinced expert. Problem was, *24 percent of the controls who did not have fibromyalgia had also sustained trauma.* On a statistical basis, the difference would be considered proof. Would it be proof to twelve reasonable men and women? Perhaps it would. But if the jury were told that in half the cases "trauma" was a surgical procedure, that there were only two patients with fibromyalgia whose remembered trauma was a motor vehicle accident, and there were two persons in the nonfibromyalgia control group who'd sustained similar accidents, what should the jury think about the relevance of whiplash to fibromyalgia?

One Tender Point Is All You Need

There's no disagreeing that some patients with fibromyalgia will attribute their condition to a motor vehicle accident or other trauma, and their medical advisers accept this explanation. Patients who develop fibromyalgia don't break out in spots or have some sudden visible occurrence that renders the diagnosis obvious. To justify the diagnosis there must be widespread pain for at least three months, that is to say, the diagnosis cannot be validated until three months after the putative traumatic event. There must also be pain to pressure at a minimum of eleven of the eighteen designated points. Some physician must make this purpose-directed examination; it is not part of a routine examination and is only performed with the intention of determining if fibromyalgia is a justifiable diagnosis. For the moment, we'll stay away from the issue of pain and consider only tender points.

The mechanism of the motor vehicle accident is such that as the vehicle's speed changes (either acceleration or deceleration), the torso, secured to the seat, moves with the altered acceleration-deceleration of the vehicle, but the head continues to travel at the original speed. The muscles and ligaments connecting the head to the torso stretch, react, and reposition the head on the torso or possibly overcorrect. The damage to the muscles and ligaments is a simple matter of physics. If the force is sufficient the subject is decapitated, not uncommon in aircraft accidents. At less force the spine may dislocate; the spine may remain dislocated (with or without spinal cord damage) or may spontaneously reduce to normal position although remain unstable. At even less force the muscles and ligaments are stretched or possibly partially torn. In simple terms of healing, the time taken and the end result depends on the damage done. It's this last group that's called whiplash. Anecdotal evidence is that long-term pain and disability is found almost exclusively with the least severe injuries. Remarkably, there's not nearly as much continuing pain with the patients whose necks were dislocated and required surgery.

Patients who have experienced this injury will be tender in the muscles and ligaments that connect the heavy head to the torso, the reason why collars are applied and the reason doctors will tell their patients to rest the head on the back of the chair when they're seated, and to use their hands to support the weight of the head when they get up from the recumbent position.

Looking at the polyspotted Three Graces that adorn every work on fibromyalgia, it's hard to think it was by accident that ten of the eighteen chosen points are in the muscles holding the head on the torso, exactly the muscles that are made sore in a whiplash accident. Without any issue of fibromyalgia, ten of the designated points can be guaranteed to become painful to pressure, and in most persons will still be tender to moderate pressure three months after the accident. And since many persons are also hurt in the low back with this accident, that adds two more spots.

So when the plaintiff's lawyer sends her for examination to his chosen expert witness in rheumatology, and she has a complaint of widespread pain ever since that accident four months ago (how do you deny a patient's pain?), all that's necessary to clinch the diagnosis of fibromyalgia is just one more tender point than would be found in the patient who is not considered for this diagnosis. And the well-educated plaintiff's lawyer knows that fibromyalgia is a lifetime condition with a diagnosis recognized by the AMA, CDC, and WHO. The case becomes indefensible in court; it's only a question of how much.

Prospective Study

Although a skeptic could claim fibromyalgia is not caused by the motor vehicle accident, there's no denying that the condition is diagnosed after the accident. Tishler (2006) conducted a prospective study, following one hundred fifty-three patients from the time they were seen in the emergency room and for fourteen months thereafter; only one patient developed evidence of fibromyalgia.

Lithuania

In Norway, insurance compensated those involved in traffic accidents; in Lithuania it did not. Malleson (2003) explains there was a "devastating epidemic" in which seventy thousand persons of a Norwegian national population of four and a half million claimed to have been disabled by whiplash. A group of Norwegian researchers examined two hundred and two persons in Lithuania who had, one to three years previously, been involved in rear-end collision traffic accidents (Schrader 1996). Neck pain was reported by 35 percent, and headache by 53 percent. Taken by themselves, that would seem convincing evidence of long-term pain attributable to the accident. Pretty convincing evidence with numbers like that?

However, they also questioned persons matched by age and sex *who had not been involved in accidents*, and found 33 percent had neck pain, 50 percent had headaches, and furthermore none of the persons involved in the accidents were considered disabled. In a later letter, the Norwegian authors stated they had not found any of the four hundred and twelve patients in Lithuania with chronic symptoms that they related to their accident (Schrader 2003).

In another work, having reviewed a thousand references in the literature, Malleson (2002) concluded in countries that do not offer compensation for whiplash, the most severe cases of discomfort and disability last no more than a few weeks and end in full recovery. It has already been pointed out that in three current texts devoted to the subject of whiplash, the potential for developing fibromyalgia is not even mentioned (Ameis 1988; Foreman 1995; Gunzburg 1998).

Arguments against Whiplash as a Cause of Fibromyalgia (Winfield 2007)

Where accident insurance is unavailable, and whiplash is not ingrained, no one develops disabling or persistent symptoms from minor motor vehicle accidents. Persistent morbidity from motor vehicle accidents decreases dramatically when no-fault liability insurance is implemented. Automobile crash tests using human subjects have never resulted in chronic pain syndromes. Some ordinary activities in life have more effect on neck strain than do minor motor vehicle accidents but do not cause persistent symptoms. Most persons developing fibromyalgia after motor vehicle accidents are accident victims and not accident causers. Stress of litigation is an important factor following minor acute pain. Patients perceive the trauma, not the pain, as the precipitating factor and as determinant for seeking compensation. Symptoms consistent with undiagnosed fibromyalgia precede the motor vehicle accident that is supposed to have caused it.

So Why Does the Pain Persist in Whiplash?

Reread what happened to Delilah, at the beginning of this book. Some unlucky patients get caught up in the cycle of endless treatments, directed, or self-directed to one therapist after another, to one examination after another, a tough test of the strongest personalities. Some fail the test and develop psychiatric disturbances and a conversion disorder (Mailis 2005); to some the mere threat of a diagnosis of permanent illness is more than their mental stamina can handle (Greenhalgh 2001).

The severity of the injury bears no relationship to the prolongation of pain. The factor that seems relevant, not surprisingly, is the character of the person injured, and their susceptibility to suggestion that they are permanently damaged, are victims of another person's carelessness or of society in general, have a "right" to be compensated and will never be able to work again. The cycle of pain and fear is the same as that for the prolongation of low back pain, described in that chapter.

The only appropriate treatment is psychologic supportive, directed at encouraging the patient to return to a productive life, and most likely to be achieved through a pain clinic where the different specialists are available. "Multidisciplinary" is a term I do not like; too often it means six people wearing different hats all doing the same thing and thereby uselessly but expensively prolonging the patient's treatment regimes.

If legal and insurance interests require the patient to be totally incompetent in order to gain the recompense she has been told she has a right to receive, she will make little progress. The person least likely to get better is the one who believes she has been victimized, then becomes mired in the victim role, sits huddled in a wheelchair in court while she and the jury listen to her lawyer recounting how she can't care for her family, will never return to work and has a lifetime of pain and drugs ahead of her. The misconception that a "green poultice" of dollar bills will cure her is unfortunately not true. She is now permanently damaged. The lawyers and all those therapists benefit from the award—she does not.

EFFECT OF FIBROMYALGIA ON PREGNANCY

Since fibromyalgia is predominantly a condition involving women, and predominantly within the childbearing and certainly child-rearing age spectrum, one would have expected that aspect to have received a good deal of attention. It does not, however, seem to have been much commented on. Blotman (2006) doesn't seem to mention pregnancy; Staud (2007) relates a single dramatic misadventure; the Arthritis Foundation's user-helpful manual (2006) doesn't mention pregnancy; Starlanyl (2001) draws attention to the need for caution when taking medication during pregnancy. In Bennett's (2007) self-reporting survey, his respondents, twenty-five hundred women, reported: 20.9 percent had more than three children; 30.5 percent, two children; 16.5 percent, one child. So 68 percent of the women completing the survey had had children. The time relationship between childbirth and onset of fibromyalgia is not mentioned, nor are the effects of childbirth and child rearing offered as subjects for comment.

Raphael (2000) reported reduced fertility rates in patients with myofascial facial pain, but one could question whether that is the same as fibromyalgia, and Bennett and associates' figures do not seem to support such a concept. What one might reasonably call "The Blogs," or in another sense, "The Agony Columns," will occasionally refer to pregnancy in fibromyalgia; the blogs are supportive; the agony columns in general describe ill experiences. The anonymous Fibromyalgia Symptoms blog has posted, "It is disheartening that there is a lack of information regarding the course of the disorder during pregnancy. Few studies have been conducted to investigate how pregnancy aggravates fibromyalgia symptoms."

Karen Schaefer, assistant professor of nursing at Temple University, mailed a questionnaire to fibromyalgia sufferers aged twenty-nine to thirty-one in their third trimester of pregnancy, inquiring about fatigue, depression, pain levels, and daily functioning. The conclusion was that fibromyalgia sufferers had a great deal more difficulty in pregnancy in comparison to women without fibromyalgia, corroborating earlier research conducted in Norway that pregnancy aggravated fibromyalgia symptoms (Aphrodite).

Pellegrino, a specialist in physical medicine with substantial experience treating fibromyalgia as well as suffering from it himself and writing about it, says he tells his fibromyalgia patients, "The potential for flaring up is there. But people that have had babies tell me they're very glad. The joy of bringing a child into the world far outweighs the pain of flares."

Mason, a specialist in high-risk obstetrics, believes that fibromyalgia affects a pregnancy,

> although there is severely limited research in this area. Some studies indicate reduced fertility rates among fibromyalgia patients. Another study followed twenty-six women with fibromyalgia and a total of forty pregnancies were studied. The women in the study found fibromyalgia symptoms to be worse in the third trimester of pregnancy (with the exception of one patient). In thirty-three of the forty pregnancies, the women ultimately returned to the same level of fibromyalgia symptoms they were experiencing prior to pregnancy. There was an increase in depression, and anxiety during postpartum for the women studied. This did not affect the pregnancy nor the health of the baby. Seventy-two percent of patients had worsening of their fibromyalgia symptoms just before menstruation. This mimics changes occurring in the third trimester of pregnancy, where the majority of women studied had increased fibromyalgia symptoms.

Certain pain relief drugs can be used during pregnancy. Narcotics can be used. Ultram also can be used. The risk for birth defects when the drugs are used appropriately is limited. Thus narcotics are generally safe in pregnancy. More controversial are NSAIDs. If they are used at all during a pregnancy, they *must* be discontinued by the end of the second trimester. Aspirin is similar to the NSAIDs. A low dose may be appropriate, but it *must* be discontinued by late second trimester. Tylenol can be used, but appropriately. Don't exceed four grams a day (which would equal two extra-strength pills every six hours per day).

Nondrug options are the best and safest pain relief solution during pregnancy. But this does not mean that patients and doctors should shy away from using medications. One weighs risks and benefits all the time. If the benefit of a medication can be life changing and life improving, then it's reasonable to use it during pregnancy.

Set hard limits for yourself. Understand pregnancy is a job in and of itself for a patient with fibromyalgia. When you are pregnant, you expend much body energy just being pregnant. You can use twelve hundred to fourteen hundred calories for basic life function before you even take a step or go to work or begin chasing your kids around the house. Being pregnant is a metabolically fatiguing stage. Limits are important, too, because it is critical that you do not push yourself past the point of fatigue. This is important for women without fibromyalgia, so it's especially important for pregnant women with fibromyalgia. If you plan to breastfeed, you will need to consider this point because it actually takes more of the body's energy to produce milk than to be pregnant.

You and your physician should be aware and should act preemptively, knowing that:

- Sixty to seventy percent of all pregnant women develop the "baby blues."
- Ten percent of women develop clinical postpartum depression.
- People with an underlying depressive disorder are at a higher risk for developing postpartum depression.

FIBROMYALGIA AND OTHER PAIN SYNDROMES IN CHILDHOOD AND ADOLESCENCE

We can't discuss fibromyalgia in childhood without first defining a child. In the medical world a child used to be a prepubescent. Then supply met demand and the upper age acceptable in the pediatricians' offices began to climb. A subspecialty of adolescent medicine developed, so who better to look after the adolescent than the pediatrician? In terms of dealing with painful conditions, puberty is a watershed. Puberty begins when a mechanism that is still poorly understood prompts the hypothalamic-pituitary axis to discharge gonadotropin-releasing hormone. This response in its turn results in skeletal growth, sexual maturation, and an increase in circulatory system efficiency. For as many as three years, the body experiences rapid growth that averages nine cm a year in females and over ten cm a year in males (Neinstein 1996). But childhood and adolescence are all lumped together in the age span of cradle to university.

The next issue is the pediatrician's warning to all students first starting on her service: "Children are not little adults." There was a time when she could say, "They're different animals altogether," but these days that would for sure get her into trouble. It's difficult to think of a child as a "small adolescent," but much less difficult to think of an adolescent as a "large child."

Pain in Children

Next, we must consider the issue of pain in childhood, since fibromyalgia is essentially a condition of chronic widespread pain. The published statistics are worrying, in that among the patients who come under the designation "pediatric," 15 to 20 percent suffer chronic pain (Goodman 1991), giving rise to concern that this may lead to chronic pain in adult life (Walker 1995). Throughout puberty, more than half of adolescents express concern about suboptimal health, including pain, and report at least one common physical ailment (Zwaigenbaum 1999).

Evaluation of a child with chronic pain must include consideration of the psychological, social, and cultural issues as well as the overt medical problem (Bursch 1998). The history of the current problem must include a description of the pain, recounting its features, such as intensity, quality, location, and duration, together with exacerbating and alleviating factors, and the effect this pain has on daily life (e.g., sleeping, eating, school, social and physical activities, family and peer interactions).

The history, evaluation, and treatment of the current pain problem in terms of its onset and development should be detailed. Inquiry should include the magnitude of distress for the child and family attributed to the pain, and the impact of the pain on cognitive functioning, anxiety, depression, and feelings of hopelessness. Assessment also should include what the child and family members perceive as the cause of the pain and how they respond to it. History of past pain problems in the child and in other family members also should be elicited. Particular attention should be paid to recent stressful events, such as deaths, marital disruption, moves, and other changes in life circumstances (e.g., a new school).

A review with the family of current treatments for the pain should include inquiry about home remedies and alternative and complementary therapies (Zeltzer 1997). The physical examination always should include observation of the child's general appearance, posture, gait, and emotional and cognitive state. Muscle spasms, trigger points, and areas of sensitivity to light touch should be assessed. It can be helpful to examine the painful area(s) multiple times during the examination.

A multimodal approach often is more effective than a single sequential treatment approach. This approach includes specific treatment targeting possible underlying pain mechanisms, as well as symptom-focused management addressing pain, sleep disturbance, anxiety, or depressive feelings. Treatment also should address pain-related disability with the goal of maximizing functioning and improving quality of life. For example, partial or complete return to school should often be an early target of treatment for children with pain-related school absenteeism. Treatment techniques include education about the pain experience and the pain problem, behavioral techniques (e.g., reinforcement), family interventions, physical interventions (e.g., physical therapy, occupational therapy), and systemic and regional pharmacological interventions (e.g., opioid and nonopioid analgesics, anxiolytics, antidepressants, anticonvulsants, hypnotics).

Whenever possible, oral routes for medication are preferable. Referral to a pediatric pain program should be considered for children with complex or refractory problems.

Fibromyalgia in Childhood

The first account appears to have been made in 1985 by Yunus and Masi, who compared juvenile fibromyalgia to the adult form.

One Canadian study showed a high prevalence of recurrent and persistent idiopathic pain syndromes, reflex sympathetic dystrophy, and fibromyalgia (Malleson 1992). The researchers found these syndromes affected up to 26 percent of children seen in rheumatology clinics and from 4 percent to as much as 15 percent of children studied outside that setting. A survey of twenty-five rheumatologic centers showed a nonrheumatologic diagnosis (including fibromyalgia, reflex sympathetic dystrophy, growing pains, hypermobility, and idiopathic or psychogenic pain) in more than 50 percent of their patients (Bowyer 1996).

From 1996 to 1997, the prevalence of fibromyalgia in children rose from 2 to 7 percent. The mean age at presentation in children ranged from twelve to fifteen years (Siegel 1998):

- 25% of new referrals to pediatric rheumatologists are musculoskeletal pain syndromes
- 7.5% of new diagnoses made by pediatric rheumatologists in the United States are fibromyalgia
- 6.2% of the general pediatric population, the incidence of fibromyalgia in children
- 6.2% of Israeli schoolchildren diagnosed with fibromyalgia
- 1.3% of Mexican schoolchildren diagnosed with fibromyalgia

Race, Sex, Age, and Onset

In the United States, fibromyalgia is less common among African American children. Even a study from New Orleans reported a predominance of "Caucasian" (Eraso 2007). Fibromyalgia is diagnosed more commonly in girls than in boys. Studies show that girls are at least three to seven times more likely than boys to be diagnosed with fibromyalgia.

Patients with pediatric fibromyalgia most frequently present in adolescence. The youngest reported case is a five-year-old child. The New Orleans report included one hundred and forty-eight children; in forty-six the fibromyalgia had started before the age of ten, at a mean age of seven and a half years (Eraso 2007).

Some authors also describe a reactive fibromyalgia, which arises after an illness or after trauma. More than 30 percent of cases involve psychologic comorbidity.

Clinical Presentation—History

Fibromyalgia is characterized by musculoskeletal pain, stiffness, and aching. Symptoms of fatigue, anxiety, and depression are reported. Adolescents with fibromyalgia often describe abnormal sleep patterns that interfere with school and family activities. Descriptions of difficulty falling asleep, frequent awakenings due to discomfort, and feeling unrested in the morning are common.

A standard personal, family, and social history is taken with special attention to the issues described and their impact on the family and schooling because these details may provide hints to other factors that either may influence pain perception or may themselves be at the root of the pain. The history taken from the child should be supplemented by the parents' knowledge. It often may mean posing open-ended questions to prompt the adolescent to give more than a vague description of his or her pain. One approach to obtaining the social history is a structured interview format, such as the HEADSS (home, education/employment, activities, drugs, sexuality, and suicide-depression screening) inventory.

Diagnostic Criteria

Yunus and Masi proposed fibromyalgia criteria that differ for children and adolescents from the adult criteria in order to take into consideration a more variable presentation along with a dependence on adult input to make the diagnosis. They proposed two major criteria and some minor diagnostic symptomatology:

- three months of widespread pain in the absence of other underlying causes for the symptoms
- severe pain in five of eleven designated tender points with palpation of less than four kg per unit area of force
- three out of ten of the following: chronic anxiety or tension, fatigue, poor sleep, chronic headaches, irritable bowel syndrome, subjective soft tissue

swelling, numbness, and pain modulation by physical activities, weather, anxiety, or stress

Clinical Presentation—Physical Examination

A standard physical examination is performed, supplemented by special examination points needed to diagnose fibromyalgia. The examination of joints in juvenile fibromyalgia reveals normal findings despite tenderness and spasms in soft tissue on palpation. The classic signs of joint swelling, heat, or redness, as in rheumatic fever or juvenile rheumatoid arthritis, are not found in juvenile fibromyalgia.

The search for tender points is performed with the thumb using a force of three kg rather than four kg in children, because their threshold is different from adults; palpation elicits tenderness in five of the eleven described locations.

Overlapping Syndrome

As with adults (see relevant chapters), fibromyalgia in children is often accompanied by other (comorbid, concomitant) conditions. Gedalia (2000) reviewed fifty-nine children with fibromyalgia and found generalized aches (97%), headaches (76%), sleep disturbances (70%), stiffness (30%), subjective joint swelling (24%), fatigue (20%), abdominal pain (17%), and depression (7%).

Siegel (1998) found at the initial presentation of forty-five children with fibromyalgia: sleep disturbance (96%), diffuse pain (93%), headaches (71%), general fatigue (62%), morning stiffness (53%), morning fatigue (49%), depression (43%), feeling worse with exercise (42%), subjective swelling (40%), irritable bowel (38%), dysmenorrhea (36%), illness changes with weather (36%), paresthesiae (24%), global anxiety (22%), lack of energy (18%), and Raynaud phenomenon (13%).

Tayag-Kier (2000) found children with fibromyalgia showed long sleep latency, shortened total sleep time, decreased sleep efficiency, and increased wakefulness during sleep, and also reported a subset of children with fibromyalgia who exhibited periodic limb movement in sleep.

Treatment

Effective treatment of fibromyalgia requires a multidisciplinary approach because of the multifaceted problems that develop. The goals of treatment are to reduce pain and depression, to decrease sleep disturbances, and to promote physical activity. Low-dose tricyclic antidepressants help decrease pain intensity and promote deeper sleep in children and adolescents. Cognitive behavioral interventions may help to improve the disorder. Supporting the child and family to maintain as normal a lifestyle as possible is important. Attendance at school and other usual activities is imperative. Modifying participation or attendance may be necessary in light of the child's ability to keep up with the expected activities.

Psychologic treatment has proven helpful in some cases. Conte (2003) compared children with juvenile primary fibromyalgia with healthy children and those living with arthritis. Findings showed that children and adolescents with juvenile primary fibromyalgia showed increased levels of anxiety and depression, greater temperamental instability, higher pain sensitivity, and less family cohesion than healthy children or those with arthritis.

Activity

Activity is a mainstay in the treatment of fibromyalgia. The goal of an exercise regime is to improve cardiovascular health and musculoskeletal fitness through nonimpact aerobic activity. Gedalia (2000) recommended physical therapy guidance to low-impact exercises, such as stretching, walking, biking, and swimming, at least half an hour per day, to improve cardiovascular fitness. Returning to normal activity is imperative for the child who has stopped sport and social activities because of pain; this helps to modulate the pain.

Prognosis

Improvement in symptoms of fibromyalgia is likely in children and adolescents. Prognosis in children is more favorable than in adults. Gedalia (2000) collected data on fifty children with an average follow-up period of eighteen months and found 60 percent had improved, 36 percent stayed the same, and 4 percent worsened. Nearly all the children needed to continue medications for up to four years after initial presentation.

Buskila (1995) studied children aged nine to fifteen years. At thirty months' follow-up, 73 percent no longer met the criteria for fibromyalgia. Symptoms among the four children who still met criteria for fibromyalgia included abdominal pain, headache, paresthesiae, morning stiffness, and sleep disturbance. Seven children were observed who did not progress to the point of meeting the full criteria over the thirty months, and all had improved.

Siegel (1998) observed thirty-three patients, with a mean follow-up of two and a half years. Improvement was observed in most patients during that follow-up time, with all patients showing some positive response to treatment.

Given these findings, the prognosis for children with fibromyalgia is for a more favorable outcome than in adults.

Other Pediatric Pain Conditions

The first documentation of growing pains was Duchamp's description in 1823 of a musculoskeletal pain syndrome that he mistakenly attributed to rheumatic fever (Baxter 1988). Estimates place the prevalence of growing pains, which are most likely to occur in early adolescence, between 4 and 34 percent (Peterson 1986). The generally accepted diagnostic criteria include limb pain of at least three months, intermittent pain with symptom-free intervals of days or months, pain not specifically related to joints, pain severe enough to interfere with regular activities, a normal physical examination and normal laboratory and radiographic findings (Baxter 1988). Growing pains are physically benign. However, because the differential diagnostic considerations include infection and tumor, further investigation is warranted if a patient has any abnormal results on physical examination.

Treatment includes reassurance, massage, application of heat, and use of nonsteroidal anti-inflammatory drugs (NSAIDs). Resolution is spontaneous but may take as long as two years.

The cause of growing pains is unclear. The "emotional theory" states that psychosocial disturbances are especially common in patients with growing pains found with headaches and abdominal pain, a spectrum of emotional disturbances that can lead to psychogenic pain (Passo 1982). For this reason, further exploration of psychosocial factors may be indicated in such circumstances.

Benign Hypermobility Syndrome

This term was coined by Kirk and colleagues to describe joint complaints in healthy patients with an extremely wide range of motion in their joints. Diagnosis is confirmed by a patient's ability to perform at least three of the following maneuvers (Gedalia 1985):

1. passive hyperextension of fingers until they are parallel to the extensor surface of the forearm
2. passive apposition of the thumb to the flexor surface of the forearm
3. hyperextension of more than ten degrees in both elbows
4. hyperextension of more than ten degrees in both knees
5. flexion at the hips, with knees extended and palms flat on the floor

Patients with this condition do not have hyperelastic skin, easy bruising, or other manifestations of collagen disorders. Over time, undue stress on the joint capsule can lead to articular pain even in the absence of joint instability (Gedalia 1993). More than 12 percent of teenagers are believed to have benign hypermobility syndrome. Treatment consists of reassurance.

The other point of view, expressed by Grahame (2008), is "an urgent need for rheumatologists to accept the challenges posed by hypermobility-related disorders."

Anyone needing experience in hypermobility should watch Indian and Cambodian women using their expressive hands in traditional dance. To the best of the author's knowledge, acquired in the countries where they dance, these women do not suffer ill effects in later life.

Psychogenic Pain

Few adolescents with pain syndromes have emotional disorders (Zwaigenbaum 1999), but somatization has an incidence of 1 percent among patients in all hospital visits (Merskey 1996).

Somatization appears to peak in early adolescence, particularly in girls who excel socially or academically. It may last more than a year and may be linked with a recent trauma or family dysfunction, such as marital discord. Often, a parent is involved in an adolescent's somatization. Typically, symptoms are unremitting and involve multiple body sites. Results of diagnostic tests are normal, and diagnosis must be one of exclusion (Dalton 1996). Pain, which is very real to patients with these illnesses, may interfere with peer and family interactions. It may be a precursor to other emotional disorders, such as depression, mood disorders, and panic attacks, which may manifest within four years of initial diagnosis (Zwaigenbaum 1999).

No pain should be labeled psychological without referring the patient for psychosocial evaluation (Merskey 1996). Adequate weight must be given to the history taking and physical examination. Many conditions need to be ruled out before concluding that the patient's pain is psychogenic.

WHAT IS MY PROGNOSIS?

Prognosis, the word derived from the Greek, is a "telling beforehand" and has been in medical use at least since the time of Hippocrates, who seemed more concerned with forecasting the future than improving the present. It's what Mark Twain would have called a five-dollar word when a perfectly good ten-cent word is available, namely, "guesswork." For that's all a prognosis is—the best guess at what will happen in the future. Some prognostications are based on sound experience—the sun will rise tomorrow. Others are not—the world will end on Tuesday.

Unfortunately, there is sound experience of the progress for fibromyalgia, which isn't good, and the prognosis (for which read "best guess") is against total resolution of the condition. But there was a time when prognosis for most medical conditions wasn't good. The problem would either solve itself, as does the common cold to this day, or would continue until overtaken by death, despite enemas, leeches, blood-letting and so on.

We need to appreciate that although we might like to think of modern medical care as so much more sophisticated than a couple of hundred years ago, in the absence of a specific therapy (penicillin for a strep throat, appendectomy for appendicitis), the principal difference lies in our mounting fees and increasing difficulty gaining access to attention.

Horizon and Weisman (2005) observe there is difficulty in following the course of fibromyalgia because the patients do not as a rule require to be admitted to hospital, and if they are, fibromyalgia is unlikely to be used as the admitting diagnosis. Nor do they die of this condition, so their fibromyalgia is unlikely to become a recorded statistic. They also observe there are differences between early fibromyalgia and the long-established form, in terms of response to therapy, and the absence of any definition for remission.

Disability, they point out, is not a valid marker since some may have changed their occupations but remain gainfully employed. Approximately one-third of patients with fibromyalgia reportedly modify their work to keep their jobs. Some patients shorten their workdays, their work-weeks, or both. Many patients with fibromyalgia have changed to jobs that are less physically and mentally taxing than their previous ones, often leading to decreased income. The same issues are true of chronic back pain, which may well resemble fibromyalgia in more than its chronicity.

There are two bits of good news. First, we're not quite as uninformed as we used to be about the extraordinary complications of the physics and chemistry of the pain process. Second, as described elsewhere, children diagnosed with fibromyalgia may recover. Granted, the diagnostic stipulations for the juvenile diagnosis are less stringent—three months' history, five tender points at three kg pressure. Granted, it might be a different disease process altogether—juvenile rheumatoid arthritis differs from the adult form. But there is hope, and if children recover, so might adults.

We'll look not only at the question of cure, but also at the lifestyle of the patient with fibromyalgia.

Cure? Improvement?

To answer the question of a cure, there's no shortage of documents to show that fibromyalgia rarely ends in total remission in the adult (Bengtsson 1986 and 1992; Cathey 1986; Felson 1986; Hawley 1988; Henriksson 1992; Ledingham 1993).

Is it cheering to a patient to tell her the prognosis describes a condition that is not life-threatening, is not deforming, and is not progressive, only to add that her symptoms will be variable, and in consequence there will be times when she'll think she's getting worse, which might be attributed to sleep deprivation and physical deconditioning? (Gilliland 2007).

Improvement generally occurs in a wide spectrum of chronic patients (Crook 1989; Whitney 1992), and as such fibromyalgia should be considered a chronic rather than an unchanging condition. Based on an eight-year prospective study employing a self-assessment questionnaire, it was concluded that once the disorder was established the patients continued to be symptomatic and did not improve; in fact, their functional disability worsened (Wolfe 1997; Russell 2004). Four years after their initial examination, 97 percent of patients still had symptoms, and 85 percent continued to meet the diagnostic criteria for fibromyalgia. Half had significant levels of functional disability. Many had abnormal scores for depression and anxiety (Ledingham 1993).

The so-called secondary fibromyalgia, related to trauma, appears to be just as chronic and perhaps in terms of symptoms, rather more severe (Greenfield 1988). Thirty-nine patients, mean age fifty-five years, fibromyalgia symptoms for fifteen years, all continued to meet the diagnostic criteria for fibromyalgia (Kennedy, in Bennett 1997):

- 55% had moderate to severe pain or stiffness
- 48% had significant sleep difficulties
- 59% had notable levels of fatigue
- 66% of these patients, however, reported that fibromyalgia symptoms were somewhat improved compared to when they were first diagnosed

Thirty-one patients were followed for fifteen years (Bennett 1997):

- 66% had some improvement; 59% had notable fatigue
- 55% moderate to severe pain and/or stiffness
- 48% had significant sleep difficulties

After a seven-year follow-up, 50 percent of fibromyalgia patients reported their health status unchanged and 59 percent rated their health as poor, which leaves the other 40 to 50 percent who are not as bad as they were (Wolfe 1997).

Although entirely reversing the allodynia and hyperalgesia in patients with fibromyalgia may not be possible, many patients improve significantly in response to therapy if ongoing stressors are relieved and self-control of pain control can be achieved. Prognosis is more guarded for patients who are highly distressed and have long-standing fibromyalgia, major psychiatric disease, an ingrained pattern of work avoidance, or established disability compensation. Prognosis is poor in patients with opioid or alcohol dependence, marked functional impairment despite multidisciplinary approaches to treatment, and severe depression and anxiety that responds poorly to treatment (Winfield 2007).

On Learning the Diagnosis

Receiving a diagnosis can be a turning point in the patient's life. A diagnosis may be significant when it provides the road to relief, understanding, or legitimization of problems.

A study was performed in Norway of the reactions of women in two fibromyalgia self-help groups to learn their reaction to the diagnosis of fibromyalgia. The social and medical meaning of the fibromyalgia diagnosis appears to be more complex, and for some the diagnosis did not seem helpful. Among the verbatim statements:

"When I came to the specialist, I was told I had fibromyalgia, but she did not like to give me such a diagnosis since there is nothing to be done about it."

"I felt happiness the day I finally got a name. For as long as I can remember, something was always wrong with me, and it was a real problem during my childhood and in my family."

"I felt paralyzed the first twenty-four hours. It was terrible, because I'd heard of this woman who was very sick with this disease. I thought my life would be turned upside down."

"It's no use telling people you have fibromyalgia since they all seem to have something similar. People have come to me and said they have a touch of it, too."

"You felt like the pain didn't get any respect. Like they didn't believe you."

The challenge for the doctor is to tolerate the uncertainty of the diagnostic concept while supporting the individual patient to create meaning in a life with chronic illness (Undeland 2007).

How Will Life Be?

If it's any comfort to the patient, the available statistical studies estimate the prognosis as it occurs averaged out for a group, and the prognosis for an individual may not be the same as that of the group (Russell 2004). There is some evidence that fibromyalgia patients seen in the community, rather than tertiary care centers, have a better prognosis (Bennett 1997). A 24 percent remission rate after two years was found in patients seen in an ambulatory care setting (Granges 1994).

Everyday activities take longer for fibromyalgia patients. They need more time to get started in the morning and often require extra rest periods during the day. They have difficulty with repetitive sustained motor tasks, unless frequent time-outs are taken (Henriksson 1994). Tasks may be well tolerated for short periods, but when carried out for prolonged periods become aggravating factors (Waylonis 1994).

Prolonged muscular activity, especially under stress or in uncomfortable climatic conditions, was reported to aggravate the symptoms of fibromyalgia (Waylonis 1994). The adaptations that fibromyalgia patients have to make in order to minimize their pain experience has a negative impact on both vocational and avocational activities.

In comparison with other rheumatic conditions, fibromyalgia patients have more comorbid medical conditions, more surgical interventions, more abnormal pain scores, more disability, more fatigue, more sleep disturbance. and more psychologic issues. In academic centers, they average ten outpatient visits per year and one hospitalization per three years (Winfield 2007).

CHAPTER SIX

MORE COMPLICATED EXPLANATIONS

HISTORY OF THE FIBROMYALGIA CONCEPT AND RELATED CONDITIONS

Nemesis, the spirit of divine retribution, sent her attendant Poena to the earth as punishment for our hubris. From Poena, via the concept of punishment, came the word "pain," and as a result, pain and punishment remain historically intertwined.

The philosophical, political, and religious meanings of pain defined the suffering of individuals for much of human history. Pain is the central metaphor of Judeo-Christian thought, as illustrated in the test of faith in the story of Job and the sacrificial redemption of the crucifixion (Meldrum 2003). For millennia, pain was equated with just retribution and suffering was a punishment for known or unknown sins. "We have left undone those things which we ought to have done; and we have done those things which we ought not to have done; and there is no health in us." Therapy was limited to penance, hacksaw, and opium; if we're honest with ourselves, we haven't gotten much further.

The unconscious mind desires to be taken seriously and not to be ridiculed. It will therefore strive to present symptoms that always seem, to the surrounding culture, to be legitimate evidence of organic disease. This striving introduces a historical dimension. As the culture changes its opinion about what is legitimate disease and what is not, the pattern of psychosomatic illness changes. Late nineteenth- and twentieth-century culture regarded physical paralysis and sudden "coma" (both common before 1900) as inappropriate responses. It is the interaction between doctors and patients that determines how psychosomatic symptoms change over the years, and the history of psychosomatic illness is one of ever-changing steps in a *pas de deux* between doctor and patient (Shorter 1992).

Neurasthenia

George Beard, an 1866 Columbia University medical graduate, became an electrotherapist and seems to have been the originator of this word, *neurasthenia*. Beard built the concept on many similar current terms in American and European medical practice, all of which implied some failure or weakness of the central nervous system, and all of those weaknesses open to improvement with electrical treatment. The symptoms covered were whatever could be imagined, both mental and physical, but primarily of a sensory nature, and so they were labeled "hyperesthesia," or feeling everything too much. Not everyone was taken in by what became known as the "American Nervousness." A German neurologist christened George Beard "The P.T. Barnum of medicine" (Brown 1980).

Neurasthenia became the catch-all disease and a specialty in itself, although the cynics designated it as a diagnostic wastebasket and a "mob of incoherent symptoms borrowed from the most diverse disorders." These symptoms were characterized by a mix of exhaustion and insomnia—"the longer they stay in bed, the tireder they feel," so "fatigue neurosis" was suggested as an alternative name to neurasthenia (Shorter 1992).

All body symptoms were regarded as a "real disease" instead of manifested in a patient's head; however, the diagnosis became so convenient, so all-embracing, that it was eventually valueless and the field moved out of the hands of the neurologists, the "nerve doctors," and into the field of psychoanalysis. In reading the reports of the distressing symptoms that became classified as neurasthenia, it is easy to think of the legitimate diagnoses we would give now, but not to the persons who, after a course of electric shocks, were restored from prostration to a full and active life.

Although the effect of the mind on the body was clearly known to the earliest practitioners of the healing and spiritual arts, the coining of the word *psychosomatic* dates to Johan Heinroth in 1818, at the time when Mesmer was holding sway with animal magnetism.

Fibrositis—Early Reports

In fibromyalgia, and with the components of Yunus's overlapping syndrome, we are now trying to come to grips with invisible pain, essentially invisible by definition. If a proximate cause can be seen, heard, or felt, then the diagnosis must be rethought, for it can't be fibromyalgia.

Dommerholt describes some of the earlier literature on trigger points, not fibromyalgia. Balfour in 1816 described, "Nodular tumors and thickenings which were painful to the touch, and from which pains shot to neighboring parts," and Strauss in 1898 described, "Small, tender and apple-sized nodules and painful, pencil-sized to little-finger-sized palpable bands."

The history of chronic pain, well described by Wallace and Clauw (2005), covers a wider field than invisible pain; among the historical features:

- Brown (1828)—"spinal irritation" in young women with tender spots when pinched
- Velleix (1841)—*points douloureaux*, painful to pressure, provoking radiating pain
- Froreip (1843)—tender areas in muscles accompanied by pain and stiffness
- Inman (1855)—spasm of muscles causing rheumatic nodules
- Helleday (1876)—neuralgic pain spreading from nodules in rheumatic muscles
- Graham (1893)—muscular rheumatism attributed to "coagulation of the semi-fluid contractile muscular substance and adhesion of muscular fibrils"
- Gowers (1904)—coined the term *fibrositis* while writing about lumbago (back pain)
- Stockman (1904)—described (incorrectly) microscopic evidence of inflammation in fibrous tissue
- Steindler (1937)—an orthopedic surgeon, described "trigger points"
- Kellgren (1938)—induced and explained "referred pain"
- Graham (1940)—first use of the term fibrositis in North America and employed the term "tension rheumatism"
- Hutchison (1942)—69 percent military rheumatology referrals for "fibrositis"
- Savage (1942)—fibrositis painful areas relieved by injection of local anesthetic
- Ellman (1942)—fibrositis definition incorporated all forms of soft tissue pains, including "psychogenic rheumatism"
- Boland (1943)—24 percent military referrals for fibrositis; strong concomitant issues in psychological profiles
- Kelly (1946)—connected visceral pain syndromes with fibrositis
- Travell (1952)—coined term "myofascial pain syndrome"
- Imboden (1959)—importance of pre-illness personality structure defined in patients with chronic fatigue attributed to brucellosis

Most, if not all, of these historical reports relate to a palpable abnormality, a localized pain, or radiating pain. A palpable mass might perhaps be what we now call myofascial pain syndrome, and localized pain with radiation on pressure might be myofascial pain syndrome or a regional pain syndrome, but "no mass felt" and "all over" are today's diagnostic criteria for fibromyalgia.

Fibrositis was a very common complaint of the twentieth century and covered everything from traumatic muscle tears to myofascial pain syndrome, but it was a localized, not a generalized, condition. Gowers had coined the term *fibrositis* in 1904, published in the *British Medical Journal*. He considered what he found to be a different form of lumbago. Interestingly, low back pain is a major concomitant symptom of fibromyalgia, and, who knows, maybe that's what Gowers found. The dual association of terms persists; Horne (2006), a psychophysiologist and expert on sleep, refers to "a type of low and middle back pain called fibromyalgia."

The Advent of Fibromyalgia

Wallace and Clauw's list of contributors to the field continues:

- Smythe and Moldofsky (1977) described "tender points" and showed electroencephalograph changes in sleep patterns. They coined the term *fibrositis syndrome*.
- Yunus (1981) accepted Hench's objection to "fibrositis" since there was no inflammation and pointed out the condition was often accompanied by other medical issues, and it appears he originated the term *fibromyalgia*.
- Yunus (1984) went on to describe the central sensitization syndrome.
- American College of Rheumatology (1990) defined the criteria for fibromyalgia.
- The World Health Organization (1992) accepted fibromyalgia as a diagnostic term.

Other points in the historical development of the concept are made by Russell (2004). Traut (1968) expanded the meaning of fibrositis to include diffuse musculoskeletal pain, multiple site tender points, poor sleep, and fatigue. Smythe and Moldofsky (1977) corroborated the expansion of symptoms to include poor sleep and fatigue with specific changes demonstrable by sleep encephalographs. With the help of colleagues, they went on to devise a set of criteria for clinical diagnosis, formalized in the ACR's 1990 statement, whose structured nature assisted in the legitimization of a questioned diagnosis.

Blotman (2006) follows the development of the variability in diagnostic criteria. Smythe and Moldofsky (1977) had proposed a condition to comprise: diffuse pain, pain provoked by palpation in the suprascapular region, difficulty with sleep, and negative findings by lab and x-ray. The location and number of tender points necessary to confirm the diagnosis remained widely variable: Bennett suggested 10 out of 25; Yunus and associates, 3–5 out of 40; Wolfe and associates, 7 out of 14; Campbell and associates, 12 out of 17.

Until the ACR's 1990 agreement, the 1981 definition of Yunus was the most widely used. It required for diagnosis:

- *Obligatory criteria:* Diffuse pain or stiffness particularly in at least three anatomic regions for a minimum of three months.
- *Major criterion:* Consistent findings of pain over at least five characteristic points.
- *Minor criteria:* At least three in a list of ten symptom components that featured later in Yunus's overlapping syndrome.

Harth and Nielson (2007) review the use of the "11 out of 18" tender point system. They believe many rheumatologists do not use the system and explore the much chewed-over conundrum of what diagnosis should be given to a person with widespread pain, but only nine tender points, or eighteen tender points without widespread pain? They suggest a cutoff point is necessary and compare this with setting a cutoff point for diagnosing hypertension. Harth and Nielson believe if they did not use the tender point count as a controlling mechanism, the patients qualifying on the basis of chronic widespread pain alone would be 15 percent of the nation's population.

Gracely (2007), a pain psychologist, in reference to the article of Harth and Nielson, expresses concern on two levels: Concern for those who are excluded from treatment because they don't meet the arbitrary standards, and concern for how these standards are applied or misapplied. Obvious to everyone, there is bound to be a cadre of persons who learn the right answers from the freely available information and pictures of the Three Graces with spots on them, and then on the other side of the coin, patients bearing a diagnosis of fibromyalgia who were often not very tender. Perhaps this is a question not of "what you have," but of "who you know." Get the right doctor—get the right diagnosis.

In view of the uncertainty of the cause of the condition currently known as fibro-my-algia syndrome, it's not unreasonable to wonder how many further changes in name await it. Since there is no component of inflammation associated with fibromyalgia, "itis" was dropped from the earlier term, *fibrositis.* Although there is no recognizable change in muscle or fibrous tissue, the anachronistic "fibro" and "my" designators are retained. It's agreed there is pain, so "algia" is all that remains appropriate.

"Algia" means no more than pain. It would not be unreasonable to rename the condition as "widespread and persisting pain not yet diagnosed," or more simply, "WPP nyd," thereby eliminating the disinformation conveyed in the current name. But, as the above authors point out, that creates a syndrome of unknown cause, and a diagnosis that's applicable to 15 percent of the US population.

MORE COMPLICATED EXPLANATIONS OF PAIN

The central nervous system (CNS) is composed of the brain and spinal cord. Within this system the cells that concern us are called neurons, and each cell has a body (sometimes referred to as a *soma*). From the bodies of the cells extend many short receiving branches termed *dendrites* and long transmitting branches called *axons*. Some axons are located within the CNS, where they collectively form a number of named *tracts* on their way to be distributed to different parts of the brain. Some axons extend from the CNS, bundled together to form *nerves,* which, once outside the CNS, are distributed to the torso and limbs, and collectively called the peripheral nervous system.

Nerve axons transmit messages going from the spinal cord, *efferent*, and to the spinal cord, *afferent*. In general terms, the afferent bear sensory impulses telling the brain what is happening, and the efferent bear motor impulses to carry out the brain's wishes. Afferent says, "My hand is burning," and efferent responds by moving it.

Anatomical Pathways of Pain

There are specialized nerve endings called nociceptors (from the Latin *nocere*, meaning to harm) located in the skin and in every other part of the body where pain can be felt. There are several types of nociceptors, which allow us to distinguish between differing stimuli such as pressure, sharp or blunt, hot or cold. From this terminal structure, the nociceptor, a signal is sent to the brain.

Nerve Fiber

The axon of the nerve cell that ends at the nociceptor is the first to get the message, so logically this cell is termed a first-order neuron. The message from the nociceptor travels toward the cell body (soma) by a combined chemical and electrical process.

Like Orwell's animals, all axons are not equal. They come in different sizes, significant to their speed of action. Of course this requires labeling, and of course that requires systems that use Roman letters and numbers, and you can't be surprised they didn't pass up the chance to toss in a little Greek lettering as well.

The nerve fibers are classified with Roman letters; the thickest is "A," twenty times thicker than the thinnest "C." Thick fibers send their signals faster, and A transmits up to a hundred times faster than C. The speed of transmission is readily measurable; the time between touching the toe with a pin and the brain knowing it's happened is about one-tenth of a second.

There are several types of A fibers, subclassified by the Greek letters alpha, beta, gamma, and delta. The variety concerned with pain transmission is A delta, written as Aδ. (Some classifications will show in Roman numerals the Aδ fiber as "III" and the C fiber as "IV," but more commonly Aδ and C are used.)

Thus the sensations of pain are transmitted from the nociceptor along the speedy Aδ fibers, conveying the sensation of sharp pain, while the less-speedy C fibers convey the sensations of burning, aching, or throbbing pains.

The signal passes in the axon, bundled up in a nerve, toward the spinal cord, as if it were traveling an electric power grid. Its cell body is located close to the spinal cord in a swelling named the "dorsal root ganglion" (taken from the Greek word meaning a small swelling), where the signal continues in the axon going on past the cell and enters into the back of the spinal cord via the "dorsal root," an aggregation of axons comparable to an extremely short and thin peripheral nerve.

A section made across the spinal cord shows it to be more or less round, with a grey, squat, H-shaped figure occupying the middle. At the top of the upper arm of the H, known as the dorsal horn, the axon from this first-order neuron interfaces with an axon of the second-order neuron, whose cell body is contained within the grey matter composing the H. Rather surprisingly, this second-order axon crosses to the other side of the spinal cord, where it joins with fellow second-order axons collectively to form a tract (also called fasciculus—think of the bundle of sticks making the fascist emblem) at the anterolateral aspect of the cord. Because of the destination to which it ascends in the spinal cord, it's known as the spinothalamic tract.

Important to a number of conditions involving the spinal cord, damage to the right side of the cord might affect the reception of sensations from the left side of the body and vice versa. There are well-known neurological and occasional traumatic conditions that characterize this apparent enigma.

At the thalamus and other parts of the midbrain (the region lying above the floor of the skull and hidden from view by the wrinkled cerebral hemispheres), the second-order neurons interface with a set of third-order neurons, which transmit the message to the sensory cortex, located as one of the major wrinkles. And all of this in a tenth of a second.

The less inquiring minds should stop here. Accept the mysterious process of transmitting a message from toe to brain. The more inquiring mind should read on.

Interface or Synapse?

Skinner (1961) describes how the word *synapse* was introduced into the medical language. Derived from the Greek for "clasp," Sherrington, a major player in the neurophysiology field, thought it an appropriate word for what has so far been passed off in this chapter as signals passing between neurons. It's not usually like an electric spark jumping a gap between wires. In fact, such a form of electrical transmission regularly occurs in the invertebrate, and to a much lesser extent, in the nervous system of animals with backbones. In most instances, in our nerve impulse transmissions, there is chemistry as well as electricity. Anyone following the stories about mythical weapons of mass destruction in Iraq will know about "nerve gases," which in effect are chemicals that block activities at synapses, and the same chemicals are commonly used in our agriculture.

So how do signals pass between nerve cells? What's the mechanism? And what does it have to do with fibromyalgia?

The neuron along which the impulse travels is designated presynaptic; it ends in a slight swelling, the presynaptic button, which contains a dense mass of assorted proteins. This button is separated by a minute gap, the synaptic cleft, from a similar swelling at the next neuron along the line, here called the postsynaptic neuron, which also has an array of proteins. An adhesive protein binds the two active surfaces of the synapse together, not necessarily end to end or axon to axon, but one axon's end glues to some part of another neuron.

Signals pass from presynaptic to postsynaptic neurons via chemical activity. The terminal buttons of the presynaptic neuron contain minuscule packets (vesicles) loaded with neurotransmitter chemicals, lined up like a row of army tanks filled with weapons, ready and waiting to use them. Each vesicle contains thousands of neurotransmitter chemicals. These chemicals, many different kinds, have been made in the body of the cell; they migrate down the axon to take their ordered place in the button, so to speak, at the front. Upon the arrival of the electric signal, the vesicles fuse with the end surface of the presynaptic button and discharge their contents into the synaptic cleft.

What happens next is determined by the postsynaptic receptor neuron, and it should be understood that there are many neurons at simultaneous play. Think of a bunch of kids at a farm gate. Some are pushing it open, some are keeping it closed. Effectively, the same may occur at the numerous synapses. Not all of the neurons are interested in transmitting the pain signal up to the brain. Some neurons have descended from the brain and their specific function at the dorsal horn is to modify the extent of the pain signal (Basbaum 1984; Staud 2005).

Not all of the neurotransmitter chemicals excite a positive continuing reaction; some are specifically inhibitory, meaning they block the action from going any further. A major excitor of action is glutamate, and the major inhibitors are glycine and gamma-aminobutyric acid (GABA). Guess where pregabalin, marketed as Lyrica, got its name?

In the same manner, while some of the chemicals released want to transmit the sensation of pain, others are trying to inhibit this sensation. How they are taken up and react with the next set of neurons determines the outcome. It's impossible to read much about fibromyalgia without having some of these chemical names thrown at you, so some of them are grouped by which side of the fence they're on: (1) acting in favor of pain transmission (pronociceptive): substance P, nerve growth factor; or (2) acting against pain transmission (antinociceptive): serotonin, norepinephrine, endorphins.

Think of a battlefield: the action's over and the protagonists are no longer needed at the front. When it's all over, some of the neurotransmitters just drift away; others are drafted back for further duty by *reuptake* (a word to remember in connection with drugs); and still others are so chewed up they're no longer fit for service.

What Does This Have to Do with Fibromyalgia?

It's generally agreed that fibromyalgia is characterized by a complaint of widespread pain. One thing physicians agree upon, whether or not they believe in fibromyalgia, is the total absence of any physical finding at the body's surface or in the peripheral nerves that could explain this pain.

Those who believe in fibromyalgia are satisfied the problem is real, not imaginary, and therefore ascribe to the idea that it must be located somewhere between the interpreting cortex of the brain and the point where the nerves enter the spine; or in a succinct but more complicated term, the pain is neuropathic.

Various imaging techniques fail to reveal any physical changes in the CNS. Although physical changes can be demonstrated when imaging various other perplexing conditions such as multiple sclerosis, they have not been shown in fibromyalgia.

What does that leave us with? Nothing? Or a change in function? Putting aside the possibility of nothing, we take up the possible change of function, which Russell (2005) illustrates with a diagram, indicating that the function of the "push-me, pull-me" neurotransmitters in widespread pain might either be excessive or insufficient—there might be excessive activity by the neurotransmitters that are pronociceptive, or insufficient activity by the antinociceptive ones.

The spinal cord is bathed in cerebrospinal fluid (CSF); chemicals that drift away from their site of action in the spinal cord can be expected to be found in the CSF. If the neurotransmitter chemicals are found in the CSF of patients with fibromyalgia in concentrations different from the normal, then perhaps that indicates an invisible difference in neurotransmission. In fact, the pronociceptive neurotransmitter, substance P, has been found in concentrations three times higher than the normal (Vaeroy 1988) and the pronociceptive nerve growth factor in concentrations four times the normal (Giovengo 1999). On the other side of the coin, the precursor chemical for the antinociceptive neurotransmitter serotonin is found at lower than usual levels in the CSF (Russell 1992).

TRANQUILITY AND STRESS

We'll start with some very basic concepts and build from there. Homeostasis (derived from Greek) was Claude Bernard's fundamental principle in physiology. The implication is that by development (or by happenstance), the human body functions in an optimal manner, and there are automatic mechanisms within the body to keep it functioning in this same optimal manner. Our body temperature is kept within a very narrow range, as are the rates of our heartbeat and our breathing.

Stress

A term used in many different ways in many different contexts, but for our purpose should be thought of as the point where resources no longer match demands. A certain amount of stress is supposed to be good for you—builds character, as Dickens' Squeers and other schoolmasters would tell you. Some of us can handle more than others; not everyone was intended to be a commando. Not every woman can get up night after night to tend to her sick mother and screaming children and go to a demanding job with a warm smile the next day.

From the early 1900s, Cannon showed that fear or injury would result in delayed emptying of the contents of the stomach. To this day, anesthetists are disinclined to put someone with a fracture to sleep until six hours after an injury, which probably does not ingratiate Cannon to the orthopedic surgeon. Selye did nasty things to rats, leading him to postulate a "general adaptation syndrome," which described the phases the body will go through when presented with continuous stressful situations: first alarm, followed by resistance, and finally ending in exhaustion. During this process, the adrenals became bigger and the stomach ulcerated.

Many cases of fibromyalgia can be traced back to a state of stress. Physicians have decided the mind is not separate from the body and are therefore not surprised that exhaustion of the mind leads to deterioration of the body's endocrine and immune systems.

Does "dysregulation" of the general adaptation syndrome result in fibromyalgia? Here's how it might happen.

Cybernetics

Although there must have been a time when it was supposed homeostasis happened by magic, or an act performed by the gods, we now expect there to be some kind of mechanism at play, and some kind of control. Unlike our external system of government where we're told what to do by higher authority, our internal homeostasis is self-controlling by a series of switch-on and switch-off mechanisms, which keep it functioning at the preordained levels, a system known as cybernetic after the Greek word for a helmsman. (How would scientists communicate if it hadn't been for the Greeks?)

Systems, of course, must go beyond the theoretical, so to put the cybernetic mechanisms into play, to stabilize our body functions, there has to be a system of messengers, which are nerve signals, followed by liberation of chemical hormones. Derived from the Greek meaning "to set in motion," hormones are the chemicals that cause things to happen; they're secreted by cells under the stimulus of the nervous system and travel in the bloodstream to their target. And if there's a system of messengers, there has to be a system of pathways. We'll discuss pathways first.

Autonomic Nervous System

The central nervous system is composed of the brain and spinal cord. The peripheral nervous system is composed of nerves and their branches running from the spinal cord. These nerves, motor and sensory, are concerned with the functions of the body's frame, the muscles, the bones, the skin, and so on. They don't concern themselves with what's inside the body, inside the chest and abdomen, namely, the heart, lungs, stomach, and gut. Whereas we can go to sleep, or be anesthetized, rendering the peripheral nervous system inactive and stopping all its activities, it wouldn't do at all if the heart and lungs were to stop. So they have a separate, "autonomic," nervous system—derived from autonomous, meaning it runs under its own control mechanism and might be thought of as either automatic or involuntary. It's possible in some instances to override the mechanism; you can speed up your rate of breathing, but you can't stop it for long—except by suicide.

There are two parts to the autonomic nervous system, sympathetic and parasympathetic. Very broadly speaking, the parasympathetic system is "sugar and spice and all things nice," keeping our systems working at a tranquil pace, whereas the sympathetic system is "slugs and snails and puppy dogs' tails," and abhors tranquility; it functions to speed everything up, very useful in an emergency, not so desirable when we'd rather be at rest.

The central nervous system is as much central to the autonomic system as it is to the peripheral system, but the connections are different. Again, very broadly speaking, the sympathetic system makes its connections at the thoracic (chest) level, while the parasympathetic system connects at either end of the CNS, cranial and sacral.

Messages are brought to the spinal cord via first-order neurons, through the posterior root, and into the H-shaped grey substance. Here the message-carrying neuron may synapse with cells of the sympathetic system, their cell bodies located in the grey matter of the cord, in the thoracic and upper two lumbar segments. The axons of these autonomic nervous system cells leave the cord via an anterior root to a synapse with a cell body housed in a chain of ganglia running close to the spine. From these ganglia, axons may join the peripheral nervous system to be distributed in company with the peripheral nerves, but going to blood vessels and sweat glands. By running along the blood vessels and forming a network around them, the sympathetic nerve fibers gain access to the entire body. Other axons will leave the ganglia, pass to other ganglia, coalesce, and form a separate array of fibers known as splanchnic nerves, going to the organs within the chest and abdomen. There are pain receptors present in this system; the two most severe pains, by physicians' reckoning, are caused by cardiac infarct and by kidney stone, both pains carried via the autonomic system.

We are more concerned, however, with the sympathetic side of the autonomic system.

Switch cameras to the brain.

Hypothalamus and Pituitary

The brain stem is the part of the central nervous system between the spinal cord and the wrinkled cerebral hemispheres. It transmits signals, has a mass of cells, and has many functions in the cybernetic field. The hypothalamus zone of the midbrain is effectively the cell station for the autonomic nervous system— parasympathetic in front, sympathetic behind. Its messages are sent either through the spinal cord by a descending tract, or through tracts in a connecting stalk (infundibulum) to the pituitary gland.

In medicine, whenever possible, we give any structure at least two names. The pituitary is also called hypophysis, because it is "growing under," but I prefer pituitary. Although the pituitary gland is located in a socket in the floor of the skull, it in fact lies immediately above the cavity of the nose, and when necessary surgeons may approach it via the nose instead of the earlier requirement to make a hole in the skull.

Called the conductor of the orchestra, the pituitary has distinct anterior (adenohypophysis) and posterior (neurohypophysis) segments, and is the source of many of the body's controlling hormones. Growth hormones and other hormones that stimulate the adrenal, thyroid, breasts, and ovaries are derived from the anterior pituitary. While the posterior pituitary circulates hormones named oxytocin and vasopressin. The two portions of the pituitary gland function independently.

Anterior pituitary hormones are selectively switched either on or off by releasing or by inhibiting hormones, passing in the bloodstream from the hypothalamus. The posterior pituitary is also activated by chemicals, but they are carried closer to their targets by a special tract of nerve fibers entering the posterior pituitary.

Switch cameras to the kidney.

Adrenal Glands

Also known as suprarenal, these paired glands sit like cocked hats on top of the kidneys. Each, like the pituitary, is in two distinct parts but has an inner medulla and an outer cortex; they're developmentally derived from different layers of the embryo and have different actions, although both cortex and medulla have roles in production of the hormones related to the problems of stress.

In the medulla are produced hormones in the chemical group collectively known as catecholamines, individually called adrenaline (or epinephrine) and noradrenaline (or norepinephrine). These are the active chemicals of the sympathetic nervous system, together with another in the catecholamine group, called dopamine, which is mostly made in cells inside the CNS.

The adrenal cortex creates cortisol, which interests us most, and other hormones of no relevance to this issue. The production of cortisol is under the direction of the hypothalamus via the anterior pituitary adrenocorticotropic hormone, ACTH. Pan cameras back to brain.

Hypothalamic–Pituitary–Adrenal Axis and the Messengers

More conveniently known as the HPA axis, this is the controlling interrelationship in homeostasis, stress, and exhaustion, and is considered by some as a major factor in fibromyalgia.

Imagine a hierarchy of hormones with the hypothalamus literally and figuratively at the top. Your unconscious activities are HPA controlled, through a chain reaction.

First, the hypothalamus forms a corticotropin-releasing hormone (CRH); this passes to the anterior pituitary, which secretes adrenocorticotropic hormone

(ACTH). In turn, ACTH stimulates the adrenal cortex to secrete the stress-resisting hormone, cortisol, which enters the circulation, locates the hypothalamus, and switches off the CRH. Unsurprisingly, there are also other hormones at play in this cycle, including serotonin, substance P, and norepinephrine.

Serum cortisol level is used as an indicator of stress. In normal release, cortisol has widespread actions that help restore homeostasis after stress. There is a normal circadian rise and fall in the typical level of circulating cortisol. The lowest levels occur a few hours after going to sleep, while the highest concentrations are found in the early morning. Changed patterns of serum cortisol levels have been observed in connection with abnormal ACTH levels, clinical depression, psychological stress, illness and fever, in association with trauma and surgery, in states of fear and pain, physical exertion, and at extreme temperatures. The consequence of chronic stress is prolonged cortisol secretion. Variations from normal cortisol levels have been reported in fibromyalgia cases (Crofford 1994), and ongoing studies have shown other aberrations in those with fibromyalgia (Russell 2005). A dysfunction of the system has been suggested as a possible cause of fibromyalgia (Marinez-Lavin 2008).

MEDICATIONS EMPLOYED IN THE TREATMENT OF FIBROMYALGIA

The Controlled Substances Act controls the availability of drugs in the United States, some of which are legally available in other countries. In particular, heroin is forbidden for use in the United States but is widely and safely used in Europe.

Schedule I drugs are not available, even with prescription, based upon the absence of currently acceptable medical use in the United States, lack of evidence for safe usage, and/or a high potential for abuse. Heroin, GHB, cannabis, ecstasy, LSD, and mescaline all fall into this category.

Schedule II drugs are available only with appropriate prescription and include drugs with high potential for abuse or psychological dependence, but have been accepted for medical usage in the United States. Narcotics and other opiates and opioids are in this group.

As with schedule II drugs, schedule III drugs are only available with appropriate prescription and include drugs with potential for abuse, but to a lesser extent than those grouped in schedules I and II. Prescriptions in this category may be refilled up to five times within six months. Anabolic steroids are in this grouping.

For schedule IV drugs, a prescription is required, but these drugs possess a relatively low potential for abuse and may be refilled up to five times within six months with a valid prescription. Grouping includes medications for sleep and anxiety such as Valium, Xanax, Ambien, barbiturates, and khat.

A prescription is needed for schedule V drugs, but there is less of a likelihood for addiction. Drugs in this category include Lyrica, cough medicines containing codeine, antidiarrhea medications such as Lomotil, and others containing opium.

Tricyclic Antidepressants

Benzene, a fundamental of organic chemistry, has six linked carbon atoms, pictured in two-dimensions as a ring. Put three of these rings together and you have a tricyclic chemical; vary this with different side chains and you've copied the 1950 accidental discovery of a large and financially rewarding group of antidepressant medications. Cyclobenzaprine (Flexeril) has a tricyclic structure but is sold as a "muscle relaxant."

As with most drugs, the exact mechanism is not fully understood, and there are probably several, the extent of each mechanism varying from compound to compound. It is believed that, to differing degrees, the effects of the neurotransmitters norepinephrine, dopamine, and serotonin are potentiated by preventing or delaying their removal from the scene of action.

Relevance to fibromyalgia. Among the members of this group, amitriptyline (Elavil) is widely used in fibromyalgia. Its original use as an antidepressant is still appropriate, but it has also been found effective in relieving chronic pain. Perhaps this is accomplished by helping the patient to sleep better, perhaps it possesses a benefit specific to neuropathic pain; however, there is no benefit to be found in using tricyclics for acute (short-term) pain. Any action cyclobenzaprine has on relaxing muscles is via its activity in the central nervous system.

Serotonin (5-HT)

Although serotonin was first discovered in the blood serum, it is now known to exist widely throughout the body; hence 5-HT, the abbreviation of its chemical name (5-hydroxytryptamine), is in preferential but not exclusive use.

Tryptophan is taken up from the intestine and passes what's known as the blood-brain barrier (not all chemicals can enter the brain). Once inside the central nervous system, some of the tryptophan is converted in stages to 5-HT, which enters the neurons, notably the dorsal horn in the spinal column, and can be discharged at the synapse interface as a neurotransmitter; although, it is suggested that most of the active 5-HT is free and diffuses in order to be taken up by specialized 5-HT receptors on the dendrites outside the nerve cell (neuron).

5-HT has metabolic functions outside the CNS. Ninety percent is found in the cells of the small intestine, and it's active in so many ways it becomes hard to define any specific action. Ecstasy (MDM), a schedule I substance, causes a mass release of serotonin, which induces a feeling of euphoria, but also releases other neurotransmitters; MDM and similar psychedelic drugs (e.g., LSD) are taken up at the 5-HT receptors.

The action of any serotonin (5-HT) that is not joined to the neurons at the 5-HT receptors is cut short by a process involving reuptake chemicals, which are carried on monoamine transporters on the presynaptic neuron. In turn, their action is blocked by reuptake inhibitors, which allow the pleasing effects of serotonin (5-HT) to continue. This wide group of medications is known variously as monoamine oxidase inhibitors (MAOIs) and selective serotonin reuptake inhibitors (SSRIs), according to their point of action. The tricyclic antidepressants are in the same group, but they also inhibit reuptake of norepinephrine. Minaciprin, a drug in the trial stages and not yet authorized for specific use with fibromyalgia, is said by its developers to inhibit preferentially norepinephrine reuptake.

Parnate is an example of an MAOI; Prozac, Zoloft, and Paxil are some of the most widely prescribed SSRIs.

Serotonin syndrome. Originally called serotonin toxicity, which better describes its origin, this condition is now known as a syndrome. It is not an abnormal reaction to serotonin but constitutes the reaction to an overdose. The overdose may be deliberate or it may be inadvertent (i.e., taking several medications, each of which affect the serotonin system). Since mental confusion is a major presenting symptom but is so common in the elderly, who are likely to be taking these medications, diagnosis might be delayed. This condition can be prevented by keeping your physician and pharmacist fully informed of all medications and supplements you are currently, or considering, taking.

Relevance to fibromyalgia. Serotonin as a neurotransmitter is involved in the pain process and particularly in central pain. Low concentrations of 5-HT could conceivably be related to the pain of fibromyalgia (Russell 2004). The mental confusion caused by serotonin syndrome should not be misdiagnosed as "fibro fog."

Opioids

Opioid Receptors. In the decades of the '60s and '70s, specific receptors for opioids were discovered. Names were allocated using the Greek alphabet, applying the first letter of the substance that was found to bind to them (ligand). The receptor for morphine, starting with "m," was called mu (μ); ketocyclazocine called kappa (κ); and the endogenous opioid delta (δ) (Corbett 2006). Since these naming conventions have undergone various changes over the years, the most current usages are shown in parentheses below (OP stands for opioid):

delta (DOP) δ found in brain; functions in analgesia, euphoria;

kappa (KOP) κ found in brain and dorsal horn of spinal cord; functions in spinal analgesia and sedation;

mu (MOP) μ found in brain and dorsal horn of spinal cord; functions in euphoria, reduced gastrointestinal mobility. Morphine and codeine bind here. Possesses high affinity for enkephalins and endorphins, low affinity for dynorphins. Three known variants are labeled mu 1,2,3. Stimulation of mu1 blocks pain, mu2 causes respiratory depression and constipation. These receptors are found in either the pre- or postsynapse, depending on the cell type; they are mostly presynaptic in the spinal cord.

Activation of receptors. This process mediates acute changes in neuronal excitability via "disinhibition" of presynaptic release of GABA. Activation is effected either by endogenous or exogenous opioids. Activation by an agonist such as morphine causes the above-listed effects.

Both in mice and in humans, the genes for the different receptors are carried on different chromosomes. Genes have been cloned, and there are now genetically modified mice for experimentation. It has been found mu and delta work in opposite ways in regulating emotions (Kieffer 2007), and the analgesic properties of morphine have no effect on a mouse without mu receptors (Matthes 1996). In mice lacking this gene, not only do they show a failure to obtain analgesia from morphine, and consequently suffer from increased sensitivity to pain, but they also exhibit altered emotional responses. In mice lacking the delta receptor, there are increases in levels of anxiety and a depressivelike behavior.

You are your own poppy. Certain peptides (a compound of two or more amino acids) formed by the human body are released by neurons and may activate the opioid receptors; they are named dynorphins, endomorphins, endorphins, enkephalins, and a few others in an actively developing research field. It took two years of work and a large quantity of pig brain before Kosterlitz had enough material to prove his belief that opium receptors in the brain and spinal cord had a normal physiologic function and were not just there to please the poppy growers. Enkephalin was named after *Kephalos*, the Greek word for head. Then a fragment of a pituitary hormone was found to have morphinelike properties and was called endorphin. The discovery of several similar naturally occurring morphinelike chemicals soon followed, including the group known as endomorphins. The physiologic role of endogenous morphine is still unclear

(Corbett 2006). Suggestions have been made they are released with analgesic effect by acupuncture and with the proclaimed "runners' high" of extreme exercise; however, neither of these suggestions meets with universal agreement. In 1917, Trendeleberg demonstrated that morphine inhibited the wave of muscular contraction in the gut (peristalsis), but it was not until many years later that the concepts of neurotransmission were understood.

Relevance to fibromyalgia. PET scan study has shown a reduced mu opioid peptide receptor (MOP) availability in the brains of patients with fibromyalgia, possibly explaining why opioids are less effective in fibromyalgia than in other pain conditions. Fibromyalgia patients who were also depressed had fewer MOPs in a region of the brain thought to modulate mood and the emotional dimension of pain (Harris 2007; Zubieta 2007).

Tramadol

This synthetic opioid, similar to codeine, is available in both oral and injectable forms and sold in the United States as Ultram, or Ultracet when combined with paracetamol. It has 10 percent of the potency of morphine (the standard marker against which analgesic medications are compared). The mode of action typically is not fully understood, but it appears not only to stimulate the mu opium receptor, as does morphine, but also to be proactive in GABA, noradrenaline, and serotonin systems. Due to its involvement in the serotonin pathway, it may provoke the "serotonin syndrome" discussed elsewhere. As with any opioid, there is a potential for abuse and addiction. Tramadol has been reported as a major suspect in epileptic seizures, in persons who had not previously suffered a seizure.

Relevance to fibromyalgia. Tramadol appears to be the most widely used opioid in fibromyalgia, possibly due to its apparent several sites of action. Antidepressants are likely to be ordered, perhaps by a different physician. In view of the dangers of the serotonin syndrome, patients should keep their physicians and pharmacists advised of all medications they are taking—prescription, OTC, and herbal.

Anticonvulsants

GABA, the manageable abbreviation for gamma-aminobutyric acid, is described as one of the workhorses of the neurotransmitter system, in which it acts, mainly but not invariably, as an inhibitor. Neurontin (gabapentin) was developed with the intention it would simulate the actions of GABA; however, like so many pharmaceuticals, its exact mode of action is not known. In 1994, FDA accepted gabapentin as an appropriate treatment of epileptic convulsions, and in 2002 it was approved for the treatment of neuralgic pain due to shingles.

It was not officially approved by FDA for a number of other uses, which in practice became a large proportion of total sales, among which neuropathic pain was just one. Lyrica (pregabalin) was designed as a follow-up to the successful gabapentin; it was also intended for patients suffering seizures and for the relief of neuropathic pain, for which it received FDA approval in mid-2005.

Relevance to fibromyalgia. In June 2007, approval by FDA was granted for the use of Lyrica in fibromyalgia. The FDA approved a second drug to treat fibromyalgia in June 2008, Cymbalta (duloxetine hydrochloride). Two pregabalin studies were conducted on eighteen hundred patients, and the results "support approval for use in treating fibromyalgia" (FDA News 2007). As with its predecessor, the exact mechanism of action is unknown, but pregabalin is structurally akin to gabapentin, and there is some knowledge of the potential mechanisms. It is not active at opiate receptors, nor is it involved in the serotonin and noradrenaline systems. Lyrica does not represent an end to the problem of pain in fibromyalgia. Although the studies showed unquestioned benefit, or the FDA would not have given its approval, 50 percent or more improvement in pain was found in 29 percent of the fibromyalgia patients, compared with 13 percent of the placebo (nonfibromyalgia) patients (Crofford 2005). Inevitably, there have been reported side effects such as dizziness, sleepiness, blurred vision, and weight gain.

Benzodiazepines

Known on the street as "benzos," this widely used group of drugs originated in 1954 and led to the development of Librium, the first of a long line of tranquilizers. Benzodiazepines have since been developed to provide rapid- and short-acting, or longer-acting, variants. In the emergency department they are used to treat epileptic convulsions, delirium tremens from alcohol withdrawal, and to sedate patients for endotracheal intubation or reduction of dislocations. They are widely used to assist patients with anxiety and difficulty in sleeping. Unfortunately, their relative safety does not preclude physical dependence or deliberate overdosing. The point of action is on the central nervous system at receptors enhancing response to GABA. Zolpidem (Ambien) is structurally different from a benzodiazepine, but they are sufficiently alike in structure and point of action that flumazenil, employed to reverse benzodiazepine overdose in the emergency department, is effective on zolpidem. It was reported in 2006 as the most widely used hypnotic in the United States. Some bizarre side effects have been reported. There are several other similar soporifics in common use (Beaulieu 2007).

Relevance to fibromyalgia. Although they are commonly prescribed for sleep disorders and may be appropriate for short-term use in insomnia, the long-term use of benzodiazepines is controversial (Beaulieu 2007). With prolonged use, they may cause a patient's insomnia to worsen rather than to relieve it; the patient's physical dependence makes it very difficult to terminate the use of what has seemed to her to be a perfectly proper medication, and, "All I'm asking is to have the dose upped."

Aspirin, Acetaminophen, and Other NSAIDs

Prostaglandins. Named after the prostate gland situated at the base of the male bladder, prostaglandins are in fact not primarily formed in the prostate; the original discovery in seminal fluid led von Euler, in 1936, to this misunderstanding. Later, prostaglandins were found to be manufactured in virtually every cell in the body using the omega-3 and omega-6 fatty acids as building blocks. They are described as fundamental hormones involved in most forms of life and "the list of functions is limited only by our ignorance of their effects" (Enig 1999). Synthesized and released on demand, prostaglandins are not stored, and are rapidly degraded in seconds to minutes after release. Cyclooxygenase (COX) acts as an essential enzyme in the formation of prostaglandin formation. Aspirin and other NSAIDs function to inhibit the action of cyclooxygenase and thereby prevent the formation of prostaglandins.

Relevance to fibromyalgia. Among the functions that are relevant to fibromyalgia are the effects of prostaglandins on the hypothalamus and on the transmission of pain sensations in the brain. Not generally understood, aspirin and acetaminophen (Tylenol) do not have identical inhibitory actions. Whereas aspirin inhibits both pain and inflammation, acetaminophen has less effect on inhibiting inflammation.

Since pain, rather than inflammation, is the primary issue in fibromyalgia, acetaminophen is more likely to be used as treatment because of the undesirable side effects of aspirin. Acetaminophen is frequently compounded with codeine or other opioids.

Cannabis

Extracted verbatim from the FDA: Marijuana is listed in schedule I of the Controlled Substances Act (CSA), the most restrictive schedule. The Drug Enforcement Administration (DEA), which administers the CSA, continues to support that placement and FDA concurred because marijuana met the three criteria for placement in schedule I under 21 U.S.C. 812(b)(1) (e.g., marijuana has a high potential for abuse, has no currently accepted medical use in treatment in the United States, and has a lack of accepted safety for use under medical supervision). Furthermore, there is currently sound evidence that smoked marijuana is harmful. A past evaluation by several Department of Health and Human Services (HHS) agencies, including the Food and Drug Administration (FDA), Substance Abuse and Mental Health Services Administration (SAMHSA), and National Institute for Drug Abuse (NIDA), concluded that no sound scientific studies supported medical use of marijuana for treatment in the United States, and no animal or human data supported the safety or efficacy of marijuana for general medical use. There are alternative FDA-approved medications in existence for treatment of many of the proposed uses of smoked marijuana.

CHAPTER SEVEN

OVERLAPPING SYNDROME

IS THERE A SINGLE, ALL-EMBRACING SYNDROME?

I t is well recognized that the patient diagnosed with fibromyalgia may have other symptoms that are not related to the essential issues of this condition, namely, widespread pain, the tender points, difficulty sleeping, and an element of fatigue. The painstaking full history and the exhaustive (and exhausting) physical examination may not provide a diagnosis of the usual kind to explain these other symptoms. It will then be concluded that the symptoms represent one or more of numerous conditions that are similar to fibromyalgia in that they are "symptoms without signs" and are indicative of other conditions of widespread and poorly explained pain.

It is not unusual for fibromyalgia patients to have an array of somatic complaints other than musculoskeletal pain (Clauw 1995; Bennett 1997).

The diagnosis awarded to the patient who has multiple seemingly unconnected symptoms is related more to the specialist consulted than to the condition itself. If the patient is sent to a gastroenterologist for her problems with abdominal pain, she will be told she has irritable bowel syndrome; if she sees an oral surgeon for her jaw pain, she will be told she has a temporomandibular joint disorder; if she emphasizes to the consulting internist that she feels exhausted all the time, she will be told she has chronic fatigue syndrome; if she is sent for consultation to a rheumatologist for her overwhelming "all-over pain," she will be told she has fibromyalgia (Wolfe 1985; Yunus 2007).

Is there any wonder that some of the experts have sought a common ground? A single unifying factor?

As far back as 1981, a triad of statistical associations was pointed out—fibromyalgia, headache, and irritable bowel syndrome (Yunus 1981). Progressively, numerous other conditions of "pain without clinical signs" were found associated with fibromyalgia. Yunus, an early player in the definition of fibromyalgia, noted chronic fatigue syndrome and the fibromyalgia syndrome overlapped by 75 percent and that in both of these conditions 50 percent of the patients would also have chronic myofascial pain. He first grouped these numerous conditions, with the aid of a Venn diagram, under the heading of a dysregulation spectrum syndrome, or DSS. Later, Yunus changed his term but retained the essential concept. He now describes a central sensitivity syndrome, or CSS, explaining his preference for *sensitivity* as opposed to *sensitization*, a word others use. He writes, "The term *sensitization* implies an active response to some peripheral or environmental stimuli. We had suggested that some persons may be genetically or otherwise intrinsically predisposed to hypersensitivity without such stimulus" (Yunus 2005).

What has become known as the First Gulf War of 1991 resulted in an investigation of unusual symptoms reported with an unusual frequency in persons of all branches of the services in all of the nationalities that had served on the allied side. I am unaware of any comparable study made of Iraqi troops serving at much greater personal risk on the other side. From these assorted complaints was devised the term "Gulf War syndrome." Extensive examination with a great deal of statistical data resulted (Fukuda 1998). The veterans reported to varying degrees suffering pains in joints, muscles, and the head. They suffered also from disturbances in sleep and mood and had cognitive difficulties.

These investigations led to the generation of yet one more term, "chronic multisystem illness," which in fact is very similar to Yunus's overlapping syndrome, but chronic multisystem illness has been given the *Good Housekeeping* stamp of approval by the Centers for Disease Control and Prevention (CDC), and of course given an abbreviation to CMS (CDC 2006).

The criteria for award of this diagnosis are one or more chronic symptoms lasting more than six months that fall into at least two of these categories: fatigue; mood and cognition, including depression, problems with memory or concentration; problems with sleep; pain or stiffness in joints and/or muscles.

It's very hard to see this chronic multisystem illness as different from the overlapping syndrome, other than that it was approached from the perspective of the Gulf War syndrome and not from the perspective of fibromyalgia. Whereas Yunus illustrated his concept with lapping circles in a Venn diagram, a similar illustration has been proposed showing overlapping circles and ovals representing fibromyalgia, multiple chemical sensitivity, chronic fatigue syndrome, and Gulf War syndrome. All of these contained within the circle of somatoform disorders except for an extruding edge of the fibromyalgia component (University of Michigan 2008).

CHRONIC FATIGUE SYNDROME

Although only recently codified by the Centers for Disease Control and Prevention, for many years similar syndromes have come and gone, the features persisting, the names changing with medical fashion. These have included poorly described disease states such as neurasthenia, Da Costa syndrome (reported after the American Civil War), chronic mononucleosis, and vapors (or to the French, *vapeurs*). Called myalgic encephalitis (ME) by the British, the current different names all suggest belief in an underlying stressor, such as inflammation, as the cause of the condition. However, no causative relation between infection and the syndrome has been definitely established, despite strenuous efforts to relate it to the Epstein-Barr virus, herpes viruses 6 and 7, enteroviruses, and many others (Tolan 2007).

Fatigue—General Statement

Fatigue is one of the most common symptoms in clinical medicine; nevertheless, fatigue may be difficult to define because it is rather loosely partitioned into physical and mental components. Fatigue often proves evanescent or, if chronic, relates to an underlying systemic illness. Fatigue may also be associated with a psychiatric disorder.

Less commonly, patients may have chronic persistent fatigue, lasting longer than six months without an apparent etiology and associated with exercise intolerance, sleep difficulties, and an inability to perform mental or physical activities in a competent fashion (Tolan 2007).

Definition of Chronic Fatigue Syndrome

A simple description: a disorder of unknown etiology comprising a state of fatigue that exists without other explanation for a year or more, accompanied by cognitive difficulties, and occurring usually in people who, from a personality standpoint, want to be fully functioning (Cunha 2007).

The more elaborate diagnosis under the aegis of the CDC was outlined in a 1988 paper and did not effectively distinguish chronic fatigue syndrome from other types of unexplained fatigue. It was decided in a 1993 meeting to revise the definition, which now sets uniformly applicable guidelines for the clinical and research evaluation of chronic fatigue syndrome and other forms of fatigue.

Because a precise etiology for the syndrome remains elusive, the diagnosis is largely made by exclusion of other medical and psychiatric disorders. Thus chronic fatigue syndrome is seen as an illness primarily characterized by self-reported symptoms with an absence of physical findings.

The CDC diagnostic criteria state: "In order to receive a diagnosis of chronic fatigue syndrome, a patient must satisfy two criteria:

1. Have unexplained persistent or relapsing chronic fatigue that is of new or definite onset (i.e., not lifelong), is not the result of ongoing exertion, is not substantially alleviated by rest, and results in substantial reduction in previous levels of occupational, educational, social, or personal activities.
2. Concurrently have four or more of the following symptoms: substantial impairment in short-term memory or concentration; sore throat; tender lymph nodes; muscle pain; multijoint pain without swelling or redness; headaches of a new type, pattern, or severity; unrefreshing sleep; and postexertional malaise lasting more than twenty-four hours. The symptoms must have persisted or recurred during six or more consecutive months of illness and must not have predated the fatigue.

A large number of clinically defined, frequently treatable illnesses can result in fatigue. Diagnosis of any of these conditions excludes a definition of chronic fatigue syndrome unless the condition has been treated sufficiently and no longer explains the fatigue and other symptoms (Fukuda 1994).

Other Symptoms and Signs

Fatigue in young people is serious when it persists for more than three months and impairs school attendance, academic results, and peer relationships. It is now claimed by some researchers to be the commonest medical cause of long-term absence from school (Tolan 2007).

Patients may present as depressed due to an inability to perform their normal duties, their problems with short-term memory, and verbal dyslexia. They suffer postexertional fatigue, are excessively tired after normal tasks, and do not arise refreshed after sleep (Cunha 2007).

There are no abnormalities to be found on physical examination that point to a diagnosis of chronic fatigue syndrome. The examination must eliminate endocrinological explanations such as abnormalities of adrenal or thyroid glands and other issues such as HIV.

Clinical Studies

A minimum battery of laboratory screening tests should be performed. In clinical practice, no tests can be recommended for the specific purpose of diagnosing chronic fatigue syndrome although the CDC recommends a "basic battery" that usually includes a complete blood count, liver function tests, thyroid function tests, erythrocyte sedimentation rate (ESR), and serum electrolyte level measurement. Tests should be directed toward confirming or excluding other possible clinical conditions.

Examples of specific tests that do not confirm or exclude the diagnosis of chronic fatigue syndrome include serologic tests for Epstein-Barr virus, enteroviruses, retroviruses, human herpes virus 6, and *Candida albicans*; tests of immunologic function, including cell population and function studies; and imaging studies, including magnetic resonance imaging scans and radio nuclide scans (such as single-photon emission computed tomography and positron emission tomography).

So many patients with a possible diagnosis of chronic fatigue syndrome present with elevated immunoglobulin G, viral capsid antigen, EBB titer, this should be considered consistent with, but not diagnostic of, chronic fatigue syndrome. Most patients demonstrate elevated IG, coxsackievirus B, human herpes virus 6, and pneumonia titers. Commonly found is a decrease in the percentage of natural killer cells. The most consistent abnormality is an extremely low ESR (0–3). Abnormalities are nonspecific but together present a pattern of normalities of viral findings. Extensive immunological testing is neither diagnostic nor specific and is not helpful (Cunha 2007).

Diagnosis

The basis of the diagnosis is unexplained fatigue for a period of one year or more, accompanied by cognitive dysfunction. Patients without cognitive difficulties should not be considered to have chronic fatigue syndrome. Then there is the matter of excluding other possible causes that meet these criteria:

- Any active medical condition that may explain the presence of chronic fatigue
- Any past or current diagnosis of a major depressive disorder with psychotic or melancholic features
- Alcohol or other substance abuse, occurring within two years of the onset of chronic fatigue and anytime afterward
- Severe obesity as defined by a body mass index

Tolan (2007) observes the CDC criteria indicate that, essentially, any chronic illness that produces extensive disability in a setting of persistent fatigue may be included in the differential diagnosis. Once such a specific illness has been diagnosed, then chronic fatigue syndrome is excluded by definition. Chronic fatigue syndrome is, in large measure, a diagnosis of exclusion.

Psychosocial assessment should include consideration of individual and family function; relationships with friends; school performance; any history of bullying, refusal to attend school, and psychiatric disorders. The most common comorbid psychological problems include depression and sleep disturbance.

Pathology and Distribution

Single-photon emission computed tomography studies have shown diminished blood flow in the fronto-parietal-temporal areas of the brain—areas possibly responsible for the reported cognitive difficulties (Cunha 2007).

In the United States, chronic pain and fatigue are extremely prevalent in the general population, especially among women and persons of less fortunate socioeconomic status; the incidence of regional pain and of chronic fatigue is given as 20 percent of the population; more common in females than males; most commonly young to middle age. Fatigue, headache, stomachache, and backache are extremely common.

This is not the same, however, as having met the criteria described or having been diagnosed as suffering from the chronic fatigue syndrome. The figures from surveys showed an overall range in Chicago of 0.42 percent, highest for the poor, the minorities, and the ill educated, and in women marginally more frequently than men (Jason 1999).

There is a marked overlap between fibromyalgia and chronic fatigue syndrome. The crossover is between 20 to 70 percent, with fibromyalgia patients marginally more likely to have chronic fatigue syndrome than vice versa (Wallace 2003).

Differences between Fibromyalgia and Chronic Fatigue Syndrome

Chronic fatigue syndrome and fibromyalgia are often found together. Seventy-five percent of chronic fatigue syndrome patients also met the criteria for fibromyalgia, but not as many fibromyalgia patients met the criteria for chronic fatigue syndrome (Goldenberg 1990). A spectrum is proposed with chronic fatigue syndrome at the extreme of fatigue, fibromyalgia at the extreme of pain and both of them involving cognitive dysfunction (Russell 2004). Three groupings of patients have been suggested: a) pure fibromyalgia; b) pure chronic fatigue syndrome; c) mixed fibromyalgia and chronic fatigue syndrome (Buchwald 1994).

Another important difference between the conditions is the response to exercise. Patients with relatively mild fibromyalgia are better able to tolerate exercise, whereas chronic fatigue syndrome patients find their condition aggravated by exercise.

Pediatric Chronic Fatigue

Large international surveys show that about 8 percent of adolescents report daily headaches; 10 percent daily backache, and 16 percent daily sleepiness in the mornings. Fatigue is even more common: about a third of both boys and girls have substantial fatigue four or more times a week (Viner 2005).

Recent epidemiological evidence suggests chronic fatigue syndrome, as defined on the basis of the criteria of the CDC, occurs in about 0.2–0.6 percent of adolescents aged eleven to fifteen years.

Pediatric patients with chronic fatigue syndrome are typically teenage females with severe school absenteeism. The clinical profile of an individual with chronic fatigue syndrome is of a high-achieving student or athlete who is usually female (80 percent), Caucasian, and in the middle-class or upper middle-class socioeconomic level. This may reflect referral bias but appears consistent throughout most studies (Tolan 2007).

Etiology

The etiology of chronic fatigue syndrome is unknown, with many hypotheses proposed. No convincing evidence exists to support persisting viral infection (Cunha 2007). Patients do show an excess of depression, other psychological symptoms, and low self-esteem, although data on the psychological and endocrine states of patients show that chronic fatigue syndrome is not merely a masked form of depression, somatoform disorder, or refusal to attend school.

Viner and Hotopf (2004) were unable to identify any association between maternal or child psychological distress, academic ability, parental illness, atopy, or birth order and increasing risk of lifetime chronic fatigue syndrome, but they found sedentary behavior increased the risk.

Chronic fatigue syndrome is likely to be a collection of different conditions and that several biopsychosocial "causal pathways" can lead to chronic fatigue.

Patients must be assessed with a combined biopsychosocial approach, once all possibility of treatable conditions has been excluded.

Rowe (1995) produced neurally mediated hypotension in twenty-one of twenty-two adult patients with chronic fatigue syndrome using the head-up tilt-table test (HUTTT), a standard orthostatic test that produces enhanced sympathetic tone while decreasing parasympathetic tone in healthy subjects. More important, treatment of orthostatic intolerance improved symptoms in many patients. These observations have focused on the neurologic aspects of orthostasis and have led some investigators to suggest an autonomic defect in chronic fatigue syndrome (see later chapter).

The finding that both children and adults with chronic fatigue syndrome maintain strong convictions that their fatigue is purely physiologic, rejecting psychological explanations, lends some support to an attributional model. A familial predisposition has been reported.

Preliminary data suggest that the illness is different in boys and girls. An allergic history is common. Milk intolerance is often reported (Tolan 2007).

Treatment, Prognosis, Controversy

Treatment can only be supportive and in response to symptoms. It should include physical therapy and modest aerobic or anaerobic exercise (if possible) to avoid cardiovascular deconditioning. Sleep may be addressed with medication, nighttime amitriptyline. Biofeedback regimens have been helpful at times, but treatment has remained controversial (Tolan 2007).

The clinical course is punctuated by remissions and relapses often triggered by intercurrent infection or stress. The course in adolescents is similar to that in adults.

There is continuing controversy over the existence of chronic fatigue syndrome, together with uncertainty and contradictory research findings about etiology and treatment, which has made the management of chronic fatigue syndrome extremely difficult for health professionals and patients alike.

CHRONIC PAIN SYNDROME

There is acute pain of short duration, and there's chronic pain of longer duration, and there's chronic pain syndrome, which is a different kettle of fish altogether.

A useful distinction is made (terminology is necessary but bothersome) between nociceptive pain and neuropathic pain.

To give an example: if a kitchen worker is stabbed in the hand, by accident, at work, it is expected there would be pain for a while—nociceptive pain, recognized by the pain sensors in the hand, the nociceptors. No big deal. Happens to every kitchen worker at regular intervals.

This pain should gradually subside, until there is a slight ache, and then the worker should after a few weeks have forgotten about it altogether. If it doesn't go away completely, various forms of treatment are likely going to be offered, not only analgesics, but therapy with heat and machines and all the lights and bells and whistles the top-of-the-line physical medicine departments have available.

But her pain gets worse instead of better.

During this time, the patient has been replaced in her employment, she finds her employer has no accident insurance; together with her older husband, now crippled by a stroke and their twin children aged six months, she's put out of her apartment. Welfare won't support her until she's drained the last dollar from her savings account and sold her unsellable car. She's in pain. Her hand won't close. She can't get a job. She gets angry. She drinks. She's thoroughly unpleasant to deal with.

Now we have a chronic pain syndrome. Agonizing pain is felt in the hand, but treatment of hand pain is no longer effective. The pain is in some way "fixed higher up." It's neuropathic pain.

Her employer is totally unsympathetic. He has a restaurant to run. Twice in that business he's gone bankrupt. Not only does he have his own family to support, he has to help his brother's family as well. His brother used to work in the same business. He hurt his back lifting. One thing led to another and his back was operated on. He got worse, not better. They operated again, this time a fusion. And once more he was even worse. With the third operation they lengthened the fusion area. He could hardly walk. His pain was devastating. They called him a "failed back," like it was the back's fault. They'd ignored the surgical axiom, "No matter how severe the pain, it can always be made worse with another operation."

Now he has a chronic pain syndrome. The pain in some way is "fixed higher up." It's neuropathic pain. The pathology, the part of his body that's gone wrong, is "higher up," in the spinal cord or in the brain, somewhere along the pain pathways.

The number of persons suffering chronic pain is difficult to ascertain, but broad figures given for the United States report 35 percent of the population have some element of chronic pain and as many as fifty million persons are partially or totally disabled by pain (Singh 2005). Not everyone likes to tack the word "syndrome" onto the end of "chronic pain." There is a pejorative connotation, making it seem as if pain was not really the problem any longer, and all attention becomes focused on the "pain behaviors," and the exploration of the cause of this behavior, like, "How many times were you molested as a child, and was it your stepfather, the priest, or both of them?"

The positive side of the concept is the conceptual switching from treatment of nociceptive pain, as if it was only due to the hand or the back, to a realization of neuropathic pain and attention to the wider range of problems, requiring more comprehensive treatment.

COGNITIVE DYSFUNCTION (FIBRO FOG)

Cognitive function can be considered the ability to think, reason, image, remember, or learn words. Decades of research have defined several memory systems: short term, working, episodic, semantic (verbal memory), and procedural (memory for different skills).

The euphemism "fibro fog" is often employed to describe the memory problems and the unclear thinking (cognitive dysfunction) reported by patients with fibromyalgia (Landro 1997). The research on cognitive dysfunction in fibromyalgia suggests that actions are faulty, which may adversely affect some patients' ability to be competitively employed (Bennett 1997).

Symptoms and Signs

Symptoms include confusion and forgetfulness, inability to concentrate and recall simple words and numbers, and transposing words and numbers; all of these are activities that had been second nature prior to the onset of fibromyalgia (Cot 1997; Turk 1997; Sarnoch 1997; Grace 2001). Cognitive functions are often so impaired that patients cannot perform the activities of daily living (ADL), getting lost in familiar places or losing the ability to communicate effectively. It is suggested that the problem is more one of slowed processing and not an actual impairment, possibly resulting from the distraction of chronic pain or chronic sleeplessness (Cote 1997).

Patients who work may be in fear of losing their jobs. Pediatric patients may drop out of school because of their inability to complete their schoolwork.

Advances in noninvasive technology have made it possible to visualize the brain. Methods such as single-photon emission computerized tomography (SPECT) have helped define some of the abnormalities linked to the cognitive dysfunction. SPECT shows decreased blood flow in the right and the left caudate nuclei and thalami of the midbrain. Functional magnetic resonance imaging (fMRI) can show brain activity by depicting increased blood flow to areas actively engaged in a task. Increased blood flow, and hence increased oxygenation, has different magnetic properties that can be detected and measured on fMRI.

Etiology

Cognitive performance of patients with fibromyalgia is correlated with their reported level of pain. The possibility is raised that they can be explained by a combination of chronic pain, sleeplessness, fatigue, and psychological distress (Sletvold, Stiles, and Landro 1995).

A dysfunction of the prefrontal cortex has been proposed, with resultant impaired function in the hippocampus, loss of memory context, and resulting confusion (Sherkey 1997). Deficit in function of the frontal lobe in the awake state (Moldofsky 1989) and failure of synaptic connections have also been proposed.

Inadequate REM sleep, leading to inadequate memory consolidation, leading to difficulties in concentration and poor initial learning, similar to chronic fatigue syndrome has been suggested (Anch 1991; Cote 1997).

Central nervous system imbalances have been linked to cognitive dysfunction. Abnormal levels of neurotransmitters such as substance P, serotonin, dopamine, norepinephrine, and epinephrine may be a cause of cognitive dysfunction. Neuroendocrine imbalance of the HPA axis (defined in another chapter) may play a role in fibro fog.

One study showed that the working memory and episodic memory scores of patients with fibromyalgia were similar to those of healthy control subjects, but who were twenty years older.

Additional research is needed to determine the brain systems involved, why fibromyalgia patients have cognitive problems, and what to do about these problems (Gilliland 2007).

Exclusive to Fibromyalgia?

But is this exclusively a fibromyalgia problem? The almost affectionate term "fibro fog" has been created for that purpose, to identify this mental confusion as a property of those who suffer the condition. One experienced author suggests they should keep a sense of humor about their mistakes and emphasizes they should get enough sleep (Staud 2007). The type of errors described, forgetting your wallet when you go to shop, forgetting where you put your keys, and so on are part of an everyday life (Starlanyl 2001). They become the center of life when they're sought, put in diaries, mulled over, and added up.

The identical problems are well known to perfectly healthy mothers, up half the night looking after a sick child, and to shift workers (Colquhoun 1976; Folkard 1979; Richardson 1989), or even to doctors undergoing the brutal initiation rights of a medical residency (Marcus 1996; Steele 1999; Geer 1997).

Mistakes are made by everyone when there's an insufficiency of sleep. Deficits in daytime performance due to sleep loss are experienced universally and are associated with a significant social, financial, and human cost (Durmer 2005). Accidents related to sleep deprivation have been estimated to have a negative impact of up to fifty-six billion dollars a year (Leger 1994), and it is believed that many motor vehicle accidents are in fact due to the driver falling asleep at the wheel (Pack 1995; Mitler 1998; Stutts 2003; Horne 2006).

There does not seem to be anything to suggest that the "fog" of cognition experienced by the insufficiently slept person diagnosed with fibromyalgia is in any way different from the exhausted surgical resident who orders an incorrect dose of medication or the truck driver who momentarily falls asleep on the road (Stoohs 1994; Lyznicki 1998; McCartt 2000).

In her column in the *New York Times*, Judith Warner (2007) describes her personal lapses of memory for which an MRI was ordered. More than one hundred and fifty comments were published, each person relating their own lapses of memory, identical in character to those described with "fibro fog." None of the correspondents suggested they had fibromyalgia.

DEPRESSION

Everyone is aware of the word "depression," and most persons will have their own understanding of its meaning. Depression, however, just like appendicitis, is a clinical diagnosis and therefore subject to being defined. As the American College of Rheumatology drew up a short list of defining characteristics for fibromyalgia, in order that all researchers would be working on a level playing field, so has the term "depression" been subjected to an exact definition.

The authorities involved here are psychiatrists, psychologists, and others working together in committee to come to agreement on terms of diagnosis. They are not involved with defining treatment, only with the definition of terms used in diagnosis. At irregular intervals their conclusions are published in a manual of nearly a thousand pages, called *Diagnostic and Statistical Manual of Mental Disorders*. The current edition is the fourth and is revised as the *Diagnostic and Statistical Manual of Mental Disorders, Fourth Edition, Text Revision (DSM-IV-TR.)*

The *DSM-IV-TR* diagnostic criteria for a major depressive disorder (MDD) are:

A. At least five of the following, during the same two-week period, representing a change from previous functioning; must include either (a) or (b): (a) depressed mood; (b) diminished interest or pleasure; (c) significant weight loss or gain; (d) insomnia or hypersomnia; (e) psychomotor agitation or retardation; (f) fatigue or loss of energy; (g) feelings of worthlessness; (h) diminished ability to think or concentrate; indecisiveness; (i) recurrent thoughts of death, suicidal ideation, suicide attempt, or specific plan for suicide.
B. Symptoms do not meet criteria for a mixed episode (i.e., meets criteria for both manic and depressive episode).

C. Symptoms cause clinically significant distress or impairment of functioning.
D. Symptoms are not due to the direct physiologic effects of a substance or a general medical condition.
E. Symptoms are not better accounted for by bereavement, i.e., the symptoms persist for longer than two months or are characterized by marked functional impairment, morbid preoccupation with worthlessness, suicidal ideation, psychotic symptoms, or psychomotor retardation.

In the primary care setting, where many of these patients first seek treatment, the presenting complaints often can be somatic, such as fatigue, headache, abdominal distress, or change in weight. Patients may complain more of irritability than of sadness or low mood.

- *Physical*. No physical findings are specific to MDD. Diagnosis lies in the history and the mental status examination.
- *Appearance and affect*. Most patients with MDD present to their physician with a normal appearance. In patients with more severe symptoms, a decline in grooming and hygiene can be observed, as well as a change in weight.
- *Mood and thought process*. Patients report a mood state, expressed as sadness, heaviness, numbness, or sometimes irritability and mood swings. They often report a loss of interest or pleasure in their usual activities, difficulty concentrating, or loss of energy and motivation.
- *Cognition*. Patients with MDD often complain of poor memory or concentration. Most commonly, no significant deficits are found on cognitive examination.

Relevance to Fibromyalgia

Narrowing this list down to a few words: the patient diagnosed with fibromyalgia will probably have five of the following six issues: depressed mood, diminished interest or pleasure, significant weight gain, insomnia, fatigue and loss of energy, diminished ability to think or concentrate. The physical appearance is unremarkable.

It is not surprising that many have considered clinical depression, a major mood disorder, as the fundamental basis of the condition called fibromyalgia.

Defining the term "depression" needed a committee to reach unified agreement. How to measure depression, or how to determine degrees of depression, has not had the same advantage. There are numerous questionnaires, some self-administered, all depending on the patient's self-appraisal. Among the commonest reported are the

Beck Depression Inventory 11 (Beck 1996) and the Hamilton Depression Rating Scale (Hamilton 1960). When there are many instruments, it usually indicates that no one of them is completely satisfactory or appropriate to all purposes.

The reason for commenting on the manner in which depression is diagnosed by the use of an inventory is the use of this technique to determine whether patients with fibromyalgia are any more prone to depression than totally healthy patients or patients with other chronic painful conditions such as rheumatoid arthritis. Hudson's (1985) study reported they were, this was criticized on the grounds of observer bias, and when repeated by Ahles (1991) in a more acceptable fashion, the study showed the incidence of depression associated with fibromyalgia was the same as with rheumatoid arthritis, namely, in the 30 to 40 percent range, although other authors put the incidence of depression with fibromyalgia as low as 20 percent (Kirmayer 1988). Some of the studies quoted in the literature were performed before the 1990 categorization of fibromyalgia (Clark 1985); in general, other studies since that time have not reinforced the notion that fibromyalgia is essentially an issue of depression.

It is accepted that patients with fibromyalgia, unsurprisingly, become secondarily depressed, but the majority of the workers in the field do not believe depression caused the fibromyalgia (Birnie 1991; Galloway 1990; Yunus 1994; Goldenberg 1989; Russell 2002).

Depression alone is not a probable cause for pain. In patients with rheumatoid arthritis, it was concluded that the depression accounted for no more than 1 percent of the pain (Ward 1944) and, arguing by analogy, it is therefore not reasonable to suppose it is the major cause of pain in fibromyalgia; nor are the multiple conditions that are comorbid with fibromyalgia (irritable bladder, irritable bowel, myofascial pain syndrome, etc.) commonly found in association with depression (Russell 2004). Although physical pain is not a common feature in depression, even when there is a complaint of pain, it is not accompanied by the tender points of fibromyalgia; there is no predilection for patients who have been indisputably diagnosed with depression to manifest symptoms of fibromyalgia.

Yunus, the originator of the use of a Venn diagram to illustrate the overlapping features of the central sensitivity syndrome, was "initially reluctant to include depression as part of the CSS spectrum, arguing that depression and fibromyalgia are different diseases. . . . A wide body of literature supports the view that depression is more significantly common in fibromyalgia and other related CSS syndromes than in control groups. . . . Depression is now added to my Venn diagram." But he does not believe depression to be the central issue or the root cause of fibromyalgia. Central sensitization (not *sensitivity*) remains at the center of the circle, with depression a satellite (Yunus 2005).

Shared Features of Depression and Fibromyalgia

In the United States, the lifetime incidence of MDD is 20 percent in women and 12 percent in men. This is a much higher incidence than fibromyalgia, and the sex ratio, female-to-male, of approximately two to one differs from the ratio of approximately nine to one in fibromyalgia.

Internationally, there are differences in the expression of psychological distress in patients from other countries or cultures. MDD may be expressed as fatigue, imbalance, or neurasthenia in patients of Asian origin. Which are all symptoms presented by patients with fibromyalgia, raising the question of the patient's interpretation of symptoms as opposed to suffering them.

Underlying Causes

Clinical and preclinical trials suggest in MDD there is a disturbance in central nervous system serotonin (i.e., 5-HT) activity as an important factor. Other neurotransmitters implicated include norepinephrine and dopamine. The role of CNS serotonin activity in the pathophysiology of MDD is suggested by the efficacy of selective serotonin reuptake inhibitors in the treatment of depression (Bhalla 2006), which is essentially the same neurotransmitter pathway postulated as an explanation for fibromyalgia and one of the treatments commonly used. But levels of cerebro-spinal fluid substance P are substantially higher in fibromyalgia than in MDD (Mastersson 1989; Russell 2004).

Is There a Subset?

Wallace (2008) has described patients with established diagnoses of both bipolar disorder and fibromyalgia.

There were unusual features: none had been benefited by the usual treatment with tricyclic or SRS medication, nor by physical therapy; seven of the ten were on opiates (the population average would be two or three); tender point examination was mild when distracted, although described as "excruciating;" eight had undergone invasive procedures including surgery and were anxious to desperate for "aggressive" treatment, even though their symptoms were vague and generalized; attribution of their problems to physical rather than psychiatric causes was important.

Treatment

Depression in fibromyalgia may be treated with a regimen that includes non-pharmaceutical therapies. Treating depression alone does not cure fibromyalgia, another indicator that depression is a secondary issue and not the prime problem. Antidepressants may help, but the clinician should also address other symptoms, such as fatigue and pain. Modifying diet and practicing good sleep hygiene are crucial. Starting a rehabilitation exercise program is important. Behavioral modification techniques and stress management may also be used (Gilliland 2007).

DIZZINESS

Dizziness is a complaint among the fibromyalgia population (Wolfe 1990), and in many cases no cause is found despite sophisticated testing (Bennett 1997). It is a symptom that needs to be evaluated, however, and the doctor cannot safely brush it aside as "just another fibromyalgia complaint." In all probability, that's what it is, but a patient with fibromyalgia is just as susceptible to one of the serious causes of dizziness as is the patient who does not have fibromyalgia.

Dizziness is one of the commonest symptoms bringing a patient to the emergency room, just as common as back pain and headache. The overall incidence of dizziness, vertigo, and imbalance is 5 to 10 percent, reaching 40 percent in patients older than forty years. Which means there is nothing unusual in being dizzy, it's not a specific symptom of fibromyalgia, nor can one reasonably say it must be due to the fibromyalgia since it's so frequently found in the same age group.

Evaluation is not necessarily a prolonged performance and does not necessarily need to have a lot of expensive equipment to be employed, but evaluation is required.

What Is Meant by "Dizzy"?

It's impossible to spend a night as an emergency physician without meeting several distressed people triaged by the admitting nurse with the single word, "Dizzy."

At one time I used to say to my patients, "Dizzy is a bad word in English," meaning only that it is so vague, so nonspecific, that in the difficult process of communication very often a totally incorrect impression is given. I had to find another way of expressing myself when the patient would apologize, thinking "bad word" implied she'd used a vulgarity. I suppose "dizzy blonde" is a vulgarity, but that's not what I had in mind when speaking to these highly respectable late middle-age ladies.

So apart from the connotation of "dizzy" as applied to fun-seeking young ladies, dizzy is used in general speech to mean anything from a minor lightheadedness when rising suddenly from a chair, to episodes when the room spins around, the patient falls to the side, vomits, and lapses into unconsciousness.

Rule number one for the doctor is never to presume to know what the patient means by the single word "dizzy," but require she explain what exactly happens. Which, after defining how she is using that word, what exactly is her symptom, opens up the rest of the W words explained in the history-taking section.

The critical distinction is to differentiate vertigo from nonvertigo. Vertigo is the sensation of rotational movement, either of yourself or of your surroundings—the sensation you provoked as a child by whirling around like a top and then stopping abruptly, allowing the world to continue rotating around you. On the other hand, nonvertigo includes lightheadedness, unsteadiness, imbalance, a floating or a tilting sensation.

This leads to the division of dizziness into peripheral and central causes; peripheral means at the "end organ," in other words the balance organ located deep in the temporal bone, known as the inner ear, whereas central is the region of the brain to which sensations from the inner ear are conducted by the eighth cranial nerve. True vertigo, the sensation of spinning, is often due to a problem located in the inner ear, whereas symptoms of nonvertigo may be due to central nervous system, or cardiovascular, or systemic diseases, or very commonly, is attributed to emotions.

A sudden onset of dizziness is usually peripheral in origin, whereas the gradual and ill-defined symptoms are most commonly of central origin. Many medical conditions and emotional factors can create a sensation of dizziness and imbalance. Hypertension, hypotension, atherosclerotic disease, endocrine imbalances, and anxiety states are common causes of lightheadedness, near syncope, and/or instability but rarely produce a sense of true vertigo.

Medication side effects are of particular significance in fibromyalgia. Dizziness is noted as an occasional ill effect when taking antidepressants or anticonvulsant medications; excessive caffeine, nicotine, and alcohol intake must also be ruled out as causes of the dizziness.

Particularly in the context of fibromyalgia, which is accompanied by so many other conditions (concomitant, comorbidity), emotional conditions must be considered when physical causes have been eliminated and the complaint is considered to be significant to the patient. Appropriate questioning will determine whether it is part of a panic attack, the parameters defined by: feeling dizzy, unsteady, lightheaded, or faint, and other symptoms such as numbness or tingling sensations, palpitations, sweating, trembling, sense of shortness of breath, feeling of choking, chest pain, nausea, feeling detached from oneself, fear of going crazy, fear of dying, and/or hot flashes.

There is an oblique connection between panic disorders and fibromyalgia in that both are sensitive to medications directed at central nervous system neurotransmitters suggesting at least a shared pathway or mechanism.

HEADACHE

The current classification of the different types and causes of headache, by the International Headache Society, is:

> Primary: migraine, tension-ype headache (TTH), cluster headache, and "others."
> Secondary: meaning secondary to known causes, such as trauma and infection.
> Third group: cranial neuralgias and face pain.

For episodic tension-type headaches (frequent), the classification criteria are (1) at least ten previous headaches, with the number of days with such headache fewer than fifteen per month and the headaches lasting from thirty minutes to seven days, and (2) at least two of the following pain characteristics:

- pressing/tightening (nonpulsating) quality
- mild or moderate intensity (may inhibit but does not prohibit activities)
- bilateral location
- no aggravation from climbing stairs or similar routine physical activity
- neither nausea nor vomiting
- absent or only one: photophobia (intolerance of light) and phonophobia (intolerance of sound)
- secondary headache types not suggested

For chronic tension-type headaches (frequent), the classification criteria are:

1. An average headache frequency of more than fifteen days per month for more than six months, with at least two of the following pain characteristics:

   - pressing/tightening (nonpulsating) quality
   - mild or moderate intensity (may inhibit but does not prohibit activities)
   - bilateral location
   - no aggravation from climbing stairs or similar routine physical activity
   - no vomiting

2. No more than one of the following: nausea, photophobia, phonophobia
3. Secondary headache types not suggested or confirmed

Clinical Presentation

The differential diagnosis of severe headache is a great problem to the physician working alone at night in the emergency room, confronted by a patient he has never previously met and who may not speak English. The range of significance varies from a transient headache of no consequence, to a subarachnoid hemorrhage requiring very early surgical treatment to preserve life, recognition of glaucoma to preserve sight, recognition of eclampsia to preserve the mother and child, and numerous other very severe issues.

The physician has to distinguish "my usual headache" from "the worst headache I've ever had." For the patient with fibromyalgia, the probable statement will be along the lines of "my usual headache" and "just as severe as I usually experience." If the patient does not say "usual" as a description of her headache, it may warrant deeper investigation.

If she experiences these headaches before the diagnosis of fibromyalgia has been suggested, the nature and character of the headaches must be investigated before dismissing them as "benign," or using one of the several terms, such as: stress headache, muscle contraction headache, psychomyogenic headache, ordinary headache, and psychogenic headache which are in convenient use to put aside the unexplained complaint.

History

Tension-type headaches (TTHs) are characterized by pain that is usually mild or moderate in severity and bilateral in distribution. Unilateral pain may be experienced by 10 to 20 percent of patients. Headache is a constant, tight, pressing, or bandlike sensation in the frontal, temporal, occipital, or parietal area (with frontal and temporal regions most common).

Eighty-two percent of TTHs last less than twenty-four hours (Ulrich 1996). The deep, steady ache differs from the typical throbbing quality of migraine headache and the prodrome and aura of migraine are absent. Occasionally, the headache may be throbbing or unilateral, but most patients do not report photophobia, sonophobia, or nausea, which commonly are associated with migraine. Some patients may have neck, jaw, or temporomandibular joint discomfort.

- *Physical examination.* Patients with TTH have normal findings on general and neurologic examinations. Some patients may have tender spots or taut bands in the pericranial or cervical muscles (trigger points).
- *Precipitating causes.* Various precipitating factors may set off a TTH in susceptible individuals. Half of the patients with TTH identify stress or hunger

as a precipitating factor. Stress—usually in the afternoon after long stressful work hours. Sleep deprivation. Uncomfortable stressful position and/or bad posture. Irregular meal time resulting in hunger. Eyestrain.

- *Lab studies.* The diagnosis of TTH is clinical. There is no specific diagnostic test. Lab studies may be required to exclude secondary headache disorders such as infections.

- *Imaging studies.* CAT scan or MRI is required to rule out secondary causes if the headache is unusual or if it is associated with any abnormal findings in the neurologic examination. CAT scan with contrast is usually more readily available but is in general inferior to MRI for viewing the brain's structure, especially at the lowest part of the back of the head (the posterior fossa).

Medical Care

The varieties of care comprise pharmacotherapy, psychophysiologic therapy, and physical therapy. Recognition of comorbid illness is essential. Migraine may be associated with TTH and management overlaps. Other associated conditions may include depression, anxiety, and emotional or adjustment disorders (Singh 2007).

Medication is used to stop or to reduce the severity of the individual attack and for long-term preventive therapy. Preventive drugs are the main therapy for chronic type-tension headache (CTTH), but they seldom are needed for episodic type-tension headache (ETTH).

These headaches (especially ETTHs) generally respond to simple over-the-counter analgesics such as acetaminophen, ibuprofen, or aspirin. If treatment is unsatisfactory, the addition of caffeine or use of prescription drugs is recommended. If possible, you should avoid the use of barbiturates or opiate agonists. Your physician should discourage you from overusing analgesics because of the risk of dependence, abuse, and development of chronic daily headache.

Fiorinal, a barbiturate compound, is not first-line therapy and carries a significant risk of abuse. Amitriptyline (Elavil) and nortriptyline (Pamelor) are the most frequently used tricyclic antidepressants. The selective serotonin reuptake inhibitors (SSRIs) fluoxetine (Prozac), paroxetine (Paxil), and sertraline (Zoloft) also are used commonly by many physicians.

Psychophysiologic therapy includes reassurance, counseling, relaxation therapy, stress management programs, and biofeedback techniques. With these modalities of treatment, both frequency and severity of chronic headache may be reduced.

Holroyd (2001) reported benefits from cognitive behavioral therapy and biofeedback therapy, which may be helpful in some patients when combined with medications.

Pain relief may be obtained by trigger point injections, nerve blocks, and botulinum toxin injection in the pericranial muscle. The results of acupuncture have been difficult to assess (Biondi 1994).

Distribution

TTH represents one of the most costly diseases because of its very high prevalence. The episodic and chronic types are considered to be of different origins, and whereas the episodic type can be a cause of some disability and expense, the chronic type is always associated with disability. According to the National Headache Foundation, more than forty-five million Americans suffer from chronic, recurring headaches and of these, twenty-eight million suffer from migraines. In the United States, TTH is the most common primary headache syndrome.

TTH can occur at any age. It can begin in childhood, but onset during adolescence or young adulthood is more common. About 20 percent of children and adolescents have significant headaches. About 70 percent of headache sufferers are women.

Pathophysiology

The pathogenesis of TTH is complex and multifactorial, with contributions from both central and peripheral factors (Singh 2007). In the past, various mechanisms including vascular, muscular (i.e., constant overcontraction of scalp muscles), and psychogenic factors were suggested. The more likely cause of these headaches is believed now to be abnormal neuronal sensitivity and pain facilitation, not abnormal muscle contraction.

Various evidence suggests that, like migraine, TTH is associated with exteroceptive suppression, abnormal platelet serotonin, and decreased cerebrospinal fluid endorphin. In one study, plasma levels of substance P were found to be normal in patients with CTTH and unrelated to the headache state. Several concurrent mechanisms may be responsible for TTH, myofascial nociception is one of them (Jensen 2001).

Bendtsen (2000) described central sensitization at the level of the spinal dorsal horn due to prolonged nociceptive inputs from pericranial myofascial tissues. The central neuroplastic changes may affect regulation of peripheral mechanisms and can lead to increased pericranial muscle activity or release of neurotransmitters in myofascial tissues. This central sensitization may be maintained even after the initial eliciting factors have been normalized, resulting in conversion of ETTH into CTTH.

Starlanyl (2001) suggests most tension headaches are caused by trigger points, a theory promoted by Travell.

Headache in Fibromyalgia

Headache has been reported as a feature of the fibromyalgia syndrome, the prevalence of attacks given as between 44 and 58 percent (Yunus 1981 and 1989; Campbell 1983; Wolfe 1983; Bengtsson 1986; Goldenberg 1987; Wolfe 1990; Paiva 1997; Moldofsky 2001; Peres 2003).

In the 2007 survey conducted by Bennett and associates, headache was the second most frequently occurring comorbid (other accompanying) symptom in the two and a half thousand fibromyalgia patients who completed the questionnaire; 47 percent of the patients reported headache. On a zero to ten scale, the average severity of headache was rated at 4.3, compared with the rating of their generalized pain at 6.4.

Headache associated with fibromyalgia can be quite severe, and because it is the tension variety, it involves also the muscles of the neck (Russell 2002 and 2004). Blotman reports approximately the same frequency, almost 53 percent in his patients in France. Marcus (2005) reported a higher incidence of headache, 76 percent, in a one-hundred-patient study group; he also separated headache as a complaint from the other issues of general pain, quality of sleep and psychological distress, finding no interrelationship.

In fibromyalgia, the primary-type headache may be a mix of tension headache and migrainous headache (Yunus 1981 and 1989). The mechanisms, origins, and consequences of headaches in fibromyalgia remain unclear (Peres 2003; Marcus 2005). Apart from the frequency of comorbidity, the similarity to the proposed mechanism in fibromyalgia should be noted: for example, interference with neurotransmitters.

The issue of sleep disturbance as a triggering factor for tension headaches (Paiva 1997) is of particular significance in fibromyalgia, where disturbance of sleep is a commonly expressed complaint (Moldofsky 1975).

IRRITABLE BLADDER SYNDROME

Painful bladder conditions affect a large percentage of women at some point during their lives and yet generate relatively little interest from the medical community. Sadly, it is not uncommon for a patient to be incorrectly diagnosed, offered no or inappropriate treatment, and to be denied referral for investigation that may lead to successful therapy. It is equally unacceptable for a woman to be labeled with a general, meaningless diagnosis such as "irritable bladder syndrome" as the endpoint of the evaluation (Payne).

In discussing the irritable bladder syndrome, Burks makes a statement applicable to fibromyalgia and all the components of the overlapping syndrome:

> I am glad that Interstitial Cystitis is a part of my practice because there is absolutely no question that this disorder has made me a better physician. The care and time and empathy I need to manage these patients, like the eighteen-year-old who's in the tenth grade because she's missed so much school because of the pelvic pain, has made me a much better physician and, frankly, a much better human being. We need to practice, not just physical healthcare, but also the healing side, dealing with the emotional issues, the social issues, and the psychological issues of chronic pain. A lot of physicians, unfortunately, don't want to deal with a problem that you can't see, is difficult to measure, and takes a lot of maintenance. But the physician who takes this on and deals with it and develops a comprehensive program is, in my mind, a better physician and a better healer.

Terminology and Symptoms

The condition is known by various names: irritable bladder syndrome and interstitial cystitis (IC) are in common use in North America; painful bladder syndrome (PBS) was urged but not accepted at a 2004 conference. In 2006 the European Society for the Study of IC (ESSIC) proposed yet another term and acronym, bladder pain syndrome (BPS), also not fully accepted.

The symptoms of irritable bladder syndrome are similar to those of an upper urinary tract infection (UTI) but can usually be distinguished by careful questioning. In both conditions frequency, urgency, and pain are present. The irritable bladder syndrome patient generally has increasing pain on bladder filling that is manifest by pressure, burning, and spasms. The pain typically decreases after voiding only to build up again as the bladder starts to fill. The sensation of a full bladder is very unpleasant, but most irritable bladder syndrome patients feel they can control their bladder and incontinence is uncommon. In contrast, the UTI patient has severe pain during and after voiding and the urge to urinate is sudden and severe and often results in leakage before the patient reaches the toilet (Payne).

Patients in this category are generally young females in their teens, twenties, thirties or sometimes even forties who have a less-than-one-year history of frequency, urgency, and pelvic pain. Usually, they have seen multiple physicians who treated their IC as if it were an infection. They are young, have no other major medical problems, and experience extreme frequency, urgency, and a varying degree of pain. They have negative urinalysis results, no infection, and no hematuria. They have negative pelvic exam results. There's nothing else in their history that could give them these symptoms, such as endometriosis or some spinal cord problem. But in these patients, IC can almost be diagnosed just from their history (Burks).

A study in 1987 in Washington, DC, found irritable bladder syndrome caused so much misery that the contemplation of suicide was four times higher than in the general population; 30 percent of the patients were unable to work full-time. Many women also suffer with other conditions such as irritable bowel disease, migraine headaches, fibromyalgia, and low back pain (Zamula).

Frequency

Although much less common than UTIs, it is estimated that up to four hundred fifty thousand Americans are affected by irritable bladder syndrome; 90 percent of these patients are female (Payne).

"IC is by no means not represented in any population I know of," said Burks. "In our practice at Henry Ford Health System, we see it across the board. In southeast Michigan, we have a large Arab-American population and a large African-American population. I have plenty of African-American, Arab-American, Asian-American, and everything-American patients with IC."

Change in Awareness of Irritable Bladder Syndrome

In the mid-1980s, irritable bladder syndrome really wasn't on the map. But thanks to Ann Landers' column in the late 1980s, things started to change. Frankly, the whole pelvis has come out of the shadows (Burks). She received ten thousand letters from patients and their families (Zamula).

In the 1980s, no one was talking about erectile dysfunction or vaginal infections. Now, bowel, bladder, and sexual function are discussed openly on television. Sometimes, it seems like every other TV commercial is about erectile dysfunction treatment. Vaginal yeast preparations are all over-the-counter now. There have been good articles in the consumer media about IC. So the word is getting out about this disorder as American society becomes more open about discussing problems related to the pelvis and as people become more informed about issues of the pelvis and pelvic function (Burks).

Course

Irritable bladder syndrome (interstitial cystitis) has a natural course characterized by spontaneous flares and remissions. It can seem like bacterial cystitis, especially if the patient is given antibiotics each time a flare-up occurs and sees gradual improvement. The urine culture shows no significant growth and the urinalysis is usually normal. The patient will not have a prompt improvement with the antibiotics, will feel only slight improvement with urinary analgesics, and will not go back to normal bladder function when the flare-up is over. The patient typically has persistently increased voiding frequency and at least some bladder discomfort. Sometimes the patient feels that the bladder is normal between flare-ups, but a voiding diary will usually demonstrate that the capacity is unusually low and careful questioning will bring out pressure and discomfort that is present whenever the patient must delay voiding. Most patients will reach their maximum symptoms in the first twelve to eighteen months (Payne).

Etiopathology

In contrast to bacterial cystitis, irritable bladder syndrome is an inflammation that is not caused by bacteria. Although some patients will date their symptoms to a urinary tract infection from which they never fully recovered, and other patients may occasionally have bacterial infections, the definition is that the patient's symptoms must occur consistently and over a substantial period of time in the absence of infection. The cause is unknown (Payne).

Bladder sensory thresholds of patients diagnosed with irritable bowel syndrome were compared with matched controls, by bladder capacity testing (cystometry). Urinary frequency and urgency and the urodynamic finding of detrusor instability were significantly more common in women with irritable bowel syndrome. The suggestion was made that both irritable bowel and irritable bladder syndromes were part of a generalized disorder of smooth muscle (Monga 1997).

Trigger points in the muscles of the low abdominal wall, pelvic floor muscles, piriformis or the upper inner thigh, have been suggested as the cause of urethral syndrome (Starlanyl 2001).

An article from France describes the urethral syndrome as "The Expression of Fantasies about the Urogenital Area" and is worth reading to learn about the physicians' mind-set, even though half of the authors were female (Chertok 1977).

Diagnosis

The history is the single most important factor in making the diagnosis of IC, and a thorough history will obviate the need for additional testing in many patients. Some cases will not be so clear, and additional testing is necessary and appropriate. It is extremely important to exclude other pelvic diseases that may cause bladder irritation, such as endometriosis, urethral diverticula, sexually transmitted diseases, as well as bladder and gynecologic cancers. Carcinoma in situ of the bladder can cause very similar symptoms and must always be considered as a possible diagnosis, particularly when the patient is a smoker or blood is present in the urine. When the history, physical examination, and urinalysis do not rule out other conditions, imaging studies such as a pelvic ultrasound and an IVP (kidney x-ray) may be useful.

The most important diagnostic test in the work-up is cystoscopy under anesthesia. In order to properly evaluate a patient the procedure should be done under anesthetic in an operating room so that the bladder can be stretched (distended), a procedure that is too painful without anesthesia. Before distention, the bladder of an IC patient generally looks normal although scarred, ulcerated areas may be visible in some severe cases. After distention, however, small bleeding points will be seen throughout the bladder surface (which represent rupture of the smallest blood vessels) and the lining of the bladder may be observed to crack with linear fissures. These characteristic bleeding points are referred to as glomerulations and are the hallmark of IC.

The bladder is usually biopsied to exclude the possibility of cancer as well as to evaluate the degree and nature of the inflammatory response. Alternatively, a bladder wash cytology (essentially a Pap smear of the bladder) may be collected during the cystoscopy to rule out carcinoma in situ without biopsy (Payne).

Interstitial cystitis does occur in men, making it difficult to rely on the diagnostic term "hysterical female condition" (Zamula), and may be misdiagnosed as the more commonly occurring prostatitis.

Treatment

There is no definite curative treatment. Most patients gain considerable symptomatic relief from either chronic or "as needed" therapy. In general, treatments are chosen to address the most bothersome symptoms and to minimize or take advantage of side effects.

Bladder distention is primarily a diagnostic maneuver, but it is the initial treatment for most patients. Approximately 40 percent of patients will have some therapeutic response. When the initial distention is not beneficial, DMSO bladder instillations are the most common therapy. DMSO is a liquid that has anti-inflammatory and analgesic properties, among others, that can be beneficial.

Amitryptiline is an antidepressant that is also widely used in chronic pain conditions. It is particularly useful for the patient with a predominant symptom of pain (Payne).

According to Burks, patients who are the worst:

have what I call a systemic disorder. Along with their bladder problem, they've got one or more of a host of other serious problems—fibromyalgia, thyroiditis, rheumatoid arthritis, inflammatory bowel disease, and so on. When I see a patient with systemic disorders, I work with other specialists, such as rheumatologists. When patients fly in from afar, sometimes looking for even fifth opinions because they are so desperate, I look at what's happened, make a suggestion, and send them back to their local urologist with a comprehensive note about what options there are. For these patients, we are now rethinking our former focus on the bladder and are focusing on the systemic disorder.

Relevance to Fibromyalgia

In a self-reporting survey of twenty-five hundred patients with fibromyalgia, 26 percent indicated they had bladder problems (Bennett 2007). A general estimate of the frequency of this condition in patients who have fibromyalgia varies between 40 and 60 percent (Clauw 1997). Bladder dysfunction is often associated with allodynia and pain sensitivity. Urinary frequency, dysuria, and nocturia are also common (Russell 2004). Some people with fibromyalgia suffer from the painful bladder condition interstitial cystitis (Staud 2007). Twenty-six percent of patients reported voiding urgency, essentially the same figure as Bennett, but whether there was pain is not described in the study from France (Blotman 2006). There are some "personal" symptoms that everyone will avoid mentioning, and it is probable that this condition will be underreported rather than the reverse.

IRRITABLE BOWEL SYNDROME AND OTHER GASTROINTESTINAL FUNCTIONAL PROBLEMS

Functional gastrointestinal (GI) and motility disorders are the most common gastrointestinal disorders experienced in society and are present in a significant proportion of the population. In fact, about 25 percent of the US population has some activity limitation and impairment of daily function due to these disorders, and the frequency of work absenteeism is second only to the common cold. These disorders compose about 41 percent of gastrointestinal problems for which patients seek healthcare. Despite their common occurrence, functional GI and motility disorders remain hidden in our society. Individuals do not commonly discuss these disorders, particularly when experiencing bowel symptoms (statement of the International Foundation for Functional Gastro-Intestinal Disorders).

Definition of the Concept of IBS

Irritable bowel syndrome (IBS) is a functional GI disorder characterized by abdominal pain and altered bowel habits in the absence of specific and unique organic pathology. Osler coined the term mucous colitis in 1892 when he wrote of a disorder of mucorrhea and abdominal colic with a high incidence in patients with coincident psychopathology. Since that time, the syndrome has been referred to by sundry terms, including spastic, irritable, and nervous colon (Lehrer 2007).

Chronic functional abdominal pain (CFAP) is the diagnosis given in the absence of any change in bowel habits.

IFD (inflammatory bowel disease) may be confused with IBS because of the use of acronyms, but IFD is as different from IBS as rheumatoid arthritis (RA) is from fibromyalgia. In IFD and in RA, there is undisputed evidence of an inflammatory process. Despite this apparent confusion, there is some thought that IBS and IFD represent the same condition at different stages (Quigley 2005), and it is found that patients diagnosed initially with IBS are, in comparison with the general population, sixteen times more likely to develop IFD (Garcia-Rodriguez 2000).

Diagnosis of IBS

Traditionally, IBS is a diagnosis of exclusion. No specific motility or structural physical signs have been consistently demonstrated, so IBS remains defined by its reported symptoms.

The Rome III 2006 consensus criteria for the diagnosis of IBS require that patients must have had recurrent abdominal pain or discomfort for at least three days each month, during the previous three months, which is associated with two or more of the following: relieved by defecation; onset associated with a change in frequency, form, or appearance of stool. Supporting symptoms include altered stool frequency or form, altered stool passage (straining and/or urgency), mucorrhea, abdominal bloating, or subjective distention.

The usefulness of subtypes is debatable; within one year, 29 percent switch between constipation-predominant IBS and diarrhea-predominant IBS (Lehrer 2007).

Functional GI Disorders—Diagnostic Criteria

The term "functional" is generally applied to disorders where the body's normal activities in terms of the movement of the intestines, the sensitivity of the nerves of the intestines, or the way in which the brain controls some of these functions is impaired. However, there are no structural abnormalities that can be seen by endoscopy, x-ray, or blood tests. Thus it is identified by the characteristics of the symptoms and infrequently, when needed, limited tests.

The "Rome Diagnostic Criteria" categorize the functional gastrointestinal disorders and define symptom-based diagnostic criteria for each category (Drossman 2006).

- *Functional esophageal disorders*—Globus: a sensation of a lump, something stuck, or a tightness in the throat; functional chest pain: the feeling of chest pain, presumably of esophageal origin; functional heartburn: persistent burning sensation; functional dysphagia: the sensation of difficulty swallowing.
- *Functional gastroduodenal disorders*—Functional dyspepsia: pain or discomfort located in the upper abdomen; aerophagia: repetitive air swallowing or ingesting air and belching; functional vomiting: vomiting in the absence of medical and psychiatric causes; rumination syndrome: effortless regurgitation of recently swallowed food.
- *Functional bowel disorders and abdominal pain*—Irritable bowel syndrome: pain associated with change in bowel habit; functional abdominal bloating: feeling of abdominal fullness or bloating; functional constipation: seemingly incomplete defecation.
- *Functional diarrhea*—passage of loose or watery stools without abdominal pain.
- *Functional abdominal pain*—Continuous or frequently recurrent abdominal pain with some loss of daily activities.
- *Functional disorders of the biliary tract and pancreas*—Gallbladder dysfunction: characterized by episodes of severe steady pain; sphincter of Oddi dysfunction: a motility disorder characterized by severe steady pain.
- *Functional disorders of the anus and rectum*—Functional fecal incontinence: recurrent uncontrolled passage of fecal material; functional anorectal pain: dull ache in the rectum that lasts for hours to days; proctalgia fugax: severe pain in the anal area of short duration; functional defecation disorders: inadequate defecatory propulsion.

Pathophysiology. Traditional theories regarding pathophysiology may be visualized as a three-part complex of altered GI motility, visceral hyperalgesia, and psychopathology.

Altered GI motility. Distinct aberrations in small and large bowel motility.

Visceral hyperalgesia. Rectosigmoid and small bowel balloon inflation produces pain at lower volumes in patients than in controls. Notably, hypersensitivity appears with rapid but not gradual distention. Patients who are affected describe widened dermatomal distributions of referred pain. Sensitization of the intestinal afferent nociceptive pathways that synapse in the dorsal horn of the spinal cord provides a unifying mechanism.

Psychopathology. Associations between psychiatric disturbances and IBS pathogenesis are not clearly defined. Patients with psychological disturbances relate more frequent and debilitating illness than control populations. Patients who seek medical care have a higher incidence of panic disorder, major depression, anxiety disorder, and hypochondriasis than control populations. An Axis I (clinical) disorder coincides with the onset of GI symptoms in as many as 77 percent of patients. A higher prevalence of physical and sexual abuse has been demonstrated in patients with IBS. Whether psychopathology incites development of IBS or vice versa remains unclear, although a "derailing of the brain-gut axis" is a picturesque explanation (Orr 1997).

A study of nearly one hundred thousand IBS patients showed frequent comorbidities of depression, headache, and fibromyalgia (Cole 2006). IBS patients are reported, in comparison with the general female population, to be twice as likely to undergo hysterectomy (Longstreth 2004).

Frequency, Mortality and Morbidity, and Etiopathology

The International Foundation for Functional Gastro-Intestinal Disorders (IFFGD) reports the prevalence of irritable bowel syndrome as 10 to 15 percent of the US population, or computed in head count, twenty-five million to forty-five million persons are afflicted with this condition. Of people with IBS, approximately 10 to 20 percent seek medical care. An estimated 20 to 50 percent of gastroenterology referrals relate to this symptom complex. In Western countries, women are two to three times more likely to develop IBS than men.

Patients often retrospectively note the onset of abdominal pain and altered bowel habits in childhood. Approximately 50 percent of people with IBS report symptoms beginning before they were aged thirty-five years.

International incidence is markedly different among countries. American and European cultures demonstrate similar frequencies of IBS across racial and ethnic lines. However, within the United States, survey questionnaires indicate a lower prevalence in Hispanics in Texas and Asians in California. Populations of Asia and Africa may have a lower prevalence.

This is a chronic relapsing condition. IBS does not increase mortality or the risk of inflammatory bowel disease or cancer. The principal associated physical morbidities include abdominal pain and lifestyle modifications secondary to altered bowel habits.

Fibromyalgia is a common comorbidity.

Causes remain poorly defined, but suggestions similar to those for fibromyalgia have been made, along the lines of a central neurohormonal mechanism.

The midbrain mediation of emotion and autonomic response enhances bowel motility and reduces gastric motility to a greater degree in patients who are affected than in controls. Limbic system abnormalities, as demonstrated by positron emission tomography (PET scan), have been described in patients with IBS and in those with major depression. The hypothalamic-pituitary axis (discussed in another chapter) may be intimately involved in the origin. Motility disturbances correspond to an increase in hypothalamic corticotropin-releasing factor in response to stress.

Treatment, Diet, Medication, and Economic Cost of IBS

A questionnaire sent to IBS patients has some significance for those interested in fibromyalgia; the issues of the inquiry were related to education and expectations. The highest level of response was an expectation that their physician should remain available by phone or e-mail after a visit (80 percent) and should be willing to listen to them (80 percent). By contrast, interest in education was less—58 percent interest in medication and 55 percent in the causes of IBS (Halpert 2006).

Changes of diet should be directed at preventing overreaction of the gastrocolic reflex to lessen pain, discomfort, and bowel dysfunction. Soluble fiber foods and supplements, substituting milk products with soy or rice products, care with fresh fruits and vegetables that are high in insoluble fiber, and eating frequent meals of small amounts of food can all help to lessen the symptoms of IBS.

Medications include antidiarrheals, or laxatives, or antispasmodics, as indicated by symptoms. Serotonin stimulates the gut motility, so serotonin agonists can help constipation-predominant irritable bowel, while serotonin antagonists can help diarrhea-predominant irritable bowel.

The aggregate cost of irritable bowel syndrome in the United States has been estimated at $1.7 billion to $10 billion in direct medical costs, with an additional $20 billion in indirect costs, for a total of $21.7 billion–$30 billion (Hulisz 2004).

A managed care company comparing medical costs of IBS patients to non-IBS controls identified a 49 percent annual increase in medical costs associated with a diagnosis of IBS (Levy 2001). Workers with IBS showed a 34.6 percent loss in productivity, equivalent to 13.8 hours lost per forty-hour work week (Paré 2006).

Relevance to Fibromyalgia

A high prevalence of fibromyalgia has been shown in patients suffering irritable bowel disease (Frissora 2005; Cole 2006; Kurland 2006). Bennett and associates' self-reporting survey of twenty-five hundred patients with fibromyalgia showed a reported frequency of 44 percent irritable bowel syndrome. Sivri (1996) reported the condition in 40 percent of his fibromyalgia patients.

Since IFFGD reports the prevalence of irritable bowel syndrome as 10 to 15 percent of the US population, the figures obtained for fibromyalgia patients would suggest therefore a prevalence of irritable bowel syndrome at three times the national average. Blotman (2006) showed a lower figure in France, nearly 30 percent. Veale (1991), recognizing the high concurrent frequency of the two conditions, has questioned whether they are in fact separate expressions of the same process.

CHRONIC LOW BACK PAIN

In the fourth week of the embryo's life, paired blocks of cells known as somites unite together to form thirty-five primitive spinal segments, which will eventually become the spinal column. Each segment splits transversely, then by joining with its neighbor, the primitive vertebral body, which will become bone, is formed from adjacent segments and becomes distinguished from the intervertebral disc lying between them. At this time in our life, the disc is as wide as the vertebral body. As we age, the disc alters (deteriorates and degenerates are the pejorative terms commonly used) so that if we're unlucky and live for ninety years, the disc is dried up and quite thin (Hall 1965).

The vertebral body is the block of bone in front of the spinal cord. Surrounding the cord is an arch of bone, most conveniently called the posterior element. Small joints on each side of the posterior element form a line of articulations from the head to the pelvis. The arrangement has been likened to a three-legged stool—the disc joins the vertebrae together in front, these little joints unite the vertebrae behind, and anything that happens to one leg of the stool will affect the other legs.

In the development state, the human spine has one long curve, but man has been condemned to the upright posture, obliging him to develop compensating concave and convex curves in his spine. The greatest deterioration in disc and joint occurs at the apex of the concavities of the neck and low back; where the mobile spine meets the immobile pelvis is the worst place of all for both disc and joint.

Back Pain

There is a tendency to talk about the back as if it were homogenous structure like a muscle. It's not. It's composed of many structures, each of which is liable to suffer its own array of problems. Furthermore, as the emergency room physician is well aware, pain presenting in the back does not necessarily originate in the spinal column but might be due to a leaking aorta or a kidney stone or some pathology in the womb, and so on. In this section, consideration will be given only to the low lumbar spinal column, only to the issue of chronic pain, and not to the structures from which it might arise, nor the nature of the conditions that might have initiated the pain.

There are particular issues associated with the spine:

- it degenerates inevitably over time;
- it is liable to injury in ordinary daily activities;
- having back pain is socially acceptable;
- technology permits us to picture the degeneration in great detail;
- a huge industry is well fed by back pain and would be sorry to see it go.

Acute pain merges into chronic pain not so much by a change of character as by convenience in terminology. No matter how they are treated, most patients with acute low back pain recover within six weeks, and 85 percent within three months (Van Tulder 2002). Chronic pain is variously described as having lasted more than three months or more than six months. Conventional wisdom is that if the patient has not recovered and returned to work within two years of the start of her pain, she will probably remain unemployed and unemployable. It's that small proportion of chronic back pain patients who eat up 75 percent of the costs (Maetzel 2002; Pai 2004). Many insurance policies are worded in such a manner that the insured is compensated while away from their regular work for two years but after two years must return to any kind of work for which they are fit. The problem here is a person earning high wages at a heavy job may be condemned to lower wages at a light sedentary task, unless she can demonstrate she is "permanently and totally" disabled. The resultant annual estimates of cost of back pain in the United States lie between twenty and fifty billion dollars (Pai 2004). The inevitable involvement of lawyers may raise costs by a multiple of eight times (Bernacki 2004) and may explain why the rate of growth in numbers of disabled Americans is fourteen times faster than the rate of the growth of the overall population. This would be an interesting field for a demographer, to show when the lines will cross.

Low Back Pain in Fibromyalgia

The generally published figures for prevalence of low back pain in the United States are somewhere between 5 and 20 percent. Bennett reported from his 2007 survey a very much higher prevalence of low back pain in fibromyalgia. This symptom headed the list of current comorbid complaints at 63 percent, although this issue gets little attention in other works on fibromyalgia. Blotman (2006) does not mention it in his patients in France; Wallace (2003) mentions briefly fibromyalgia may be overlooked in the diagnosis of low back pain; Starlanyl (2001) indicates trigger points as a cause, so presumably is considering myofascial pain syndrome and not fibromyalgia. Perhaps these authors thought back pain is so much part of everyday life that the complaint in fibromyalgia is irrelevant; Bennett and associates' figures suggest otherwise.

The Pain Cycle

In Bennett and associates' 2007 survey, 21 percent of the respondents did not remember a triggering factor that set off their "primary" fibromyalgia; the others had various issues of illness and trauma, either emotional or physical, that triggered their "secondary" fibromyalgia.

Not all back pain is traumatic in origin. Sometimes it "just happens—like a bolt out of the blue." It is perhaps not unreasonable to suppose that the following suggestions for the development in chronicity of back pain could be applied to "secondary" fibromyalgia, if not the "primary" sort, recognizing that this distinction is considered invalid anyway.

Linton (2005) describes a "fear-avoidance" model to conceptualize the development of chronic pain that takes into account the emotional, cognitive, and learning aspects of the process: Pain gains attention; it is interpreted according to the subject's emotional state and beliefs; which gives rise to coping strategies; which create experience by learning. If the experience has created fear of pain associated with an activity, this may provoke catastrophizing such as "I could end up in a wheelchair," leading to vigilance to avoid the activity, initiating more fear, creating a vicious cycle of avoidance of activity and chronic pain.

Such fear-avoidance beliefs in the circumstances of acute back pain have been linked to the persistence of disability a year later (Sieben 2002).

MULTIPLE CHEMICAL SENSITIVITY SYNDROME

Other terms for this disorder include environmental illness, multiple chemical sensitivity, idiopathic environmental illness, twentieth-century disease, universal allergy, total allergy syndrome, allergic toxemia, toxic injury (TI), chemical sensitivity (CS), chemical injury (CI), twentieth-century syndrome, environmental illness (EI), sick building syndrome, idiopathic environmental intolerance (IEI), and toxicant-induced loss of tolerance (TILT).

Morris, an allergy specialist in a famous London hospital, writes:

Doctor Theron Randolph, an allergist, described in the 1940's a condition he called "Environmental illness," postulating the human body was like a "barrel filling up with chemicals" until a critical point was reached after which it reacts to any further exposure.

In the 1980s, Cullen coined the term "multiple chemical sensitivity," which enjoyed wide acceptance as a medical condition in the popular lay media, among alternative practitioners, and in those individuals with nonspecific symptoms who self-diagnosed themselves with MCS.

Up to 16 percent of the general population report some form of "unusual sensitivity" to common everyday chemicals (a phenomenon that is culturally restricted to North America and Europe). This prompted the National Institute of Environmental Health in the United States to develop a consensus statement in 1999. The NIEH defined multiple chemical sensitivity as a "chronic recurring disease caused by a person's inability to tolerate an environmental chemical or class of foreign chemicals" and proposed the preferred medical term: idiopathic environmental intolerance (IEI).

Symptoms

The presenting symptoms are essentially anything that the patient finds distressing and chooses to attribute to this cause. A partial list of common symptoms include anaphylactic shock, difficulty breathing, chest pains and asthma, skin irritation, contact dermatitis, and hives or other forms of skin rash, headaches, "brain fog" (short-term memory loss, cognitive dysfunction, including attention deficit), neurological symptoms (nerve pain, paralysis, weakness, trembling, restless leg syndrome, etc.), tendonitis, seizures, visual disturbances (blurring, halo effect, inability to focus), extreme anxiety, panic and/or anger, suppression of immune system, digestive difficulties, nausea, indigestion/heartburn, vomiting, diarrhea, food intolerances, which may or may not be clinically identifiable (e.g., lactose intolerance, celiac disease): commonly wheat and dairy, joint and muscle pains, extreme fatigue, lethargy and lassitude, vertigo/dizziness, abnormally acute sense of smell, sensitivity to natural plant fragrance, pine turpines, insomnia, dry mouth, dry eyes, and an overactive bladder (Gibson 2003).

The frequency reported of these symptoms is headache 55%, fatigue 51%, confusion 31%, depression 30%, shortness of breath 29%, arthralgia 26%, myalgia 25%, nausea 20%, dizziness 18%, memory problems 14%, gastrointestinal symptoms 14%, respiratory symptoms 14% (Venturupalli 2005). Most patients (85 to 90 percent) complaining of MCS syndrome are women. Most present between the ages of thirty and fifty years (Magill 1998). The typical patient is a middle-age, well-educated female in a white-collar profession (Venturupalli 2005).

Overlapping Syndrome

Overlap has been proposed with other environment-linked conditions such as sick building syndrome (SBS), food intolerance syndrome (FIS), and Gulf War illness (GWI). Those affected may also be prone to chronic fatigue syndrome, fibromyalgia, irritable bowel syndrome, connective tissue disorders after silicone breast implants, reactive hypoglycemia, drug-induced hepatitis, reactions related to living near toxic waste dumps and electromagnetism from power lines, dental amalgam disease, and reactions to the petrol additive MTBE.

Cause—Possibly Psychogenic

There appears to be no convincing evidence in the medical literature for the existence of multiple chemical sensitivities or idiopathic environmental intolerance. The underlying cause for the IEI symptom complex is unlikely to be a direct reaction to everyday chemicals, but rather a masked stress disorder with heightened olfactory awareness and associated behavioral conditioning.

Many physicians believe that the symptoms of IEI are psychophysiological in nature and those affected are prone to panic responses that enhance their symptoms. Individuals with self-identified chemical sensitivities responded with typical panic attacks when challenged with intravenous lactate, in a similar manner to individuals with an underlying panic disorder (Binckley 1997).

In one study, all the MCS patients who responded to a challenge with their trigger substances developed symptoms and signs of acute anxiety with hyperventilation and a rapid fall in $pCO2$, although their lung function remained normal (Lenzoff 1997).

Psychological conditioning has been proposed as the underlying abnormality in IEI but is complicated by a high incidence of premorbid psychological trauma (including childhood physical and sexual abuse). This may lead to profound long-term effects on mood and affect, cognitive processing, hypervigilance, and entrenched beliefs of victimization (Staudenmeyer 1997).

The Department of Psychosomatic Medicine at the University of Tokyo found that patients experienced symptoms only when they themselves initiated the challenge tests. When they were given random prompts, there was no difference between MCS patients and controls in terms of physical and psychologic symptoms (Saito 2005).

About one half of the patients with MCS in various studies meet the criteria for cooccurring depressive and anxiety disorders (Lax 1995). Though these psychological conditions have alternative causes, it has been suggested that MCS is simply a physical manifestation of a psychological disturbance (a psychosomatic illness) that should be treated with psychotherapy and antidepressants. A study showed psychotherapy resulted in significant, long-term improvement in MCS symptoms, although criticized on the basis there was no control group with which to compare results (Lacour 2002). Using standard structured interviews, it was concluded, the similarity of idiopathic environmental intolerance and somatoform disorders regarding symptoms and psychological features of somatization support the hypothesis that IEI is a variant of a somatoform disorder (Bailer 2005).

The Minnesota Multiphasic Personality Inventory 2 (MMPI-2) was administered to fifty female and twenty male personal injury litigants, with a conclusion they "expressed distress through somatization and used a self-serving misrepresentation of exaggerated health concerns" (Staudenmeyer 2007).

A "Real" Condition?

The cause and existence of MCS are disputed. Doctors disagree about whether symptoms are physiologically or psychologically generated or both. United States courts and several medical organizations reject MCS as a physiological disease. Critics of clinical ecology, a controversial field of medicine that claims to treat MCS, charge that no diagnostic tests have been substantiated (Staudenmeyer 1995) and not a single case has been scientifically validated (Barrett 1998).

MCS is specifically *not recognized* as an established organic disease by the American Academy of Allergy, Asthma, and Immunology, the American Medical Association, the California Medical Association, the American College of Physicians, and the International Society of Regulatory Toxicology and Pharmacology (AMA 1992; Gots 1995; Magill 1998).

The National Institute of Environmental Health Sciences (a division of the NIH) defines MCS as a "chronic, recurring disease caused by a person's inability to tolerate an environmental chemical or class of foreign chemicals" (MCSS fact sheet).

Clinical ecologists claim that MCS causes negative health effects in multiple organ systems, and that respiratory distress, seizures, cognitive dysfunction, heart arrhythmia, nausea, headache, and fatigue can result from exposure to levels of common chemicals that are normally deemed as safe (Gibson 2003; Rea 2006).

Detractors describe MCS as "a label given to people who do not feel well for a variety of reasons and who share the common belief that chemical sensitivities are to blame. . . . It has no consistent characteristics, no uniform cause, no objective or measurable features. It exists because a patient believes it does and a doctor validates that belief" (Gots 1993). An editorial in the *Journal of Toxicology* stated, "It may be the only ailment in existence in which the patient defines both the cause and the manifestations of his own condition" (Gots 1995).

Significance to Fibromyalgia

Slotkoff (1997) reported a 52 percent overlap between fibromyalgia and IEI; Buchwald (1994) reported overlapping between fibromyalgia, MCS, chronic fatigue syndrome, and other conditions. No satisfactory explanation has yet been found. There is strong evidence that IEI is a somatoform disorder, which has not been shown with fibromyalgia. However, a common feature is the intense reaction to any suggestion their complaints might be psychogenic. Glenn (2002), interviewing doctors who worked in the allergy field who had become involved with IEI patients, records one as saying, "I regret it. Scientists in this field are subject to intimidation in a very broad sense. There can be harassing phone calls and e-mails at home, derogatory postings on the internet, and demonstrations at lectures. Then there are the frivolous but aggravating complaints to employers or medical boards. Even when proven groundless, every complaint takes a tremendous amount of time and energy to refute."

MYOFASCIAL PAIN SYNDROME

As described elsewhere, the usual time sequence in applying a name to a medical condition is to have first a presentation of a symptom, such as, "I hurt in my leg," then if it's found later that a lot of people with leg pain also have pain in other parts of the body and several other frequently reported symptoms, the condition becomes termed a "syndrome." If an explanation for all these different symptoms grouped together as a syndrome becomes available (as it did for Cushing's syndrome) then it moves up the medical terminology scale a notch and is termed a "disease."

Myofascial pain syndrome is an exception. It progressed from "muscle knots" as a symptom, to "myofascial pain syndrome," and is now termed "chronic myofascial pain" by Starlanyl (2001), who declares it to be a disease, so "syndrome" is dropped. No explanation is forthcoming for this disease, so for the purpose of this book we'll stick with the more usual "myofascial pain syndrome."

Commonly in the medical field the conditions we know by one name are renamed, but in the process no further understanding is obtained. We are no closer to any truth, but our filing and index systems suffer enormous cost. Muscle knots must have been known since time immemorial (see section on history). There are really very few new medical realities. Although every decade we seem to develop a set of new diagnoses, we're usually just reinventing the wheel, giving it a different name, switching from Greek to Latin to French and then to pseudoscientific double-Dutch.

Historical Perspective

In an extensive review (two hundred and fifty-two references) of myofascial trigger points, Dommerholt (2006) describes the genesis of the term. He quotes references going back to the sixteenth century: German descriptions at the end of the nineteenth century of palpable bands and a German text on trigger point treatment published in 1931, long before Travell popularized the condition in the United States.

Travell, initially a cardiologist, took up musculoskeletal pain as a treatment area, following interest in the work of Kellgren (1938 and 1949) and wrote articles on injections. She continued a primary interest in subluxations of the sacroiliac joint, a condition beloved of physiatrists and physical therapists and virtually unknown to orthopedists.

John Kennedy had undergone back surgery in 1944 and again in 1954; his pain persisted. They did not use the term in those days, but he would now be called a "failed back," and doubtless his persisting pain would be labeled "neuropathic." This did not prevent him from becoming a senator, when Travell started to treat him in 1955 (McParland 2004), or later the president of the United States. Whether the world was ready for it, or JFK's back is the cause, injection of trigger points of myofascial pain syndrome never looked back.

What Is the Myofascial Pain Syndrome?

Since this book is about fibromyalgia, we'll start with a negative aspect to the definition by saying quite clearly what it isn't. The myofascial pain syndrome is definitely not the same condition as fibromyalgia.

Although the myofascial pain syndrome may seem akin to the fibromyalgia syndrome, the 1990 ACR definition of fibromyalgia clearly explained the difference: Fibromyalgia is "all-over body" pain, four quarters plus axial. Myofascial pain syndrome is regional pain, which may be diffuse, but is not "all over."

Fibromyalgia and myofascial pain syndromes may both be found in the same patient and may both occur at the same time (comorbid, concomitant). Starlanyl (2002) writes movingly of her problems and treatment for these conditions, both of which she suffers. Bennett (2007) reported 46 percent of his patients surveyed had "muscle spasms," not a condition due directly to fibromyalgia, but possibly due to myofascial pain syndrome.

There are several other major differences, which clearly distinguish between them:

- Fibromyalgia affects mostly women; MPS is equally divided, men to women.
- Fibromyalgia is associated with general fatigue; MPS is not.
- Fibromyalgia is associated with multiple nonmuscle conditions; MPS is not.
- Fibromyalgia "tender" points are not recognizably different to the touch; MPS trigger points can be identified by touch as different from the surrounding muscle.
- Fibromyalgia "tender" points do not provoke referred pain when compressed; MPS "trigger" points cause pain locally and pain may be referred elsewhere.
- Fibromyalgia is not improved by localized therapy; MPS is relieved by direct treatment.

Patient's History

On her first presentation to the doctor, the patient will commonly describe a poorly localized diffuse pain in one particular part of the body. This is a critical difference from fibromyalgia. The pain may wax and wane, it may be diffuse within that part, but it is limited to one region, for instance, the neck and shoulders, or the arm or the leg. It is not widespread through four limbs and the axial spine.

For every patient, there has to be a first time, and the same for every doctor. But since the condition tends to recur, the patient will soon be able to tell the doctor what is wrong, and since the condition is common, the doctor will not need to be in practice for very long before she recognizes the symptoms and can make the diagnosis.

There may also be a "subjective" sensation of numbness—subjective meaning to the patient there is a numbed feeling, but when the physician touches the part the actual ability to respond to the sensation of touch has not been lost. They may or may not be aware of weakness in the affected muscles. They may have a tendency to drop things.

Any movement that stretches the muscle will increase the pain, and for that reason the patient may present with a postural problem—the head twisted, the arm bent, the shoulder shrugged.

There may be an account of unusual activity—just taken up an exercise program, decided to spring clean, or "I must have slept in a draft" are common if unrealistic explanations. As a rule, the patient is not physically very active and is not particularly well muscled, but there is a subcategory of athletes who over-exert or who don't warm up properly before commencing their routine.

Physical Examination

This is one of the not uncommon situations in clinical practice where if the doctor doesn't know what she's looking for, doesn't know where to look, and doesn't have a systematic approach to the search, she may find nothing. And that would be a pity because the source of the problem is there to find, and proper technique will reveal it.

There are many references to this and just about every other subject, complaining, "Most medical school and residency training programs do not cover this common condition adequately," and doubtless that's true. It implies that the young doctor has to be taught, which is unfortunate. The responsibility of the young doctor is to learn, not to wait to be taught. And doctors learn from seeing patients, lots and lots of patients, and learning from the patients. There's a lot more to be learned from listening to the patient than there is from listening to the professor—virtually all she has to say can be read in a book or on a laptop!

The essence of medical teaching lies in telling the student to keep her hands in her pockets, or at the very least behind her back. First she uses her ears and listens to the patient who will tell her where she hurts, for how long, and how often. Statistics being on the side of the diagnostician since this is a recurring condition, given half a chance (with her hands still behind her back) the doctor will be told by the patient the several different names she's been given for her condition, the several different treatments she's received, which ones hurt the most and which ones worked, as well as the ones that were not only ineffective but also painful and expensive.

All of this can be with the eyes closed or over the telephone. Then with the eyes open the doctor will see the patient's posture, note the contracted (spasm) muscle, and note the point of maximum tenderness as indicated by the patient.

Only after exhausting all that can be learned by eyes and ears will the doctor take her hands out of her pockets, where she's been purposefully warming them, and she'll begin a very gentle palpation of the area. Gentleness is probably an inborn characteristic. I've never convinced myself it could be taught. Violence can be restrained, but a natural sensitivity with the hands is just that—natural. Often the strongest persons are the most gentle. There's an ability to think at the level of their fingertips that the ungentle person lacks. And it's by no means tied to one sex. There are some very rough female doctors, which is perhaps the reason the iconic teacher of modern medicine, William Osler, is supposed to have said, "There are three sexes, men, women and female doctors."

Be that as it may, the gentle touch exerts virtually no pressure and starts at a distance from the point the patient said was maximally tender. The muscle should be caressed in the direction of its fibers, effectively longitudinally in a limb. With this gentle touch a band will be felt in the muscle, and then, coming to the point the patient indicated as painful, a knot will be encountered in the band.

Pressure on this knot is not only painful in itself but causes a radiation of pain through the area, called "referred" pain. This explains why the knot itself is called a "trigger point," with the inevitable reduction to initials "TrP," which must not be confused with the so-called tender point of fibromyalgia, designated "TP" or "TeP."

This pressure on the trigger point may also stimulate the autonomic nerves, which cause in the region of the referred pain a rising up of the skin hairs (pilo-erection), sweating, and flushing. Pressure on the trigger point will not only reproduce the pain, it will commonly provoke a "jump sign," which is held out as characteristic of this condition, but in fact is to be found in every painful condition, not just MPS. There should be no need to go to the library to look up the diagrams in the two bulky volumes by Travell.

Having located the offending trigger point, the physician or therapist should continue a search for lesser trigger points in the same limb or region. There is a theory that "latent" trigger points are lurking in the muscles, just like anthrax spores in the field, waiting for the right moment to become activated. It's hard to prove or disprove a negative, and it's left to the proponents of this theory to come up with their proof.

Treatment

Does every diagnosed condition have to be treated? Sometimes the patient wants no more than to be told what's wrong, to be reassured it will not shorten her life or turn into something worse. "Do I have arthritis? Is it cancer?" The best patients are delighted to be told their problems are self-limiting, just like the common cold.

Obviously people have been getting knots in their muscles for about as long as there have been people, or at least people who weren't physically active, which is a much shorter time. No one comes to the surgeon with a fixed deformity due to a shortened muscle as a result of a muscle knot or a trigger point. There is a very sad congenital condition called arthrogryposis where such contractures occur and require surgical release. Although surgeons may treat trigger points (Cabot 2007), they never have cause to operate on them. It is therefore quite safe to reassure the patient he'll recover spontaneously and prescribe an analgesic to take during the recovery period. One has to bear in mind that muscle pain is extremely common, and almost everyone develops a trigger point at some time but probably calls it a "knot." It's reported in the United States 14 percent of the general population suffers from chronic musculoskeletal pain, and 25 to 55 percent of asymptomatic individuals can be found to have these latent trigger points (Finley 2006).

Other patients may not wish to await nature, or may not be able to work and may want something done about their problem. A perfectly legitimate request.

If the patient is a self-reliant, self-motivated type, and particularly if this is a recurring problem, she can be taught to treat herself by pressure on the knot, applying no more pressure than reasonably tolerable, and at the same time stretching the affected muscle by straightening the neck or limb.

Alternatively she can be sent for treatment by one of many sorts of therapists or might seek treatment as a "walk-in" client. Physical therapists employ "spray and stretch," numbing the area with a vaporizing fluid then gently stretching the affected muscle. They will probably give a series of treatments. Physical therapists have also at their disposal numerous gadgets for passive treatment, including various forms of hot and cold, wet and dry application, and numerous electrical machines, such as electrical muscle stimulation (EMS) using interferential current (IFC) or functional electric stimulation (FES) or transcutaneous electrical nerve stimulation (TENS), as well as ultrasound (US). And if all these pieces of equipment are owned by the clinic, why not put them to use?

For these patients the physician will employ a direct attack on the painful nodule by injecting a local anesthetic into it, like the dentist uses in your mouth, and then stretching the taut muscle band. (It's not always understood that muscles are effectively a bundle of cells and that each cell runs the full length of the muscle.) Sometimes the doctor will insert a needle but not inject an anesthetic; perhaps she'll inject water, perhaps nothing—so-called dry needling. Botulinum toxin is becoming fashionable, perhaps because it's very expensive.

Persisting Symptoms

For the patient with recurring problems some thought should be given to causation. Is there something about her work or her workplace that would merit the advice of an occupational therapist or ergonomics expert?

"Leg length inequality" is dearly loved by the hands-on branch of the medical world, the physiatrists, physical therapists, chiropractors, and so on; it is offered as an explanation for virtually every physical condition including MPS and keeps the orthotists busy. Any orthopedic surgeon will tell you how hard it is to determine true leg length (a special x-ray measurement is needed) and will tell you patients with undoubted leg length discrepancies do not present with these problems.

When an inexplicable problem keeps coming back despite resolution from treatment, when a person becomes disabled as a consequence, it is proper first to consider very carefully whether the correct diagnosis has been made, second, whether there are recognizable factors that are causing this recurrence, and last of all, whether nonphysical issues might be involved. There is an enormous "treatment industry" out there. When there is a demand, there will be a supplier. The patient might in all innocence have been caught up in this. Or the patient may simply enjoy the attention. Or the patient may have more complicated emotional problems common to all the pain syndromes.

Investigations, Causes, and Pathophysiology

None are justified unless some occult cause is seriously suspected. A number of tests and imaging studies have been performed out of research interest but have no place in clinical practice. Among these are electromyographic studies, which have shown spontaneous electrical activity in the tender nodule; infrared thermography may show increased blood flow sometimes noted at trigger points. Imaging studies are only of use to rule out other sources of pain.

The simple and honest answer to what causes myofascial pain syndrome is the same as that for fibromyalgia: we just don't know. And the more we know about it, the more certain we become that we don't know its cause. If you read somewhere a clear and simple explanation, check out the author's credentials. Finley (2006) is probably correct when she writes, "The pathogenesis likely has a central mechanism with peripheral clinical manifestations."

Once again, we are uncertain what changes, if any, occur in the muscle. There are speculations on structure and chemistry, but no single agreed fact.

Fascia and Ground Substance

There are some very strange things written on the subject of fascia and ground substance. As an anatomist and histologist I taught about it for a number of years. As an orthopedic surgeon I've spent hours cutting and stitching all the different elements of fascia in the body. I can't fairly claim to be unique, but I doubt if there are many persons who wrote their PhD thesis on ground substance (Hall 1961).

I quote the opening of my own long put-aside thesis:

> Connective tissue derives its name from its function of uniting . . . the other tissues of the body. . . . Its density varies from that of bone to loose areolar tissue.

... It forms a continuum throughout the body ... leading to the synonym "supporting tissue" ... the amorphous component commonly known as ground substance is composed mostly of water, in this are the components of the tissue fluid.

When I read (Starlanyl 2001), "Ground substance can resemble gelatin that has not yet set ... or even harder, like sprayed-on Styrofoam insulation. When the ground substance hardens, it is as if it has turned to glue or cement ... it won't reverse ... without outside intervention," the most polite thing I can say is, "Lady, that simply ain't so."

CERVICAL MYOFASCIAL PAIN

Myofascial pain as a specific condition is dealt with elsewhere in this book. Cervical myofascial pain is essentially the same condition in terms of its character. It is its location that justifies dealing with it as a separate issue.

To say "the head is heavy" would seem to be no more than stating the obvious. It's the usual and obvious that's taken for granted, and only when the unusual happens do we turn our thoughts to the usual. In ordinary life today, going out on the road and sitting in a car is probably the most dangerous experience most of us undertake. Accidents are frequent, the so-called whiplash injury is common. Only when the muscles of the neck have been made sore does the owner of those muscles begin to appreciate how hard he has to work to stop his head from falling forward. Only after the whiplash injury do you appreciate how those muscles are working all the time to hold your head upright; and the only relief is to rest the head on the back of the chair or a pillow so the muscles can stop working for a while. Watch the tired surgeon sitting in a boring lecture; as soon as he gets sleepy, his muscles relax and his head drops forward, only to be snapped upright as he wakens from his Stage 1 sleep (look for that in another chapter as well).

Polio, fortunately, has been virtually eliminated from the Western world, but despite UNICEF's efforts it's not yet totally eliminated from the globe. Severe polio may cause paralysis of the neck muscles, and without support the head droops to the side. The same is seen with those persons unfortunate enough to have sustained an injury to the upper cervical spine, with paralysis of the neck muscles, or one of the several neuromuscular conditions that result in paralysis, requiring a brace to hold the head upright.

In the days when the study of muscle activity by electromyography (EMG) was a new and exciting technique, Basmajian (1962) showed that as we stand, the muscles in the front of the spine and the muscles at the back of the spine work alternately, keeping us swaying gently and maintaining the upright position. It's the same for the head—as long as we're upright. We keep our head in minimal motion, nodding imperceptibly backward and forward, giving the muscles at the back and at the front of the neck fractions of a second in which to relax. But it's not the same when we're leaning forward, typing, or operating, or looking down a microscope, or changing a diaper. During that period of time the muscles at the back of the neck are continuously contracted to prevent the head from falling forward—like the surgeon who's gone to sleep in the boring lecture.

The experienced keyboard operator knows to sit upright and touch-type. The inexperienced worker has his head forward, the muscles at the back of the neck stretching over the shoulder blades become fatigued, ache, and "go into knots." It was these knots, recognized more than a century ago, that gave rise to the concept of "fibrositis." Their treatment is discussed in the more general section on myofascial pain.

The unique aspect of cervical myofascial pain is the likelihood of spread of the pain through the base of the skull, generating headache and into the shoulder blade area, occasionally down the inner arm, following the distribution demonstrated in the 1930s by Kellgren (Hall 1965), whose suggested regions of the body (sclerotomes) had migrated from their original positions during embryologic development but had continued with the same nerve root supply.

NEURALGIA

In itself "neuralgia" means no more than "nerve pain" and the term has been very vaguely applied to pain in any area of the body supplied by a single known nerve. Because it is so vague it is more likely now to be used by the lay public than by a medical professional. There are, however, specific forms of this single nerve pain that are worth describing.

A particular difficulty in persuading skeptics that fibromyalgia is a real disease is the absence of anything that can be seen, the absence of any visible pathology, the absence of any clearly defining objective tests. There are forms of neuralgia that cover the fields of the clearly obvious because there is something to see, the less obvious but surgically treatable, and the very much less obvious, less treatable, and in that sense, more akin to fibromyalgia. Neuralgia has also historically been the model for the discovery and employment of some of the types of medication currently offered in the treatment of fibromyalgia.

Postherpetic Neuralgia—The Obvious Neuralgia

Popularly known as "shingles" from the Latin word for a belt, *cingulum,* still found in use in the equine world as the "surcingle" (Skinner 1961). The varicella-zoster virus (VZV) causes chickenpox, demonstrated by a diffuse blistered rash and occurring annually before vaccination was started, in four million children in the United States.

After the infection is established, when the disease appears to be terminated and the patient (usually a child) seems to have recovered fully, the virus may still be present in the body, having moved into sensory nerve fibers, tracked backward along them to its origin in the dorsal root ganglia near the spinal cord, and then "holed up" in a ganglion, waiting for an opportunity to show itself again.

In older life, commonly age fifty or older, when resistance is lowered by age, by stress, or other issues such as HIV, a chickenpox blister rash appears again. But now it's confined to the area of skin supplied by a particular sensory nerve (defined as a dermatome) and is frequently seen in an intercostal nerve as a band around the chest, hence the concept of a belt.

In childhood, after the annoyance of the rash and the considerable itching that accompanies it, there are usually few other problems (*usually* is an uncomfortable word in the practice of medicine, for it leaves open the possibility of catastrophic exceptions).

Not until adulthood does the shingles strike, affecting as many as half a million persons each year in the United States. Often after an attack of shingles there is a period of a few weeks when pain is distributed in approximately the same region as the blisters. Occasionally there is pain without any blister having appeared or having been noticed if it did appear. The blisters carry the chickenpox virus and the patient is infectious.

Usually this pain, called postherpetic neuralgia, fades after a few weeks.

But in a fifth of the cases it may persist much longer, may be severe, and may be described with many of the terms used in the pain vocabulary (see the chapter on pain). The older the patient, the more likely is this postherpetic neuralgia to occur and to persist.

Thus when first seen at the postherpetic neuralgia stage, the physician encounters a patient with a complaint of severe persisting pain, and physical examination at this stage is unremarkable. Because the pain is in a band, however, and because she was a careful physician who knew what questions to ask, the prior history of the blisters is elicited, the history of chickenpox in childhood is confirmatory, and postherpetic neuralgia is diagnosed. There is no question of "all in your head" or somatoform disorder (SFD). The doctor may not be able to do much for the pain, but she has confirmed it as "real." There were signs to match to the symptoms; patient and doctor are mutually satisfied with the diagnosis.

Trigeminal Neuralgia (Tic Douloureux)

"Trigeminal" means no more than "triplets." This nerve is so named because of the three divisions of the fifth cranial nerve that supplies sensation to the face: the ophthalmic division going to the face above the eye, the maxillary to the cheek and upper lip, and the mandibular to the lower lip and area below the mouth.

Whereas shingles may involve any nerve and the cause of postherpetic neuralgia is understood, the cause of neuralgia in the trigeminal nerve is far from clear. There are no preceding blisters. There is nothing for the observer to witness other than the facial grimaces of a patient apparently struck with severe pain as if by lightning. Like lightning it may be very brief, or like a thunderstorm it may recur in episodes. The pain is usually on one side of the face, most often in the maxillary or mandibular branch, and may be so severe and so disabling some patients contemplate suicide. Because of the facial contortions, the term "tic" was applied. Because of the pain accompanying the tic, it became known to the French as *tic douloureux*, which is also commonly used in English doctor-speak.

As with shingles, trigeminal neuralgia occurs most often in the middle-aged or older patient. An area of the face or inner head with sensory supply by the trigeminal nerve becomes supersensitized (see chapter on Pain), and when touched or stimulated by as little as a current of air, lightning-lancinating pain is caused. It is believed that in some cases the problem is caused by a blood vessel irritating the nerve at its origin within the skull, and this has given rise to several different procedures for surgical correction (Cole 2005; Pollock 2005).

Before surgical treatment was undertaken, medical treatment was employed, ranging from the philosopher Locke ordering bowel laxatives for the ambassador's wife to probably the first use of anticonvulsive agents for neuralgia (Cole 2005). Later, carbamazine and gabapentin were found modestly effective.

Relevance to Fibromyalgia

The relevance of this condition to fibromyalgia is twofold. There are no objective physical signs, but because of the limited distribution of the pain and the character of the pain, any reasonably competent physician has no difficulty in making the diagnosis. That is to say, the condition in the physician's understanding is "real" and although she may say "it's all in your head," this is meant in a fully literal sense.

Treatment is less satisfactory but has responded to the same type of medication now licensed by the FDA for fibromyalgia.

Persistent Idiopathic Facial Pain (PIFP)

This pain (in the territory of the trigeminal nerve) has features that do not correspond to the typical trigeminal neuralgia (Pascual 2001; Krolczyk 2007). The character of the pain is a persistent severe ache, not lancinating and not brief as in tic douloureux.

As in trigeminal neuralgia, there is no known precipitating cause and there are no objective findings.

The physician has only the history to guide her to a diagnosis, and with this one, after all possibilities have been ruled out, the patient is likely to be told, "It's all in your head," both literally and figuratively, and treatment with medication and psychotherapy has not been promising. Surgery will have been avoided in the absence of any clear-cut indication.

Relevance to Fibromyalgia

The relevance of this condition to fibromyalgia is the vague distribution of the persisting pain, the rather vague description of the character of the pain, and the failure to respond to known treatment measures. Does that make it any less "real"?

NEURALLY MEDIATED HYPOTENSION

We've all seen people turn white, collapse suddenly or slowly, fall to the floor, recover, stand up, and then fall again. Commonly known as "fainting," this was a required skill at one time for all delicately reared young ladies, to be exercised at the least hint of any male vulgarity. In London the queen attends annually a celebration known as Trooping the Colour, performed by her personal soldiers, the Brigade of Guards. This requires these soldiers, selected for their height, to stand stiffly for long hours in the sun. It's expected by the crowd that at least one of them will fall, ramrod stiff and still "at attention."

For those in the medical profession, a fainting spell has since the fifteenth century been known as a "syncope" (Skinner 1961). For those who knew that the blood pressure and the actions of the heart were controlled in part by the autonomic (automatic is a fair explanation) nervous system, of which the vagus nerve carried the slowing down component, a common faint used to be called vasovagal syncope. But we're still making progress, so we've changed the name once more and it's now a neuroregulatory or neurogenic syncope.

Despite changing the name, the basis of the problem is still agreed. In a faint, or syncope, there is a sudden decrease in blood pressure, which deprives the brain of oxygen, temporarily causing dizziness (presyncope) or an actual loss of consciousness (syncope).

Underlying Mechanism

The postulated cause is an overshoot of a normal response to lowered blood pressure (hypotension). The upright posture causes blood to pool in the legs, resulting in a diminished volume of blood returning to the heart. Early signs of hypotension are sensed by a special organ in the neck, the carotid body, and signals are sent to increase the heart's rate and strength of contraction. Conflicting signals from the heart, however, cause the rate to slow, resulting in a sudden fall of blood pressure and the fainting spell.

Tilt-Table Test

To test whether change of posture provokes this hypotension, the patient is strapped onto a horizontal table. The table, mounted on a swivel, is slowly tilted upright, raised gradually to the vertical while the patient's legs are held straight by straps. Muscle action is the normal mechanism for pumping blood back up to the heart and head; immobilization on the table prevents this. A test is "positive" when the patient becomes lightheaded; the table is then lowered to resolve her symptoms.

Relevance to Fibromyalgia

Bou-Holaigh (1997) found 60 percent of fibromyalgia patients who spent forty-five minutes at seventy degrees tilt had a drop in blood pressure, whereas none of the persons used as controls showed any drop. Of twenty of these fibromyalgia patients who tolerated seventy degrees for more than ten minutes, eighteen had an increase in widespread pain, which was not experienced by any of the controls.

Perhaps this dizziness of presyncope is what Bennett and associates' (2007) respondents meant when they reported dizziness as a significant issue, but Bennett does report neurally mediated hypotension occurring in as much as 60 percent of the fibromyalgia population, referring to the studies of Bou-Holaigh (1997). Russell (2003) recognizes neurally mediated hypotension as a comorbid symptom of fibromyalgia and recommends testing with a tilt-table, increased salt intake, support garments, and some physical maneuvers to relieve it. Winfield (2007) also associates neurally mediated hypotension with fibromyalgia and implies there may be some common pathways.

NONARTICULAR RHEUMATISM

What is rheumatism? What is nonarticular rheumatism? What is a rheumatologist? According to Skinner, the word is derived from the Greek and means a liability to flow (with reference to the humors of the body). Hippocrates wrote of both "rheuma" and "catarrh," the latter word retaining more of the original meaning of running down from the head. Guillaume de Baillou introduced the word "rheumatism" (Garrison 1929), the earlier use of the word rheumatism in English seems to have been related to rheumatic fever and its complications (Major 1945); the term rheumatoid arthritis was not coined until 1857, by Garrod.

Consultant specialists in the field of internal medicine began increasingly to subspecialize after World War Two, and in major centers there could be found a specialist, a rheumatologist who was particularly interested in rheumatoid arthritis, and to a lesser extent, in aging or degenerative arthritis, generally known as osteoarthritis. Since we've already pointed out "-itis" is a reserved modifier for inflammation, and since inflammation is not much of a component, on the Continent at least they prefer to call osteoarthritis an arthrosis. The rheumatologist had little to offer his patients beyond aspirin and physical therapy. Then in the early 1950s came cortisone with its magic benefits and all its complications. "Connective tissue diseases" became the field added to the rheumatologist's specialty, since he was the person who best understood what was meant by terms like autoimmune. Then as more rheumatologists became available, and the primary care physician increasingly practiced what one of my colleagues has called "travel agency medicine," directing all his patients to different specialists, the scope of practice of the rheumatologist expanded.

The Royal College of Physicians and Surgeons of Canada (RCP&SC) is the body that oversees training programs and licensing of specialists; standards in the United States and Canada are essentially the same, with joint accreditation boards. Their statement in regard to the subspecialty of rheumatology is: "On completion of the educational program, the graduate physician will be competent to function as a consultant rheumatologist. This requires the physician to be effective in the assessment, investigation, management, and rehabilitation of patients with acute and chronic forms of arthritis, soft tissue rheumatic disorders, collagen-vascular diseases and vasculitides, spinal, and regional pain problems and the musculoskeletal manifestations of systemic disease." Most medical specialties are devoted to a particular portion of the body, such as the central nervous system, the alimentary canal, and so on, but the rheumatologist takes care of conditions that affect tissues throughout the body. And as such "widespread pain" of fibromyalgia falls into his field of expertise, although everyone agrees it is not a problem of joints and there is no inflammation.

Muller (2007) writes, "nonarticular rheumatic pain syndromes can be classified into five general categories: (1) tendonitis and bursitis, such as the common lateral epicondylitis (tennis elbow) and trochanteric bursitis; (2) structural disorders, such as pain syndromes resulting from flatfoot and the hypermobility syndrome; (3) neurovascular entrapment, such as the carpal tunnel syndrome and thoracic outlet syndrome; (4) regional myofascial pain syndromes, with trigger points similar to fibromyalgia but in a localized distribution, such as the temporomandibular joint syndrome; (5) generalized pain syndromes, such as fibromyalgia and multiple bursitis-tendonitis syndrome." He makes a fundamental statement, "The more generalized and chronic the syndrome, the more difficult it is to treat."

There are "territorial issues" here, and it is a regrettable fact that not all branches of medicine approve what the other fellow believes. Anything ending legitimately in "-itis," an inflammation, is going to be treated by physiatrists, physical therapists, chiropractors, some orthopedic surgeons, and a host of assorted therapists. Each will have their own method of treatment, and in many cases it becomes a demonstration of the power of the human body to improve spontaneously, no matter what abuse it's subjected to during the time of its self-healing.

Most of these conditions, if they arrive "spontaneously" without known trauma, are found in persons of middle age. Fibromyalgia falls into the same age group. Muller (2007) gives a figure of four thousand cases of "soft tissue" rheumatism per hundred thousand population, so it's to be expected that there will be many persons who experience fibromyalgia and non-articular rheumatism. It has always been a principle of the diagnosis of fibromyalgia that it does not exclude the patient from having other conditions at the same time, such as rheumatoid arthritis.

CHRONIC PELVIC PAIN

The pelvis has been likened to Grand Central Station. All tracks converge. It's the end of the line. From there, everything is discharged.

The intestines end at the rectum and anus. The kidneys discharge through the ureters to the bladder and the bladder discharges through the urethra. The vagina, uterus, tubes, and ovaries are contained within it. The nerves and blood vessels for the pelvic contents are distributed within it; nerves and blood vessels for the legs lie there against the lumbar spine and sacrum. All are supported and prevented from falling from the body by a complicated set of muscles constituting the floor of the pelvis. A lot of structures in a tight space. A lot of structures means the potential for a lot of pathology, and there is no shortage of that.

Cancer is well known in the rectum, bladder, uterus, and ovaries. Infections of various kinds occur in the uterus and the tubes. Cells from the lining of the uterus may end roaming loose in the pelvis, setting up clumps called endometriosis. Painful cysts occur in the ovaries and may twist or may bleed with life-threatening consequences. Fertilized eggs sometimes fail to pass down the tube to the uterus; the embryo enlarges until the tube bursts—another life-threatening emergency. And then there are all the problems that occur in the bones, joints, and discs of the lumbar spine, the sacroiliac joint, and the little block of fiber and cartilage that unites the bones of the pelvis in the front and so conveniently loosens at childbirth.

Despite the reality of frequent unquestioned pathology in the pelvic structures, the complaint of pelvic pain for which no explanation can be found is so common it has earned its own designation as "chronic pelvic pain."

In being a common problem, it presents a major challenge to healthcare providers because of its unclear etiology, complex natural history, and poor response to therapy. It is poorly understood and poorly managed. The pathophysiology is complex, multifactorial, and unclear. A significant number of the patients may have various associated problems, including bladder or bowel dysfunction, sexual dysfunction, and other systemic or constitutional symptoms. Other associated problems, such as depression, anxiety, and drug addiction, may coexist (Singh 2006).

Definition, Frequency, Age, and Cause

The American College of Obstetricians and Gynecologists defines it as "Noncyclical pain of at least six months' duration involving the pelvis, anterior abdominal wall, lower back, and/or buttocks, and serious enough to cause disability or to necessitate medical care."

Approximately 15 to 20 percent of women aged eighteen to fifty years have this chronic pelvic pain lasting for more than one year. In the United States it affects 14 percent of women (Mathias 1996). In a study made in the United Kingdom, twenty-four thousand cases were identified, with a prevalence of thirty-eight per thousand women, as common as migraine and back pain (Zondervan 1999).

Of cases referred to gynecologists, 10 percent are for chronic pelvic pain (Reiter 1990) and more than 40 percent of laparoscopies are performed with this nonspecific diagnosis (Singh 2006). As in spinal imaging, some abnormality can usually be found, but as in spinal surgery, treating that visualized abnormality may not resolve the symptoms of pain (Mailis 2005).

Chronic pelvic pain is not reported as more common in any particular ethnic group or socioeconomic stratum. It's most common in the twenty-six-to-thirty age group (Jamieson 1996), but Zondervan (1999) found the prevalence to increase with age, from eighteen per thousand at age fifteen to twenty, and increasing to twenty-seven per thousand at age sixty and older.

Specific causes may include endometriosis, interstitial cystitis, or irritable bowel syndrome, but examination and testing are often nondiagnostic. Because negative work-up does not rule out physical causation, it does not negate the significance of a patient's pain (Barclay 2004).

Presenting History and Physical Examination

A full general and specific gynecologic history must be taken; in particular, history of sexual abuse as child or adult should be questioned; this has been reported as high as 50 percent (Lampe 2000; Barclay 2004).

The standard general examination is made. Then a very full gynecologic examination. Singh suggests a particular search for trigger points using a cotton-tipped swab. Jantos (2007) also suggests a search for trigger points, although he writes from a psychology department, and Starlanyl (2001) devotes several pages to the search for trigger points around the pelvis.

In evaluating women with chronic pelvic pain, transvaginal ultrasound can be useful. At least 40 percent of gynecologic laparoscopies are undertaken where the ultimate diagnosis is chronic pelvic pain.

Treatment—Exercise, Surgery, Psychotherapy

Both medical therapy and surgical procedures have been shown to help patients with chronic pelvic pain, but therapy must be individualized given the multiple possible etiologies and treatment options associated with this pain.

There is insufficient evidence to recommend the use of antidepressants; however, tricyclic antidepressants have been proven to aid other pain syndromes. Opioids may reduce chronic pelvic pain but do not improve functional or psychologic status. Only limited data show that combined oral contraceptive pills are effective for chronic pelvic pain. They are effective for primary dysmenorrhea. Gonadotropin-releasing hormone agonists have been shown to be effective in treating endometriosis. In addition, these agents have also been shown to be effective in women with pelvic pain secondary to suspected endometriosis that was not confirmed with surgery. Vitamin B_1 and magnesium are the only nutritional or herbal remedies that have been demonstrated to help women with chronic pelvic pain.

Injections into appropriate affected pain areas have shown a response rate of 68 percent. Psychotherapy has not been demonstrated to help women with chronic pelvic pain, but some physical therapy techniques have been demonstrated to improve symptoms.

Endometriosis: Forty-five to 85 percent of women with endometriosis will have significant pain relief for up to one year after conservative surgical treatment. However, there is a high recurrence of endometriosis after surgery.

Hysterectomy: Three to 9 percent of women develop new pelvic pain during the two years after hysterectomy. At least 75 percent of women with chronic pelvic pain will have improved for up to one year after hysterectomy.

Adhesions: Only women with dense adhesions involving the bowel benefit from adhesiolysis for chronic pelvic pain.

Presacral neurectomy: Can be effective for central pelvic pain, but pain in the lateral pelvic area is not as effectively treated with this technique.

Uterine nerve ablation: Less effective than presacral neurectomy.

Counseling may be effective to help patients with chronic pelvic pain, especially if there is a history of abuse.

Association with Other Conditions

The most common diagnoses associated with chronic pelvic pain are endometriosis, adhesions, irritable bowel syndrome, and interstitial cystitis. Adenomyosis, intrauterine devices, and cervical stenosis have been linked with chronic pelvic pain, but evidence for causality among these latter conditions is not as strong.

Gastrointestinal and urinary tract diagnoses can be more common than gynecologic diagnoses in women with chronic pelvic pain. Twenty-five to 50 percent of these women have more than one diagnosis (Barclay 2004). Eighteen to 35 percent of women with pelvic inflammatory disease go on to have chronic pelvic pain. Approximately 33 percent of women with endometriosis have chronic pelvic pain, and 38 to 85 percent of women with chronic pelvic pain have interstitial cystitis. Symptoms of irritable bowel syndrome are present in up to 80 percent of women with chronic pelvic pain. Peripartum pelvic pain syndrome, thought to be due to a strain on ligaments in the pelvis and lower spine, can lead to chronic pelvic pain.

Economic Costs and Relation to Fibromyalgia

In the United States, estimated direct medical costs for outpatient visits for chronic pelvic pain (women aged eighteen to fifty) is approximately $881.5 million per year (Mathias 1996).

In the study made by Bennett and colleagues (2007), pelvic pain as such does not seem to have been a proposed question, but 17 percent of the respondents reported pain with sexual intercourse, and 27 percent reported pain with menstruation.

RESTLESS LEG SYNDROME AND PERIODIC LIMB MOVEMENT IN SLEEP

There are two similar conditions, restless leg syndrome (RLS) and periodic limb moment in sleep (PLMS). Although these two syndromes are often considered together, and although they may have a common genetic basis, there are some significant differences.

Clinical Description of Restless Leg Syndrome

Horne (2006) describes this condition as appearing in wakefulness, particularly in the evenings, when it is experienced as an unpleasant creeping-crawling sensation deep within the knees, thighs, or calves, brought on by sitting or lying. Some people liken it to "insects within the legs." Typically it produces an irresistible urge to stretch and move the legs about or a need to get up and walk.

Periodic limb movement in sleep (PLMS) disorder is unique in that the movements occur during sleep (MacFarlane 1996; Anderson 2007), whereas other movement disorders manifest during wakefulness. The unconscious movements may cause poor sleep and subsequent daytime somnolence. PLMS disorder may occur with other sleep disorders and is related to, but not synonymous with, restless leg syndrome (RLS), a less specific condition with sensory features that manifest during wakefulness. The majority of patients with RLS have PLMS disorder, but the reverse is not true. Prevalence increases with age. The idiopathic form is rare before age forty years. Often the presenting complaint is poor sleep and daytime somnolence. Occasionally, a bed partner may provide the history of limb movements.

The movement simulates triple flexion as in kicking a ball, with hip and knee flexion, ankle dorsiflexion, and great toe extension; it lasts approximately two seconds with periodicity ranging from twenty to forty seconds, involving one or both limbs. Horne (2006) describes PLMS as if it was the continuation of RLS after the patient goes to bed.

History and Etiology of PLMS

Ekbom coined the term "restless legs" in 1945. Symonds first described PLMS disorder in 1953 (Anderson 2007). The original name, "nocturnal myoclonus," does not describe the condition accurately, since the movements are slower than are those of myoclonus, and that name is seldom used today.

The etiology of the primary form of PLMS disorder is uncertain. Disinhibition of the descending inhibitory pathways may be a factor. Some evidence supports neuronal hyperexcitability with involvement of the central pattern generator for gait as the pathophysiology of PLMS (Vetrugno, D'Angelo, and Montagna 2007), which results in decreased dopamine transmission, potentially supporting the use of dopaminergic therapy to treat the condition. A genetic basis with familial association is suggested (Jeffrey 2007).

Studies differ regarding the frequency of polyneuropathy in cases of PLMS disorder. Martinez-Mena and Pastor (1998) found that only one of nine patients had signs of neuropathy. Horne (2006) reports possible associations with iron deficiency, raised serum urea, heavy smoking, excess caffeine, use of antidepressants and antihistamines, all of which are likely to be encountered in the general population of older persons, but a low iron level may interfere with the function of the dopamine system.

There are secondary forms of PLMS disorder associated with diabetes mellitus, spinal cord tumor, sleep apnea syndrome, narcolepsy, uremia, or anemia (Anderson 2007).

Investigation, Treatment, Prognosis, and Patient Education

Lab studies: Because anemia, uremia, and the use of tricyclic antidepressants or antidopaminergic or dopaminergic medications can lead to a secondary form of PLMS disorder, laboratory screening studies should be obtained to rule out anemia or significant metabolic abnormalities. The serum iron level should be determined.

Other tests: Definitive diagnosis requires polysomnography; observation in a sleep laboratory allows documentation of the movements and rapid diagnosis.

Because the etiology is not clear, treatment is primarily directed at symptoms and does not modify the disease. Patient reassurance is essential. Treatment involves either dopaminergic medication in an attempt to modify activity of the subcortical motor system or, more commonly, sedative medications to allow uninterrupted sleep. The arsenal of medication options is expanding and includes antiepileptic agents and even opioids, although the controlled substances may not be appropriate first-line agents.

The Restless Legs Syndrome Foundation suggests that "medications should be used in the lowest effective dose and dosage should be titrated slowly upward." A dopamine agonist, used in the treatment of Parkinson's disease, ropinirole, has been approved by the FDA since 2005 for treatment of RLS.

The idiopathic form of this syndrome may be chronic. Relapses and remissions may occur, but treatment does not appear to modify the disease. The secondary form of this syndrome may cease with treatment of the underlying cause.

Informing the bed partner of the condition is important so that the potential of inadvertent and forcible physical contact may be explained on a neurological (rather than an intentional) basis.

Relationship to Fibromyalgia

Both syndromes have been reported to be found in 31 percent of patients with fibromyalgia compared with an incidence of 2 percent in the control group (Yunus 1996).

Bennett and colleagues record in their self-reporting survey of twenty-five hundred persons with fibromyalgia that 46 percent suffered from muscle spasms, 32 percent suffered from "restless legs," and 79 percent found their symptoms worsened by sleeping problems.

RAYNAUD'S DISEASE AND PHENOMENON

It is not particularly remarkable to have a pathological process called after the man who first described it (eponymous naming), but it is remarkable that Raynaud made his description in his graduating thesis, part of which is given (in translation) by Major (1945).

In this thesis, Raynaud described different severities of apparently the same condition: one was a twenty-seven-year-old woman with spontaneous gangrene in four extremities; second was a twenty-six-year-old woman whose fingers became numb and white when cold, sensation returning painfully when the fingers were warmed.

Terminology and Clinical Appearance

We now distinguish between mild and severe forms, based on an improved but far from complete understanding of their causes. However, we still employ a multiplicity of confusing words, and these several terms have led to much confusion. The mild form is known as Raynaud's disease, or primary Raynaud, or idiopathic Raynaud. The more severe form is known as Raynaud's phenomenon, or secondary Raynaud.

When the person involved puts his hands in cold water, some or all of the digits undergo a color change, initially turning white and becoming numbed. When warmed, the fingers turn red and are painful, sometimes extremely painful. The underlying change is due to a spasm of the small blood vessels supplying the digits. Metabolic chemicals accumulate and then flush the digit when the vasospasm is released. Persons with this problem may also be given to fainting easily, as can be demonstrated by tilt-table testing. Or it can be a purely local issue, affecting only the fingers.

In the secondary form of the condition, the word "secondary" is employed to indicate the condition follows another labeled disease process. The vasospasm may not resolve; the tissues may remain without blood supply and may die. Death is seen as blackened skin. The digits, fingers and toes, are most commonly affected, but the nose and the ears, just as in frostbite, may also be involved.

A number of different problems can be the underlying cause of the secondary form, ranging from changes in the chemical or physical character of the blood, to changes in the blood vessels or changes in the skin. Many of these fall into the class of autoimmune and connective tissue diseases in which the rheumatologists are the experts. Some prescribed medications such as birth control pills and chemotherapeutic agents used in the control of cancer may cause this vasospasm, as will the nonprescribed ergot.

Although in most cases the two conditions, Raynaud's disease and Raynaud's phenomenon, are essentially different processes, over a period of time the milder form may become the more severe connective tissue disease variant.

The primary form is reported as occurring in 5 to 10 percent of the US population, the secondary form in 50 percent of those using vibrating tools (Lisse and Oberto-Medina 2006).

Relevance to Fibromyalgia

Bennett (1997) reported 30 percent of patients with fibromyalgia suffered cold intolerance. This was also noted in the original article at the time "fibromyalgia" became the accepted term (Wolfe 1990) and earlier noted by Bengtsson (1986). In his survey Bennett (2007) records 46 percent of respondents with "tingling," 44 percent with "numbness." The question of Raynaud's disease does not seem to have been posed, but Bennett (1991) had written elsewhere on the relationship of Raynaud's with fibromyalgia, choosing to employ "syndrome" rather than distinguish between "disease" and "phenomenon."

Staud (2007) records "Raynaud's phenomenon is associated with fibromyalgia . . . often Raynaud's phenomenon is diagnosed while the fibromyalgia is not."

REFLEX SYMPATHETIC DYSTROPHY (RSD), A.K.A. COMPLEX REGIONAL PAIN SYNDROME (CRPS)

Given its variable character, the word "complex" is aptly chosen as the name for the condition. Bonica's description remains appropriate: "characterized by diffuse limb pain, maximal distally, developing following injury, with allodynia and hyperalgesia, and is commonly associated with vasomotor, sudomotor, swelling and trophic changes."

Weir Mitchell, during the American Civil War, was put in charge of a ward devoted to nervous problems in the Union Army hospital in Philadelphia. He described a condition he termed "causalgia," a combination word he cobbled together to indicate the burning nature of the pain he'd found in association with war-incurred peripheral nerve injuries.

Skinner speculates that Mitchell, a well-traveled and well-educated physician, may have been aware of the secondary meaning of the term he used, indicating a polishing with hot wax, since the skin in causalgia develops that polished, shiny appearance.

Mitchell is rightly credited with the description and wrote a book on his experiences. However, Scarpa had described the same findings forty years prior to Mitchell (Garrison 1929).

Mitchell wrote, "We are driven in every case to treat the pain alone, without true knowledge of its immediate cause. . . . It was our custom in the US Army hospital to resort to repeated leeching, which proved the most potent remedy." All of which raises an interesting point: Did the men say they were better when they weren't because they didn't like leeches? Or was this the placebo effect? Or are leeches really useful in the treatment of pain, and we've forgotten how to use them?

Wartime gives occasion for many surgical advances, but the next names attached to the condition were probably unrelated to the Franco-German War of 1870. Sudeck in 1900 and Kienböck in 1901 described acute inflammatory bone atrophy. Kienböck's contribution has been forgotten in the Anglophone world, but Sudeck is still remembered in the term "Sudeck's atrophy," describing the radiologic washed-out appearance of acute osteoporosis that occurs with this condition.

Leriche, in France, had occasion to treat large numbers of soldiers in the First World War. He studied the possibilities of surgical relief of pain in causalgia and was the first to use sympathectomy for causalgie. He continued with this interest and wrote books on the surgical relief of pain. He is well known for his axiom, "Physical pain is not a simple affair of an impulse traveling at a fixed rate along a nerve. It is the resultant of a conflict between a stimulus and the whole individual."

Leriche had another axiom, compatible with what has been written here on the placebo effect: "The individual on whom we operate is more than a physiological mechanism. For him nothing will replace the salutary contact with his surgeon, the exchange of looks, the feeling that the doctor has taken charge, with the certainty, at least apparent, of winning."

The name of causalgia was gradually amended, taking it from a descriptor of the pain's character to an attempt at understanding its cause. De Takats termed the condition "reflex dystrophy," and Evans with further experience gained in World War Two expanded this to reflex sympathetic dystrophy, commonly abbreviated to RSD. We now rest with complex regional pain syndrome, the name it most recently gained after one of those "wise men" conferences (Stanton-Hicks 1998). But the change does not meet with general approval. It is not fully accepted (Hord 2006), it is leading to greater confusion in the diagnosis and treatment (Kozin 2005), and 40 percent of the patients with diabetic neuropathy would meet the criteria (Galer 1998). Remarkably, the International Association for the Study of Pain (IASP), responsible for the change in the name of the condition, continued to use the older term in the title of their book (Jänig 1996).

IASP Classification

There were more changes than the name; two "types" were separated, essentially on the basis of whether there was an injury to a nerve, as Weir Mitchell had described, and "the others." Type I (represents "the others")—it does not have a known basis of injury to a nerve, and it is also known as reflex sympathetic dystrophy, Sudeck's atrophy, reflex neurovascular dystrophy, or algoneurodystrophy. Type II (does have a known injury to a nerve)—it is also known as causalgia.

Distribution—Who Has It?

1. War-injured veterans—causalgia occurring after a peripheral nerve injury: 1% to 5%
2. Civilian injuries—

   - following all fractures: 1% to 2%
   - following Colles (wrist) fracture: 7% to 35%
   - following peripheral nerve injuries: 2% to 5%
   - following hemiplegia (stroke with paralysis): 12% to 21%
   - following various traumas, analysis of cases in order of diminishing frequency: sprain 29%; surgery 24%; fracture 16%; contusion 8%
   - unknown or assorted other injuries 20% (Allen 1999)
   - 50% report RSD resulted from injury at work (Hord 2006)
   - 5% no recognized antecedent cause for RSD

3. Age: any age, more common 40–60 years; mean 40–42 years; increasingly prevalent in children and adolescents
4. Race: nil noted
5. Sex: more common in women, in ratio 1.6:3.1 (Allen 1999)

Presenting History and Physical Examination

Symptoms may start immediately or days or weeks after the putative injury. Although "burning" is the classical description, the pain is reported as "burning" in only a quarter of the cases. The remaining three-quarters are reported variously as aching, throbbing, tingling, but usually whatever the character of the pain, the time-nature described is "continuous."

The pain originates near the site of injury, then spreads proximally to involve the entire limb, occasionally the opposite limb as well (Kozin 2005). The strikingly noticeable features are:

- the severity of the pain is totally out of proportion to the injury
- the distribution of the pain is far beyond the territory of a single nerve
- moving or touching the limb cannot be tolerated by the patient

A variable feature is a history of edema, skin blood flow abnormality, or abnormal sweating in the region of the pain since the inciting event. Classically, the part is initially hot and red, later becoming cold and white, but that sequence is not invariable; Breuhl (2002) found no validity in this staging. The location of the pain is usually a limb, but it can be anywhere, including the genitalia or the nose. Hord (2006) describes other features:

- paresis, pseudoparesis, or clumsiness present in 80–90%
- tremor in 50% in late stages
- muscle spasms in 25% in late stages
- hypoesthesia, glove or stocking distribution 70%
- pain to be touched (allodynia) 70–80%
- exaggerated response to touch (hyperpathia) 70–80%
- abnormal sweating (hyperhidrosis) 50%
- edema secondary to autonomic dysfunction
- altered skin color due to vasomotor changes
- atrophy of tissues
- rapid fatigability is almost invariable in the later stages

Changes in skin leave it "shiny," as described by Skinner's suggestion of "polished," and the nails are brittle and cloudy white (Birklein 1998).

Use of Affected Part

The patient may have difficulty using the limb, either due to "cognitive neglect," in which the limb feels foreign to her, or "motor neglect," when direct mental and visual attention is required to move the limb (Galer 1995). To the inexperienced, this does not seem "real," but the same problem occurs after a stroke; the patient can move his arm if instructed but has lost the wish to use it for practical purposes. When asked to make a drawing of himself, he may subconsciously leave out the involved limb, suggesting a central defect.

Diagnosis and Tests

Diagnosis can confidently be made if the patient shows (Veldman 1993) that (1) at least four of five symptoms/signs are present (unexpected diffuse pain, altered skin color, altered skin temperature, edema, reduced active range of motion), (2) the symptoms are aggravated by activity of the involved extremity, and (3) symptoms are present in an area much larger than, and also distal to, the primary injury.

There is no specific test. Pain out of proportion to the injury is the primary diagnostic feature, however, pain-free cases have been reported (Eisenberg 2003) and this diagnosis seems acceptable to the experts (Kozin 2005). Although there is no specific test, some tests are of value as confirmatory documentation in a medico-legal or insurance context (Kozin 2005).

Thermography: difference of one degree centigrade is considered significant; the affected limb may be either warmer or cooler; the value of such findings is questionable.

Blood flow: various techniques available to document changes, e.g., doppler ultrasound.

Sweat: abnormal sweating detected by ninhydrin powder changing color; does not allow for quantification. There are quantitative tests (Sandroni 1998). Abnormal findings highly predictive of positive response to sympathetic blocks.

Imaging: x-rays as early as two weeks may show patchy osteoporosis; bone scan may detect changes even sooner, but false positives are not unknown (Kozin 1993). Densitometry is used, both to detect and to follow progress.

Electromyography (EMG): only if there is a nerve injury (Type II).

Treatment

There is a lack of specific treatment. "For the most part we resort to symptom control" (Kozin 2005). The usual range of medications for chronic pain is employed: antidepressants, NSAIDs, corticosteroids, vasodilators, pregabalin. Steroids are found helpful in early cases, and opioids are effective in both early and late cases. An implantable drug pump putting a continuous measured dose of opiates into cerebrospinal fluid may be used (there are hazards of overdosage if not very carefully monitored). Studies have confirmed relief of pain and improved quality of life but no improvement in function after the use of neurostimulators implanted into the dorsal column of the spinal cord; this is considered cost-effective (Kemler 2002) and the relief of pain is effective (Mailis 2005). Elevation of the affected part and early active exercise is indicated. If necessary, passive movements are made under light anesthesia to prevent contractures.

Peripheral nerve blockade is often the first management. Sympathetic plexus block by injection is followed by sympathectomy if pain relief obtained was at one time the standard of care (Stanton-Hicks 1998). This has now fallen into disfavor since very few subjects obtained long-term relief (Kozin 2005).

Various forms of psychotherapy might be offered, recognizing the severity of the pain and the probability of associated depression. Relaxation techniques and hypnotherapy have been tried with varying degrees of success.

Prognosis and Pathophysiology

Some patients improve without treatment; 80 percent are cured within eighteen months (Hord 2006), with or without treatment; only 20 percent return to normal function (Subbarao 1981).

Among the suggestions (Kozin 2005; Hord 2006) are:

- dysfunction of the sympathetic component of the autonomic nervous system, resulting in sympathetically maintained pain
- dysfunction of the peripheral nerves, resulting in vasodilatation, increased sensitivity to circulating catecholamines
- dysfunction of the central nervous system, resulting in alteration of central autonomic control. This suggestion meets the evidence best. Only a central alteration could explain an increase in sweating, and there is experimental evidence that substance P is involved.

Relationship to Fibromyalgia

There are common features: in both conditions there are complaints of excessive pain and tenderness, consistent with central sensitization. Fibromyalgia and myofascial pain syndrome may develop in persons suffering reflex sympathetic dystrophy (Kozin 2005), and it has even been suggested that fibromyalgia is in fact a form of reflex sympathetic dystrophy (Martinez-Lavin 2002).

TEMPOROMANDIBULAR JOINT DISORDER

The jaw joint seems simple enough but is among the most complicated in the body. Troubles with this joint form a complete specialty within the oral surgery field. There are surgeons who treat only this joint, abbreviated as TMJ. The lower jaw is called the mandible and the bone of the skull with which it articulates is called the temporal. Why is the bone called "temporal"? A complicated and probably incorrect answer suggests a blow on the side of the skull formed by this bone might terminate life (Skinner 1961).

In its simplest concept, the TMJ has a ball and socket arrangement, the ball (or head) is at the upper end of the mandible and the socket is a rather shallow depression in the temporal bone. But among the numerous features that make the joint a lot less simple than it might seem is a disc separating it into two compartments, a little similar to the incomplete discs in the human knee known to the trade as menisci and to the public as cartilages. These structures in the knee are widely known to get torn and damaged in various ways. The same can happen in the TMJ.

Another unusual feature of the TMJ is the sliding forward of the ball, moving out of the socket, a unique feature in human joints but well known in the world of snakes. This can readily be appreciated by putting the fingers in front of the ears, opening the mouth, and feeling the mandibular head rocking forward. The forward movement of the ball is arrested by a protruding mass of the temporal bone placed well in front of the socket. If the ball jumps forward of this limiting mass, it can't readily get back in place; the jaw remains dislocated and has to be forcibly replaced just as in any other dislocation, for instance, the shoulder.

Disorders of the Joint

All of this has relevance in fibromyalgia and other painful disorders. We don't as humans have the powerful bone-crushing jaws of some of the other animal predators, but our jaw muscles are nevertheless very strong. Think of the daredevil who swings from an aeroplane, saved from falling hundreds of feet to the earth by a piece of leather clenched between his teeth, attached to the plane by a rope. Then think that the weight of the body is transmitted through the small joints of the jaw.

Clinical problems associated with the TMJ are divided into those within the joint itself, the same kind of problems found in the knee or the hip, and the problems occurring in the muscles that are used in chewing (mastication) and to clench the teeth. Our concern in fibromyalgia is less with the inner structure of the joint than with clenching the teeth. The muscles used in this action are readily felt, masseter at the side of the jaw in front of the ear and temporalis at the side of the head, above the cheek bone (zygomatic arch).

When feeling nervous, perhaps part of the adrenaline-inspired fight or flight mechanism, our muscles go tense. We hold our hands clenched. We clench our teeth. When really worried we clench our teeth really tightly, keeping the masseter and temporalis muscles constantly contracted in knots. Headache ensues, eased by rubbing these muscles into a relaxed state. Those who suffer chronic pain are even more likely to be holding their jaws clenched and even more likely to suffer pain in this region as a consequence, which becomes a secondary part of the "pain all over."

Terminology, Distribution, and Treatment

The general condition was at first called TMJ syndrome, then later TMJ disorder, abbreviated to TMJD (McCain; Eriksson; Blasberg; Block). Problems with the TMJ are extremely common in the general population, estimated to be ten million people in the United States and that 25 percent of the population have had or will have TMJ problems at some time in their lives (Parnes 2006). A five-year study of TMJD showed a third of the cases resolve spontaneously, a third had intermittent episodes, and a third had continuing pain (Rammelsberg 2003).

Treatment must be directed at the primary problem, the cause of the clenching of the teeth, and at the secondary problem, the result of clenching the teeth. The local pain may be treated by simple analgesics, by discontinuing the teeth-clenching habit once the patient has been made aware of it, by muscle relaxants and antidepressants, or by a mouthguard for nocturnal teeth grinding. If trigger points are identified, local needling with or without local anesthetic might be used.

Relevance to Fibromyalgia

Wolfe (1955) reported a disproportionate number of persons with fibromyalgia having TMJD. It was his experience that in a rheumatology clinic, fibromyalgia was to be found in almost all the patients with TMJD (excluding those with rheumatoid arthritis).

Symptoms of fibromyalgia appear to be common in TMJD (Fricton 1985; Wolfe 1992). Some overlap in the two conditions has been shown and similarities have been drawn between the two conditions. In one dental clinic eight patients suffering also with fibromyalgia were examined, and of these six had severe mandibular dysfunction (Eriksson 1988). Pain in the jaw has been reported in 35 percent of fibromyalgia patients in Switzerland (Muller) and 18 percent in the United States (Leavitt). In Wolfe's view the association between TMJD and fibromyalgia was probably not fortuitous, and he suggested possible explanations for this association:

1. Decreased pain threshold of fibromyalgia results in facial and TMJD pain and symptoms.
2. Fibromyalgia and TMJD are linked to psychological distress.
3. The psychological distress noted in some fibromyalgia patients leads to increased somatic concern, medical visits, and diagnostic prevalence of TMJD.

4. All pain disorders are associated in an increased prevalence of fibromyalgia.

In his self-reporting survey of twenty-five hundred persons with fibromyalgia, Bennett (2007) found 29 percent had pain in the jaw. Blotman (2006) noted jaw joint problems as a characterizing feature of fibromyalgia, as did the Arthritis Foundation (2006) and Starlanyl (2001), who illustrated trigger points in the masseter.

VULVODYNIA

The vulva is the external part of the female genitalia. The outer and inner lips of the vulva are called the labia majora and labia minora. The vestibule surrounds the opening of the vagina and the urethra. The openings to Skene's and Bartholin's glands are located within the vestibule. The perineum is the area between the lower vulva around the anus and back to the coccyx.

The International Society for the Study of Vulvovaginal Disease (ISSVD) definition: "Vulvar discomfort, most often described as burning pain, occurring in the absence of relevant visible findings or a specific, clinically identifiable, neurologic disorder." Although the condition had been described in the textbooks for more than a hundred years, it did not achieve the status of having its own name, vulvodynia, until 1976 (Moyal-Barracco 2004). Metts (1999), describes it more in terms of its effects on the person as a "Syndrome of unexplained vulvar pain, frequently accompanied by physical disabilities, limitation of daily activities, sexual dysfunction and psychologic distress." Problems due to the pain and tenderness are created with any physical contact with the vulva, including undergarments, use of tampons or pads, and any form of sexual contact.

Frequency

In a survey of nearly one thousand women, conducted by the University of Michigan, researchers had not set out to explore vulvodynia but found 3 percent of women reported experiencing pain—"That's millions of women across the United States." Fifty percent had experienced dyspareunia at some point in their lives, 30 percent reported vestibular pain, and 3 percent reported pain lasting more than three months. Of those currently experiencing pain, 80 percent reported their pain as severe. The problems were as common among women of African heritage as European (Barclay 2004).

The problem is sufficiently significant that a branch of the National Institutes of Health, the Office of Research on Women's Health, has issued a pamphlet

(NIH 2007). They refer to the research of Harlow and Stewart in Boston and Bachman's group, who concluded 18 percent of women will at some time experience vulvodynia, with greatest frequency between the ages of eighteen to twenty-five, and decreasing after the age of thirty-five. They reported that 40 percent of the women suffered silently and did not seek care; of those who sought medical care, 60 percent had seen three or more doctors. Although the incidence of the condition was found equally distributed between white and black populations, it was 80 percent more frequent in women of Hispanic origin.

Statistical surveys vary in their results, for reasons best left to the statisticians to explain. A telephone survey of more than two thousand households found vulvar pain of six months' duration in nearly 4 percent of the respondents, 45 percent found interference with their sexual lives, and 27 percent with lifestyle (Arnold 2007).

Physical Examination

A full general examination is required to eliminate systemic disease. The pelvic examination is usually unremarkable visually, though pain may be caused by the examination. Areas of extreme tenderness, amounting to pain, may be located using very gently the tip of a cotton swab. Essentially, the diagnosis of vulvodynia is only valid when no pathology can be found that can better explain the pain. Reed (2006), from the surveyed University of Maryland group, concluded vulvodynia could be accurately diagnosed from the self-reported history but needed to be confirmed as such by later physical examination.

Cause

The cause is unknown. All known causes must be eliminated to justify the residual diagnosis of vulvodynia, which in other terminology would be "vulvar pain nyd (not yet diagnosed)." Reed (2006), involved in the University of Michigan study, reported current research using functional MRI (fMRI) to assess brain changes when pain in the vulva is provoked. It is to be expected that an inheritance, genetic basis, would be postulated (Gerber 2003), and alteration of pain sensitivity would be considered (Bohm-Starke 2001; Pukall 2002).

Treatments

The American College of Obstetricians and Gynecologists suggests, treatments should first be tried topically with gentle care of the vulva (Spitzer 2006).

The list of don'ts: no undergarments at night, no use of douches, no vaginal wipes, no bubble baths; no scented soaps, no pads with deodorants; no exercise that pressures the vulva, such as bicycling or horse riding. The list of do's: only cotton underpants, mild unscented soap, cooling gels on the vulva; lubricants with intercourse.

Improvement will be slow. If required, and under medical direction, treatment may include oral medication, local injection at trigger points, biofeedback, physical training, diet, cognitive behavioral therapy, and sex counseling. The University of Michigan study reported success with gabapentin and amitriptyline, which is in itself suggestive of a neuropathic involvement, not necessarily the primary cause. Surgical treatment is sometimes undertaken to excise the painful area; unsurprisingly there is wide variation in reports of benefits obtained.

Psychological Implications

Persistent pain; serious interference with personal, family, and professional life; a failure to obtain a satisfactory explanation; and a failure to receive satisfactory treatment can reasonably be expected to aggravate the patient and lead to a secondary depression (Metts 1999).

Bodden-Heidrich (1999) compared patients with chronic pelvic pain (CPP) to those with vulvodynia (VD); although the more severe cases in both groups showed signs of depression, there was evidence of somatization with CPP but not VD and it was concluded they are two distinct and different conditions.

After examining the women in the University of Michigan study, Reed (2000) concluded those suffering vulvodynia were not distinguishable from the general population in terms of history of abuse, and there was no evidence for a primary psychological cause for vulvodynia.

From a self-reporting Internet survey recognizing that some patients may have had conditions other than vulvodynia, Gordon (2003) found a wide range of comorbidities including irritable bowel syndrome, fibromyalgia, and interstitial cystitis; their sex lives, self-esteem, and relationships had been severely adversely affected.

It is inevitable that molestation or other violence in childhood should be considered as a possible cause of vulvodynia. Harlow and associates (2005) thought there was inconsistency in prior studies; they found patients with vulvar pain were two and a half times more likely to have been deprived of affection in childhood, and there was strong association with childhood sexual abuse, particularly by a member of the family.

Mascherpa (2007) viewed the characteristics of vulvodynia to be consistent with a somatoform disorder and was of the opinion that a full psychological and sexual evaluation should be undertaken when this diagnosis is made.

CHAPTER EIGHT

TODAY AND THE FUTURE

THE ECONOMIC BURDEN

Some words can be used carelessly, and it doesn't really matter. Others have exact legal definitions and must be employed cautiously. *Disability* and *impairment* are fine examples. Since the awarding of pensions hangs on the meaning of the words, one would expect each to have a single exact and unwavering definition; unfortunately we find each word has acquired several exact definitions. It's all a little like Alice, who when told she should say what she meant, replied she meant what she said and "that's the same thing you know." Even the March Hare knew it's not.

The medical community, the public, and the scientific literature commonly misunderstand the distinction between disability and impairment. Agencies and authorities do not agree in their definitions. The patient, the doctor, and the legal representative must be aware of the definition that's in use by the particular authority with which they are dealing (Holmes 2007).

Impairment

The World Health Organization (WHO) defines impairment as "Any loss or abnormality of psychological, physiological or anatomical structure or function." One thinks this definition must have been composed by human rights plaintiffs' lawyers—nothing has been overlooked. If you're shortsighted, you have an abnormality in your anatomy. If you're anything less than carefree, you have an abnormality in your psychological function; if you're too carefree, well, the same. No need to belabor the point. The definition is so all-embracing, it's useless.

The American Medical Association publishes *Guides to the Evaluation of Permanent Impairment,* and this guide is widely but not universally accepted. The AMA defines impairment as "An alteration of an individual's health status; a deviation from normal in a body part or organ system and its functioning."

Both the WHO and the AMA definitions are wide-open, and in that sense they underscore the difference between impairment and disability. Understanding the origin of the word *impairment* helps to understand its meaning, since it has the same derivation as *pejorative* and implies making something worse by diminishing it in quantity or value. And that's where the assessment stops. Stops at the statement of loss and deliberately refrains from making any comment on the significance of that loss.

Each state has its own workers' compensation system with its own definition of impairment, but in general they are consistent with the definition expressed in the AMA guides, and most private carriers of workperson's disability will accept them.

The US Federal Government Social Security Administration (SSA) defines a medically determinable impairment as, "An impairment that results from anatomical, physiological, or psychological abnormalities which can be shown by medically acceptable clinical and laboratory diagnostic techniques." The SSA further states that a physical or mental impairment must be established by medical evidence consisting of signs, symptoms, and laboratory findings, not only by the individual's statement of symptoms. Clearly, this definition is much more restrictive. What are the laboratory tests to confirm the schizophrenic's statement, "I hear voices telling me to kill myself"? Or the woman suffering from the pain of tic douloureux described elsewhere?

According to the AMA guides, a permanent impairment is one that has reached maximum medical improvement (MMI), has stabilized, and is unlikely to change substantially in the next year, with or without medical treatment. Commonly an assessment of a work-incurred injury is not made until two years after the injury, by which time the treating physician can reasonably judge whether the patient has recovered or to what extent she will never do so.

Disability

There are legal definitions of disability and there are sociological definitions. *Disability* is something that results from an *impairment.* The extent and significance of the disability will depend on the particular impairment and cannot be determined without first defining that impairment, which is likened to the stone thrown into a placid pool—the series of ripples the impairment creates is the disability that affects many strata of the society around the patient.

It must also be borne in mind that disability is not a free-standing characteristic. It must be used in conjunction with the word *from*. The classical comparison is made between the surgeon, the typist, and the concert pianist, each of whom has lost a couple of fingers from her nondominant hand. To the surgeon this is an irritation but would not interfere overmuch with the ability to work normally; to the typist it's an aggravation, not an insuperable problem. But to the concert pianist it's the end of her career and is personally and socially devastating. The issue is *from*. What is the impaired person disabled *from* doing?

Then once having determined what the person is disabled from doing, the opposite side of the coin must be assessed. What is the residual ability?

The AMA guide defines disability as "An alteration of an individual's capacity to meet personal, social, or occupational demands because of an impairment." Impairment ratings derived from the AMA guides are "not intended for use as direct determinants of work disability." Many states, however, utilize the impairment ratings determined by the AMA guides as direct measures of disability, despite this disclaimer. Pretty much the same as the ACR guidelines for defining fibromyalgia; the object lesson is that guidelines become cast in stone. Did Moses really intend to be taken that seriously?

WHO defines disability as "An activity limitation that creates a difficulty in the performance, accomplishment, or completion of an activity in the manner or within the range considered normal for a human being. Difficulty encompasses all of the ways in which the performance of the activity may be affected." Once again, that's so all-embracing, so vague, that it's hard to attach any level of significance to such a definition that employs the word *difficulty*.

Workers' compensation legislation concerns loss of ability to work resulting from an injury, illness, or occupational disease attributable to employment. This now considers *from*, effectively stating "*from* an ability to work."

The Americans with Disabilities Act (ADA) defines disability as meaning: a physical or mental impairment that substantially limits one or more of the major life activities of the individual; a record of such an impairment; or being regarded as having such an impairment. Under the broad definition of the ADA, almost any medical condition, under the right circumstances, could be proposed as a disability. No wonder this nebulous description is the source of so much work for lawyers.

SSA defines disability as, "The inability to engage in any substantial, gainful activity by reason of any medically determinable physical or mental impairment(s), which can be expected to result in death or which has lasted or can be expected to last for a continuous period of not less than 12 months." The

SSA disability program deals with two choices: the claimant is considered either entirely disabled or not disabled—no partials permitted. To determine whether a claimant is qualified for benefits, the SSA uses a medical consultant to determine physical and mental capacity to perform basic work activities. An adjudicator determines whether, with the residual functional capacity assigned, this person can return to his or her past job or to any other job taking into account age and education in the vocational analysis.

Numbers and Dollars—General Population

Some researchers have estimated that there are forty-three million persons in the United States alone who have a disability according to the ADA definition. These numbers suggest an estimated economic cost of approximately one hundred and seventy-six billion dollars.

According to the 1990 Centers for Disease Control and Prevention (CDC) data, the inability to perform work as a result of a physical, mental, or other health condition costs approximately one hundred and twelve billion dollars each year in the United States. According to self-reported data of the 1990 US Census, an estimate of nearly thirteen million persons aged sixteen to sixty-four years had a work disability; six and a half million of these disabilities were described as severe, and just over six million were described as nonsevere. As of June 2001, only slightly less than seven million individuals were receiving cash and medical benefits under the SSA disability insurance program, totaling over fifty-nine billion dollars that year. In 2004, the number of disability claim applications allowed benefits was nearly eight hundred thousand. The sheer volume of disability claims evaluated becomes evident, given an approval rate well under 50 percent of applicants (just over 37 percent in 2004). In the same year, SSA paid out over seventy-eight billion dollars in cash disability benefits alone, with nearly eight million persons in payment status (Holmes 2007).

Pain as a Cause of Disability

Annually, ten million visits are made to physicians based on a complaint of pain. Fifteen percent of patients who visit their doctors complain of being tired. Eighty-five billion dollars is spent each year in the United States in the diagnosis of pain. Thirteen billion dollars is spent annually in the United States on "alternative" therapies, a euphemism that implies the physician would neither have ordered them, nor would she have agreed willingly to their use.

An inability to perform normal tasks, as measured by self-reporting, is common in the fibromyalgia population (Wolfe 1995). This is supported by the abnormal scores in the widely used Health Assessment Questionnaire (HAQ), as reported in the United States (Hawley 1991) and the United Kingdom (Ledingham 1993). HAQ scores and the ability to perform work tasks were statistically correlated (Cathey 1988).

Work Disability

The definition of disability from work and employment compensation differs in each country and with each of the many social systems. Despite the superficial appearance of normality many fibromyalgia patients have difficulty remaining competitive in the workforce (Bennett 1996). Most report that chronic pain and fatigue adversely affect their quality of life and negatively impact their ability to be competitively employed (Hawley 1991; Henriksson 1992 and 1995). The extent of reported disability varies greatly from country to country, probably reflecting the differences in political philosophies and socioeconomic realities (Bruusgaard 1963; Bengtsson 1986; Ledingham 1993; Bennett 2008).

A survey of fibromyalgia patients seen in six US centers reported that 42 percent were employed and 28 percent were homemakers. Seventy percent perceived themselves as being disabled. Twenty-six percent were receiving at least one form of disability payment (Wolfe 1997). Sixteen percent were receiving Social Security benefits, compared to just over 2 percent in the overall US population.

In Sweden, after an average of seven years, 55 percent of persons with fibromyalgia were unable to do their necessary household tasks, and 24 percent were receiving disability pensions (Bengtsson 1986).

In the United States, separate reports from the same centers over a two-year period showed a disability rate between 6 and 9 percent (Cathey 1986 and 1988); of these persons, over 5 percent were receiving disability pensions; 30 percent had changed jobs; and 17 percent had retired because of fibromyalgia.

In another US center, 22 percent were reported as disabled, and 33 percent had changed jobs due to fibromyalgia (Mason 1989).

In a 1990 multicenter study of 620 patients, 15 percent had received disability payments. Nearly 9 percent of these were Social Security payments.

In a 2007 self-reporting survey of twelve hundred fibromyalgia patients, mostly living in the United States, the respondents were nearly equally divided regarding their ability to maintain gainful employment. Those who were still working felt their symptoms compromised their ability to be productive due to frequent absences and reduced work hours. Approximately 20 percent of the respondents had filed some form of disability claim and 6 percent received worker's compensation (Bennett 2007).

Approximately one-third of patients with fibromyalgia reportedly modify their work to keep their jobs. Some patients shorten their workdays, their work-weeks, or both. Many patients with fibromyalgia changed to jobs that are less physically and mentally taxing than their previous ones. This change often leads to decreased income and increased financial burdens. One report suggests that approximately 15 percent of the people with fibromyalgia are receiving disability benefits. Disability rates as high as 44 percent are reported (Gilliland 2007).

Utilization of Healthcare Services

In the 2007 survey (Bennett), responders reported over the past year for their fibromyalgia visits to healthcare providers (96 percent at least once, 44 percent one to four visits, 33 percent five to eight times, 14 percent nine to twelve visits, 13 percent more than twelve visits; the questions this provokes: Did the patient initiate the visit? Or was she told to return? Did she need frequent visits to renew a prescription for a controlled drug?). Responders also reported on their visits to emergency departments (29 percent on at least one to four occasions) and hos-pitalization due to fibromyalgia (3.5 percent). Another perspective on outpatient visits showed an average ten trips to the hospital per year (Wolfe 1997).

This is a chronic, relapsing condition: in academic centers, patients average ten outpatient visits per year; one hospitalization per three years. Health status unchanged after seven-year follow-up; 50 percent dissatisfied with their health; 59 percent rated their health as poor. In comparison with other rheumatic condi-tions, fibromyalgia patients have more comorbid medical conditions, more sur-gical interventions, more abnormal pain scores, more disability, fatigue, sleep disturbance, and psychologic issues (Winfield 2007).

A Canadian study reported the average number of annual visits to healthcare providers was 11.6, to the emergency room 0.6, and hospital inpatient days were 2.1 (White 2002).

Numbers and Dollars—Fibromyalgia

One report suggests that approximately 15 percent of people with fibromyalgia are receiving disability benefits; others give a higher figure of more than 25 per-cent receiving disability or compensation payments with disability rates as high as 44 percent reported (Winfield 2007); however, Horizon (2005) gives a figure of only 10 percent receiving disability payments.

Approximately 70 percent of the 2007 self-reporting sample had medical insurance. Most responders had out-of-pocket expenses related to management of their fibromyalgia. For instance, 74 percent of responders reported spending between one hundred and five hundred dollars each month on over-the-counter products, whereas 61 percent spent the same amount on prescription medications (Bennett 2007).

An estimate of the overall annual cost of this disease to the American economy is over nine billion dollars (Gilliland 2007).

Fibromyalgia is estimated as between two and five times more common than rheumatoid arthritis (Wolfe 1995). Therefore, it can be anticipated medical costs for fibromyalgia will be at least double those for rheumatoids, although there is an important difference in that fibromyalgia patients are not expected to show joint destruction and are not likely to need an arthroplasty (Russell 2004).

Studies from the United States (Wolfe 1997) and Canada (White 1999) showed annual direct medical cost per individual was $2,275. If multiplied by the 2 percent prevalence in the population (Croft 1994; Wolfe 1995), overall costs in the United States can be estimated at twelve to fifteen billion dollars annually (Russell 2004).

These costs can be apportioned in three equal categories: hospitalization, outpatient visits, and medication (Wolfe 1997). There is very little justification for the management of pain in hospital except sometimes to exclude other diagnoses, which could have been done better on an outpatient basis (Wolfe 1982; Baker 1988; Erhardt 1989; Mitchell 1989). Early consideration of fibromyalgia in the differential diagnosis should be in place, lessening hospitalization, not considering fibromyalgia as a last resort, as an exclusion diagnosis, but one that should be made early on as a positive diagnosis.

In Canada the annual costs generated by fibromyalgia patients are twice those of chronic widespread pain patients (White 1999).

Medical/Legal Pitfalls

Although no basis for many of the multiple symptoms of patients with fibromyalgia will be found on physical examination or laboratory testing, the physician must remain alert for organic illness (e.g., colon cancer in a patient with irritable bowel syndrome).

Secondary gain becomes a major perpetuator of illness in people with fibromyalgia if there was an injury at work or involvement in a minor motor vehicle accident that is inappropriately identified as a trigger of their illness. Well-meaning physicians, unaware of the biopsychosocial nature of fibromyalgia and current clinical and epidemiologic research data that, in the aggregate, fail to support trauma as a cause or trigger of fibromyalgia, unwittingly create legal imbroglios that adversely affect the patient's long-term prognosis. Associations of events do not establish causality.

The ACR criteria for classification of fibromyalgia have created a major pitfall with respect to diagnosis. These are classification criteria, not diagnostic criteria, that have not been validated in compensation settings. Pain at tender points is subject to manipulation by the patient. The ACR criteria have no place for diagnosis in clinical settings (Winfield 2007).

Canada's Supreme Court ordered Sun Life Insurance to compensate Ms. C F, 38, accused of faking symptoms of fibromyalgia and chronic fatigue syndrome "despite lacking adequate medical evidence to back up the conclusion." She was cut off benefits in 1998, although her policy entitled her to benefits if she was "unable to do any job" (*Globe & Mail*, Toronto, June 29, 2006).

Prevention of Disability

There is no dispute that constant pain, inadequate sleep, and severe fatigue individually and collectively constitute an impairment. But need that impairment be the cause of a disability?

Most fibromyalgia patients are not disabled but are differently "able" (Wallace 2005). No one is better off financially or emotionally by being declared unemployable. Every effort must be made through all aspects of the medical and social systems to keep the patient in a form of gainful employment. Time away from work must be minimized. It is well known to all experienced physicians that the longer a patient is away from work, the harder it will be to return to any employment. Therapy will play a role in rehabilitation, but the patient should not be kept away from work in order to be treated.

IS FIBROMYALGIA A REAL DISEASE?

"Question everything," Euripides said. Of course, that's not all he had to say, but it's a useful beginning to set the tone for the argument we're about to construct. Professor Blotman in his excellent, attractive, and informative book names professors Hadler, Ehrlich, and others of the same ilk as "fibroskeptics" for holding to an argument along the lines of "the pain is real, fibromyalgia is not." Professor Wallace (2004), author and editor of excellent books, urges "fibromyalgia nihilists" to stop pontificating and notes the type of complaints presented by fibromyalgia patients "date back to biblical times, and will not go away."

Professor Wolfe cannot have been warned by his mother of the dangers of talking to journalists. Although he was the lead author of the 1990 American College of Rheumatology text that defined the criteria for fibromyalgia, although he is the author of many papers in this field, and although he is sought after to write chapters in textbooks, he is quoted in the *New York Times* as saying he has become cynical and discouraged about the diagnosis (and) considers the condition a physical response to stress, depression, and economic and social anxiety (Berenson 2008).

Professor Clauw, author of many articles and director of advanced research, describes the articles of his older colleagues, with whom he would seem to disagree, as "pejorative," "uninformed," and "false." Professor Bennett, author of many articles and much research, freely quoted in this book, disagrees in more professional language: "The symptoms of fibromyalgia are common and real." The number of letters written by leaders in the field suggest an organized campaign "to get out the troops." Ms. Matallana in the same series of responding letters describes her personal problems with fibromyalgia, bedridden for two years, which led her to found an Internet site, and to this site were addressed numerous indignant and infuriated letters. Dr. Lapp, not yet risen beyond the assistant consulting professor stage, advises the *New York Times* readers, "Skeptics will always exist."

Whether these respected professors appear as expert witnesses in court is not known; if they do they will doubtless be aware of the rhetorical difference between *ad rem* and *ad hominem.* When the advocate does not have valid evidence permitting him to attack the subject, he will resort to an attack on the messenger.

These various responses to an article that was making a reasonable attempt to explore an important issue characterize certain features of the condition that, only since 1990, is officially designated as fibromyalgia. There is vituperous and intense hostility directed at anyone who raises any questions about the condition or who writes or says anything other than in its praise. Anyone who has doubts about this should type "fibromyalgia blog" into Google's advanced search. It seems to have been elevated to the level of religious dogma—put beyond question. The diagnosis has become infallible. The diagnosticians have become infallible. Some claim for themselves that degree of infallibility, where they are not merely exempt from error but have exemption from the possibility of error. And there can be few other conditions where the majority of books on the subject are written by persons who suffer the condition. A description of overwhelming personal disability is a *sine qua non* for the preface.

"Become cynical and discouraged about the diagnosis," Professor Wolfe says about himself. May we quote Ambrose Bierce? "Cynicism is that blackguard defect of vision which compels us to see the world as it is, instead of as it should be" (Fitzhenry 1986). Is that defect of vision inappropriate in a professor?

Skeptic? Why should it be used as a term of abuse? "A person seeking the truth, an inquirer who has not yet arrived at definite convictions" is what the *Oxford English Dictionary* says—doesn't sound like a bad fellow at all. Aren't all doctors seeking the truth? Pyrrho, who started the idea, seems to have been a bit confused over what he meant, so we'll give him a pass; too much armchair thinking would leave us no further than Descartes with his *cogito ergo sum*. In our self-congratulatory era of scientific thought, we physicians remain partial skeptics—no more than semi-skeptics. We don't go so far as to deny the existence of whatever we can't prove by argument, all the while standing on a cold porch in the rain, but we accept "best evidence" and remain open to further examination. Or if we turn our minds back twenty-five hundred years, *we question everything*.

Enter the Devil's Advocate

A committee wrote the King James version of the Holy Bible (Nicolson 2003). They wrote it in English, contrived from multiple items in several archaic languages. They can never have expected it would later be held to be the direct word of God, who so conveniently spoke to them in the vernacular English, nor that every word they wrote must later be accepted without question.

The American College of Rheumatology in 1990 was confronted with multiple views on how many tender points were needed to justify a diagnosis of fibromyalgia. One has to wonder if any member of the committee asked, "How many thousands of spirits can dance upon a needle's point?" (Cudworth 1678). After 1990 it was decided eleven out of eighteen was the right number for research purposes (the different views on this number have been described). And this too became Gospel. Like it came down from on high. But it was no more than the work of a well-meaning human committee, the lead author of which now says he's become "cynical and discouraged about the diagnosis."

Pope Sixtus V in 1587 conferred the title *Promotor Fidel* (Promoter of the Faith) on an officer of the church whose function was to look under every stone, search for every negative reasoning that might be offered against conferring on a seemingly worthy individual the title of saint. With a touch of irony, the holder of this office became known as *Advocatus Diaboli*—the Devil's Advocate.

We use the principle of *Advocatus Diaboli* to determine whether fibromyalgia, effectively beatified in 1990, is worthy of being canonized. In making his examination, there was no intent to belittle or besmirch his subject, nor did the Devil's Advocate suffer abuse in the performance of his task. It must always have been Advocatus' expectation that the subject would in fact be worthy of the honor to be bestowed, but it was his task to prove it, or to display the reasoning why it should not be granted.

Professor Blotman quotes Kahn in requesting a cease-fire between the two sides until more information is available, but here the Devil's Advocate does not "take sides," he merely explores the groundwork for a decision.

Define the Issue

We need first to be sure we're all talking about the same thing, all of us on the same wavelength. First, what do we mean by a disease? And then, when is a disease "real"? Are there "unreal" diseases?

"Disease" is easy enough. Although it's used in a restricted sense in pathology, it has its origins from the French, meaning "away from ease" and initially meant no more than "uneasy." Only in later centuries was it given a medical connotation, which can just as well be replaced by "condition" or "disorder." There's no question that persons with fibromyalgia are not at their ease, and anyway, we've already explained why "syndrome" is preferred at this stage of our knowledge to "disease." Professor Yunus, who has written much in this field, has explored the "nosology for fibromyalgia and the overlapping conditions." He rejects "disease-illness" and prefers "syndrome" (2008).

So, yes, call it syndrome, condition, disease, or what you please—the person diagnosed with fibromyalgia is not at her ease.

Are There "Unreal" Diseases?

There are instances when the person is consciously pretending to have symptoms that are created for a purpose—to avoid school, an unworthy preference not to be killed in the war, or to get a disability pension. The process is conveniently called "malingering" and is mentioned only briefly in DSM to ensure it is not confused with a true psychologic disorder. Occasionally one will meet a doctor who declares, "There's no such thing as a malingerer," and one will also meet persons who've never been outside central Africa who'll tell you there are no people in this world with blue eyes—it's all a question of exposure and experience.

But there is no suggestion that the person with fibromyalgia is malingering. Prudent physicians follow the basic rule in the practice of medicine, "She has as much pain as she says she has." The only question that arises is whether the diagnosis she's been given is appropriate. For a woman who's told her pain is due to a prolapsed disc, and then she passes a kidney stone, although the severity of her pain was never in doubt, the diagnosis she was given was not appropriate.

An "unreal" disease is not a wrong diagnosis. It's like the Loch Ness monster—created to impress, to explain what is not understood, and not without coincidence, to profit from the facile explanation. There are many historic examples described by Professor Shorter, such as the paralyses and convulsions cured by magnetism, and the "colitis" Axel Munthe conjured from his imagination to satisfy a patient suffering (to him) bizarre pains. So yes, there are "unreal" diseases.

A Modern-Day "Unreal" Disease

This whole domain of illness without disease, the real essence of functional has always been a sandbox for theory builders (Shorter 1992).

Professor Wallace (2005) quotes Meador (1965), "When a specific disease is suspected but not found, the patient has a particular nondisease," and he recognizes "a minority of distinguished rheumatologists have published that fibromyalgia is a nondisease, a medically unexplained syndrome that does not exist" (Meador 1965; Bohr 1996; Wessely 2001; Ehrlich 2003; Hadler 2003; Butler 2004), and he has challenged their statements (Wallace 2004).

There is a common modern condition, in which the typical patient is a middle-age, well-educated female in a white-collar profession. The frequency of the various reported symptoms is: headache 55 percent; fatigue 51 percent; confusion 31 percent; depression 30 percent; shortness of breath 29 percent; arthralgia 26 percent; myalgia 25 percent; nausea 20 percent; dizziness 18 percent; memory problems 14 percent; gastrointestinal symptoms 14 percent; respiratory symptoms 14 percent. No single widely accepted test of physiologic function can be shown to correlate with the symptoms, and typically the patients with this condition do not have any defining abnormalities on physical or laboratory examination. Substantial controversy exists about this condition, including whether it's a primary psychiatric disorder or a combination of psychiatric and organic medical syndromes (Venuturapalli 2005).

No, this one's not the fibromyalgia syndrome; it's the previously described multiple chemical sensitivities syndrome. "Unreal" in what sense? Not unreal to the person with all those complaints, but unreal to the justice system of the United States and unreal to all major medical bodies since, unlike what Koch was able to show, there is a lack of evidence of cause and effect. Probably someone came out with the *shibboleth*, "absence of evidence is not evidence of absence," but as of now MCS as a medical entity does not exist. It's a "nondisease."

What about a disease whose diagnostic criteria are: a physical complaint of six or more months that cannot be fully explained by any known condition; the complaints and impairment are grossly in excess of what the history, examination, and lab findings would indicate?

No. Once again, this is not fibromyalgia. This one's accepted as a "disorder," the undifferentiated somatoform disorder, previously described. That's an emotional disorder, and it seems that if the proponents accept the inexplicability of "no physical signs" as emotional, then it passes muster; but try and say it's a physical problem even though there are no physical signs, and it's left out in the cold, turning slowly in the breeze.

When Is a Disease Real?

"Real" must mean there's a consensus among the knowledgeable members of the profession who say that such-and-such a condition is found, or is there to be diagnosed. They find signs and symptoms that characterize it. They write papers about it. Since they want it to be generally accepted they take it to official bodies for their stamp of approval, a bit like getting your vineyard accepted. Unlike getting a drug approved by the FDA, no tests are required to get a disease approved, it just needs the right people sitting on the right committees putting their project to the right other people sitting on all of their committees, and they're all part of the same university medical specialty-circuit coterie. There's nothing wrong with that. They're all honorable professionals giving their time, and usually without reward, to further their patients' interests.

Other examples have been cited in this book. The entire DSM is composed of committee decisions classifying the various mental conditions. Committees classified the many sleep disorders and the many forms of functional gastro-intestinal disorders. But the acceptance of the name of a disease or condition does not prove anything beyond a consensus of involved and knowledgeable persons supporting it. Quinter and Cohen (1999) go to lengths to point out that the effect of a condition should not be confused with the name of the condition, that fibromyalgia cannot be both the result of widespread musculoskeletal pain and the cause of that pain.

The skeptic believes he doesn't know the whole truth, or that there is any final truth. Isn't that what doctors are supposed to believe? After all, they say the half-life of medical knowledge is only five years, and it's a pity we don't know which half until it's too late.

There are some absolute truths in medicine. The cause of tuberculosis was "miasma" until Koch showed them the tubercle bacillus. Even then there were debunkers. How could a little thing like a bacillus devastate a strong and healthy man? they asked. You might just as well think the bird sitting on the pile of horse manure had caused it, they said. But Koch used his time-honored postulates, had evidence to prove his points, and his explanation for the disease has remained "real."

Is It All or None?

Saints aren't born as such, they have to work up to their full status, and it takes time. It's the same with medical conditions. Maybe, if it's a fracture or a gun-shot wound, one second you don't have it, and the next you do, but medical conditions don't happen that way. Some brew rapidly, like a strep throat, some brew slowly, like tuberculosis. Some grind away at a low chronic level like blockage of a coronary artery; at first it's mild angina with effort, then it's angina without any effort, then it's overwhelming pain with an infarct.

What reason do we have to suppose fibromyalgia is different? As already observed, you don't suddenly break out one day in those fibromyalgic spots. Doesn't going from doctor to doctor (some persons report they saw more than twenty doctors) imply the gradual development of the syndrome? Agreed, some doctors are a bit slow on the uptake, but the condition is well known to the profession, the report of seeing numerous doctors so common, that progressive development of the condition is a more rational interpretation for the late diagnosis than is widespread obduracy and stupidity in the medical profession. It is simply not rational to suppose that the patient had on the first day of her condition widespread four-quarter-plus axial pain, and all the tender spots, nor that she went to her first contact doctor and said, "I hurt in my neck and my back, I hurt in both arms and in both legs, and I hurt in all these places when you press on them."

We have a wealth of information about the patient when she's been diagnosed with fibromyalgia, but there's insufficient information about the progression of the condition from its first stirrings.

Pain Clinic Viewpoint

There are those who specialize in arthritis, and for whom half their patient load might be persons whom they have diagnosed with fibromyalgia. On the other side of the coin are the specialists in the treatment of pain, pain as a field in itself, not pain due to a specific condition. What are their views?

Angela Mailis (2003) writes as director of the pain clinic in the same University of Toronto hospital in which Smythe and Moldofsky had in 1977 coined the term "fibrositis syndrome." Her views are, "As a lifelong student of chronic pain, I have had a hard time accepting fibromyalgia as a specific, definable and hopeless entity, and I am not alone. . . . All the symptoms attributed to fibromyalgia do not necessarily constitute a condition that is scientifically specific. . . . The vast array of symptoms shared in all these overlapping disorders makes none of them specific, unique, or well defined. . . . Certain abnormalities in neurotransmitters have been found, but are these the cause or the effect of chronic pain? . . . Many studies show significant psychosocial and environmental issues in patients diagnosed with fibromyalgia . . . have led other researchers to attribute the abnormal sensitivity to pain . . . to psychological factors, which result in switching attention more easily toward 'detecting pain.' . . . Ignoring the psychological and socio-environmental contributors, is short-sighted and undoubtedly leads to failed management."

Mailis also draws attention to the difficulty in making a diagnosis of fibromyalgia, recording the experience of Smythe (1997) in a self-imposed test, diagnosing 15 percent of real patients with fibromyalgia as "fakes" and up to 40 percent of the "fakes" as having fibromyalgia.

History of the Diagnostic Tender Point Count

The conceptual origin of "tender points" is reviewed by Quinter and Cohen (1999), who go back in time to Beard's concept of neurasthenia, a diagnosis that took the place of "muscular rheumatism," whose sufferers "were rarely free of tender spots" (Head 1922). Neurasthenia as a "real disease" did not carry any suggestion of deliberate misrepresentation (malingering) but the term fell out of favor. In 1976 Moldofsky and Scarisbrick postulated that neurasthenic-type symptoms might be due to sleep disturbance; a year later "fibrositis syndrome" was introduced by finding tender points in the muscles of these sleep-disturbed patients. Since it was known there was no local pathology to be found in these tender areas, it was necessary to postulate a central pain amplification mechanism (Smythe and Moldofsky 1977). The tender points were considered an essential aspect of the diagnosis but incidental to the pain experienced—two propositions that are mutually incompatible.

The intended purpose in defining the condition in this manner was to defend sufferers of chronic pain from accusations of psychiatric problems (Smythe 1979; Yunus 1981), but if the patient didn't have the requisite number of tender points, she failed the test and didn't get that distinguishing diagnosis of fibromyalgia. If she, however, was to get that diagnosis anyway, with fewer than the requisite number of defining points (Wolfe 1996), then the original purpose to distinguish a worthy group of patients from neurasthenia has failed, and "the diagnosis of fibromyalgia is out of control" (Wolfe 1997). Beard would be happy to know that neurasthenia is alive and thriving, even if masquerading under another name.

The American College of Rheumatology (ACR) 1990 committee reviewed data and selected two hundred and ninety-three patients and two hundred and sixty-five controls. The patients with putative fibromyalgia were divided into "primary" who had no other condition and "secondary" who had another painful condition of a musculoskeletal nature such as rheumatoid arthritis. Controls were divided into two similar nonfibromyalgia groups. Twelve pairs of tender points were selected; three of these pairs were later rejected as unsuitable. The reason for selection of the residual points was unclear. "Blinded" examiners, basing their conclusions exclusively on the tender point examination averaged 84 percent correct diagnoses. Viewed from the other direction, 16 percent of their tender point examination conclusions did not coincide with their clinical diagnoses.

Quinter and Cohen posed three difficult questions: If 19 percent of those with eleven or more tender points were judged not to have fibromyalgia, then what condition did they have? How are patients with widespread pain but less than eleven tender points to be diagnosed? What is the correct diagnosis for people with a high tender point count but without widespread pain?

Two years after the 1990 ACR classification criteria were promulgated, they were disputed at the 1992 European League Against Rheumatism (EULAR) meeting, the approximate European equivalent of the ACR (Harth 2007); the objections raised were:

- The number and location of the tender points is arbitrary.
- Control points were mentioned in the ACR paper (but not required), and they could also be found to be painful.
- Eleven or more tender points can be found in 5 percent of Healthy Normal Controls.
- Tender points were interpreted at this meeting as representing psychologic distress.

Wolfe, the lead author of the ACR 1990 paper, in hindsight (2003) wrote, "The idea that fatigue, sleep disturbance and pain alone could represent illness was new to rheumatology—fibromyalgia was fought bitterly in those days by the same persons who now compete for NIH grants to study it. . . . The criteria were a working tool for studying this diffuse and hard to characterize syndrome. . . . They ignited the fibromyalgia wars. . . . It was OK science but it was bad reality."

Significance of Tender Points

This is an issue of substantial importance to the question of fibromyalgia as a specific condition. The "tender points count" is the feature that distinguishes fibromyalgia from chronic widespread pain (CWP), accepting that less-well-defined condition to mean a distribution in four quarters of the body plus axial, as defined for fibromyalgia. If the tender point count is invalidated as a reliable test, then there is no justification in separating fibromyalgia into a unique compartment. That is not to suggest fibromyalgia is not "real," it is to suggest it is no more and no less real than other cases of chronic widespread pain. Quinter and Cohen (1999) discounted the essential significance of the tender points but postulated the patients have a "mechanical allodynia" not confined to the tender points, that they have lowered pain thresholds, resulting in altered pain recognition (nociception), all consistent with Yunus's central sensitization model.

In fact, Professor Wolfe (1997) later suggested tender points should be considered only as indicators of distress, and that numerically they indicated the extent of distress. Using an index (RDI, Rheumatology Distress Index) developed from measures of sleep disturbance, fatigue, anxiety, depression, and global severity, he found a direct relationship between this index and the number of tender points. Professor Harth (2007) believes that in their clinical practice many rheumatologists do not use tender points in their diagnostic decision, as had already been suggested by others (Katz 2006; Hughes 2006).

Professor Croft, director of a primary care musculoskeletal research center in an English university, has interested himself in this issue (Croft 1994). Clinical examination of patients who responded to a questionnaire and who also completed extensive questionnaires regarding sleep, fatigue, depression, and so on, of the type described elsewhere in this book, led him to the same conclusion as Professor Wolfe. He found most people with chronic widespread pain did not have high tender point counts, and conversely most people with high tender point counts did not have chronic widespread pain; he noted also that tender points were often found at locations other than those proposed by the ACR. His conclusions were, "Tender points are a measure of general distress" and "Fibromyalgia does not seem to be a distinct disease entity." As would only be expected, his methods, and therefore his conclusions, have been challenged (Harth 2007). But Professor Croft (2004) reasserts his position, stating, "No one knows what tender points actually mean," and adds, tender point counts are higher in persons with other symptoms such as fatigue and poor sleep but can also be found in persons who have no pain. He refers to a German study (presumably Schochat 2003) that demonstrated the higher the number of nonpain symptoms, the higher went the tender point count. The same conclusions as Wolfe and Croft that a high tender point count should be interpreted as an indicator of distress were reached. Unsurprisingly, their methodology also is challenged (Harth 2007).

Gracely (2007), a pain psychologist, draws attention to the obvious but generally unspoken fact that it is all too easy to fake a positive tender point, possibly inadvertently, possibly due to an overenthusiastic examiner. In a group of ninety-seven patients diagnosed in their clinic with fibromyalgia, only one-sixth were noticeably tender (Giesecke 2003). He suggests the possibility that the ACR line between widespread pain and tenderness is fallacious, and that the two may occur independently of each other, tenderness having no bearing on the diagnosis and treatment of fibromyalgia; in chronic widespread pain, although sensitivity to physical stimulation may be relevant, other symptoms such as mood or cognitive function may be more closely aligned with spontaneous pain and thus more important for diagnosis and treatment.

A study from Sweden also suggested there are separate groups of chronic widespread pain and fibromyalgia patients. Questionnaires with "pain mannequins" were sent to nearly ten thousand persons. The drawings revealed three hundred and forty-five persons with widespread pain, of whom one hundred and twenty-five were examined for tender points. The researchers concluded chronic widespread pain without tender points was present in 4.5 percent of the population, fibromyalgia in 2.5 percent, and that the fibromyalgia patients had a higher pain severity and more severe symptoms affecting daily life (Cöster 2008).

The unreliability of tender point counts was demonstrated by comparing three groups, one composed of fibromyalgia patients, a second healthy group prepared to simulate fibromyalgia, and a third healthy nonsimulator group; simulators could not be discriminated from genuine fibromyalgia patients by tender point examination; simulators were misidentified as fibromyalgia in one-third, and fibromyalgia misidentified as simulators in one-fifth of the persons examined (Khostanteen 2000).

What If There Weren't a Tender Point Examination?

It is reported that some diagnosticians are labeling their patients as "fibromyalgia" without doing a tender point count and that this is happening regularly in clinical practice (Hughes 2006; Katz 2006) to such an extent that 40 percent of the patients diagnosed with fibromyalgia prior to referral for management at one particular clinic did not meet the ACR criteria when examined there by the consulting specialists (Fitzcharles and Boulos 2003). According to Wolfe (2003), "Perhaps tender points as the essential criterion was a mistake. By ignoring the central psychosocial and distress features . . . we allowed fibromyalgia to be seen as mostly a physical illness. . . . We removed all traces of the most central features of the illness. . . . It was as if we were to define diabetes by requiring diabetic coma." If the tender point count was officially ignored, and if attention were paid only to chronic widespread pain, the approximate proportion of the population involved would be raised from the current 5 percent to twice or three times that number (Clauw 2003).

Suffering Victims

All the best saints have suffered and have been rejected. Certainly on those grounds the Advocatus would have to accept fibromyalgia. The fibromyalgia patients suffer. They suffer pain. They suffer rejection, rejection by many physicians. They suffer disbelief of their condition, labeled as "unreal" by a substantial portion of the profession.

There are of course some saints who were universally adored during their lifetime, but the ones we remember most were victims of the society in which they lived. Which raises an extremely touchy issue. Because in our modern society the victim is by mere virtue of her victimization raised to the level of sainthood. Put beyond any doubts. It is unthinkable and totally unacceptable ever to question whether the saint needed to provoke society to the extent she did. One must never ask, "Why did they choose her to be chained to the rock to make the dragon's tasty morsel?"

In our current brutal society, what are the demographic features that typify the victims? Certainly the weak have little opportunity to take advantage of the strong. And the weak? Who are they? Women, minority groups, and the financially disadvantaged are the usual victims. And what are the demographic characteristics of the fibromyalgia patient? Ninety-five percent women is the most obvious and universally reported feature. And the explanations usually offered to explain why that should be so are very thin indeed.

There's no doubt whatsoever—ask a policeman—that females are the victimized group in our society. Both when they're children and when they're adults. The remarkably high incidence of physical abuse in childhood has been noted already; this cannot take account of the unreported, denied, or "yet to be remembered" abuse, but it is beyond doubt that not everyone is going to talk about the nasty incidents of her childhood, particularly when the perpetrator is likely to have been a member of the family or a trusted, "highly respectable" person.

What happens to the child victims when they become adults? Most must put the incident behind them and out of their minds. Some cannot. Perhaps some choose to use it as their excuse for failing in society. Perhaps they failed because of their unerasable memories. A subject far too deep and socially difficult to enter here, but there is a "victim psychology" out there, and statistically fibromyalgia fits the demography of our society's most likely victim.

The Viewpoint of the Nonbelievers

"Chronic persistent pain is an ideation, a somatization that some are inclined towards as a response to living life under a pall . . . that these people choose to be patients because they have exhausted their wherewithal to cope. The complaint of persistent widespread pain should initiate a treatment act quite different from that leading to labeling as fibromyalgia. The symptoms of persistent widespread pain should be heard as likely surrogate complaints for psychosocial confounders to coping" (Hadler 2004).

"No one has fibromyalgia until it is diagnosed. Chronic pain remains chronic pain . . . until a doctor diagnoses fibromyalgia. Then support and advocacy groups aggravate the problem, disability is certified, a hopeless prognosis is offered. . . . Thus we have turned a common symptom into a remunerative industry. In Western cities, fibromyalgia tends to be diagnosed when no other reason is found for the pain. Giving a name to the pains has spawned the very symptom amplification and imitative behavior the rheumatologic profession should be combating. Is it any wonder that most treatments, at least the drugs and the obscene neurosurgical interventions, don't really work? One cannot really treat nondisease" (Ehrlich 2003).

The Viewpoint of the Reluctant Consultant

"I do believe there are patients who have widespread musculoskeletal pain attributed to a syndrome we call fibromyalgia. However, I do not believe rheumatologists should be the primary caregivers for these patients. . . . The main reason for my stance is the lack of any credible evidence supporting fibromyalgia as a rheumatological condition other than the existence of chronic pain. . . . With the burgeoning entrepreneurial specialty masquerading as 'pain management' my opinion is that these patients would be best served by those who claim to be pain specialists—if only we could get them to put their needles down long enough to actually treat the pain and the patient. . . . Labeling patients with fibromyalgia potentially encourages them to 'grow into' the label and remain unwell" (Luetkemeyer 2005).

An editorial in the respected *Journal of Rheumatology* observed, "Many physicians express frustration directed not only at the fibromyalgia construct, but also at the patient. This hostility seems related to the fact that patients with fibromyalgia display very much more psychological distress than other patients. All this is further compounded by the lack of effective treatment for it and the fact that many patients have a record of adversarial interaction within the health-care system. It is not so surprising that some rheumatologists will not see patients that are referred to them for fibromyalgia and others will only see the patients for a one-time assessment to exclude other conditions, but not provide ongoing care" (Graham 2003).

In the Alternative?

Professor Harth regards the tender point count as a convenience that is hard to relinquish, but he has pointed to its many defects in construction and practice. He suggests an alternative would be to redefine fibromyalgia based on a combination of underlying pathophysiological processes such as pain threshold, affective distress, and fatigue; this would allow consideration of typical fibromyalgia symptoms that are now only incidentally recognized.

The same approach was suggested in the Canadian study reported by Russell (2004).

ADVOCATUS' CONCLUSION: THE ENVELOPE, PLEASE

This is what has been established so far:

- There are five million persons in the United States bearing the diagnosis of fibromyalgia.
- They are nearly all women, although there is a juvenile form.
- The criteria for diagnosis were promulgated in 1990. They were disputed at the time and remain in dispute.
- The purpose in defining criteria was to set an agreed base point for research into the issue of patients with widespread pain and to set criteria to separate "real" clinical cases from "unreal" neurasthenics.
- Not intended by the members of the 1990 committee, these criteria have become fixed and unwavering determinants for who does and who does not qualify for a "real" diagnosis, named fibromyalgia.
- The diagnosis of fibromyalgia has become representative of a permanent and disabling condition and a foundation for disability awards, including civil litigation.
- The only required feature of the history is the patient's unverifiable report of chronic widespread pain.
- The only required feature of the physical examination is the patient's unverifiable complaint of pain when four kg pressure is applied by the thumb at eleven of eighteen designated points. Ten of these designated points are above the nipple line.
- The position of these "tender points" is displayed in pictures of spotty ladies, widely available on the Internet and in popular books and magazines.
- The choice of the points was arbitrary, both in location and in numbers. These points are tender to everyone, but were expected from experience to be more tender than usual, in fact painful, to someone with fibromyalgia.
- The test was for an abnormal sensitivity to pain, or lowered pain threshold. There is no known abnormality in the tissues that are compressed, nor was it ever supposed that there was a tissue abnormality.

- Chronic widespread pain is now known to occur in the absence of tender points. No diagnostic term was applied to this state, which has remained up in the air as a complaint and not designated as a disease.
- Tender points are now known to occur in the absence of chronic widespread pain. No diagnostic term was applied to this state, which has also remained up in the air as a complaint and not designated as a disease.
- In practical "real-life" terms, it is reported that many physicians, perhaps most outside university clinics, make their diagnosis on the basis of the history and either do not perform the tender point examination or may discount the results.
- It is suggested by the lead author of the 1990 report that the tender point examination is irrelevant to the diagnosis.
- Others, including that author, equate the tender point examination with the degree of the patient's distress.
- To some, the diagnostic approach has come full circle. The intention was to separate "real" from "unreal" and although most gave weight to the history, a physical test was devised as a *sine qua non*.
- It is now known that this physical test is unreliable, in that there are false positives and false negatives, and it excludes from an important diagnosis a significant element of patients. In fact, this was known at the time, or shortly after, the test was established.

WHAT IS CONTENDED?

Three issues need to be addressed:

1. Persons diagnosed with fibromyalgia resent intensely and even abusively the removal of the physical construct of the diagnosis, with the thought that fibromyalgia is consequently designated as "other than physical," which is to say "it's all in your head."
2. Is fibromyalgia a unique disease, in and of itself?
3. If it is agreed the tender point examination, worthy intention though it might have been in 1990, is not a valid indicator of a separate condition, what Pandora's box does that open? It is estimated that if history alone were the basis, the number of persons qualifying for the diagnosis would be raised by two- or three-fold.

Persons Diagnosed with Fibromyalgia
Reject Removal of the Physical Confirmation

If there is no physical sign, if there are symptoms but no signs, then to some persons the condition cannot be a physical one. It can be no more than emotional, which to some persons is tantamount to calling them a mental case. This conclusion ignores the invisibility of the pain associated with numerous conditions such as postherpetic neuralgia, tic douloureux, causalgia, diabetic neuropathy, and many others that have the advantage of social acceptability.

It is widely accepted that chemical and possibly physical changes occur in the central nervous system, neuroplasticity, resulting in an altered state of function called neuropathy. These changes are signaled by sophisticated tests that show the presence of neurotransmitter chemicals to be found in patients suffering from fibromyalgia in quantities that differ from those found in unaffected persons. Other sophisticated tests show altered functioning activity in the brains of persons with fibromyalgia, demonstrating their difference from healthy normal controls. There is no reason to suppose these changes cannot be reversed.

One can understand the urgency with which the patients insist their problem is physical and not emotional, but the weight attached by some researchers in the field when their conclusions are challenged, when they come to a forceful defense of their patients' viewpoint, is more suggestive of self-interested polemic than science.

These same researchers would serve their patients well if they were to go on the warpath on the bizarre modern concept of separation of mind and body. The ancient Chinese, Indians, and Greeks knew better, even today the witch doctor in central Africa knows better, but many Western physicians continue with this misapprehension. These biochemical tests of neurotransmitters measurably demonstrate the physical connection between mind and body. With PET scans and fMRI the lucky few can actually watch the mind in action. There is no longer any defense for arguing whether a symptom is "only in the mind."

Is Fibromyalgia a Unique Disease, in and of Itself?

There's a kind of a selfish streak to fibromyalgia. It seems almost as if sufferers are saying, "This is our disease—others keep out." Even the books written for the consumer talk "family" as do the networks and the blogs. Much of the research seems to be directed at proving a point, not at exploring a field to find what's there, but in proving a hypothesis that fibromyalgia is in some sense unique, leaving the work open to the criticism that the results are intended to please the customers—the customers of course being the researcher's own patients and the network supporting him. *(Noticeably a "him." Is this paternalistic?)*

The "tender points" was a well-meant idea, but a *faux pas*, a false step, conceptually fallacious, finding tender points in normal tissues and basing a diagnosis on finding pain where by definition there was no cause for pain. It's led the researchers into an impasse in both the French and the English meanings of that word. Some are unwilling to turn around and leave this blind alley. Others are reviled for doing so. But it makes no sense, and clinging to the well-intended mistake will not bring respect and will inevitably retard progress.

So what does that leave? It leaves all the symptoms of fibromyalgia, the distress, and the association with multiple other conditions as outlined by Yunus. These are sufficient for Wolfe to make his diagnosis; they're sufficient for many clinicians to make their diagnoses.

But is chronic widespread pain and distress unique? Is it peculiar to fibromyalgia? We know it's not.

The researchers have shown changes in neurochemistry and brain function in a small number of patients with fibromyalgia. People are funny. They're a bit reluctant to have needles stuck into their spines, so the ability to study cerebrospinal fluid and its circulating neurochemical transmitters is limited. MRI machines are expensive and usually they're expected to be revenue-earning; not many people have the luxury of using them for time-consuming research. So progress in learning is slow. And when opportunities are restricted, they'll be limited to a target group. We'll not know whether the observed neurochemical and brain-function changes are unique to fibromyalgia until it is shown they are not to be found in other cases of chronic widespread pain, nor in reflex sympathetic dystrophy, nor the multiple other forms of regional pain.

We do know changes of this nature are produced by both placebo and nocebo effects—further physical evidence of the mind-body inseparability. We have also learned over time that the alpha/delta sleep wave anomaly encountered in patients with fibromyalgia is in fact neither unique to that condition nor diagnostic of it.

So, no, nothing unique has been shown about fibromyalgia, except perhaps the expressed severity of the pain. But any clinician knows severity of expression has almost an inverse relationship to severity of pain. Some clinicians report how severe distress can be seen in the face of the patient with fibromyalgia. No doubt about that at all. But there's distress to be read in the face of the woman who walks the desert to bring her starving and emaciated child to a feeding camp in Ethiopia and the man who carries in his son whose feet were blown off by a landmine in Afghanistan. They have distress. You can see it in their faces. They don't have fibromyalgia.

If Tender Point Examination Is Not a Valid Indicator of a Separate Condition, What Pandora's Box Does That Open?

The original premise pursued by Smythe was to separate the worst affected patients from others who could or would be classified as neurasthenics and seemingly less worthy of a diagnosis. This skimmed the top off the iceberg, granting the status of "real disease" to a minority (who jealously guard that privilege) and leaving the majority out in the cold without so much as a name to put to their symptoms, beyond one supposes, "all in your head." Essentially this was the grossest form of discrimination, taking the loudest or most visible complainers, giving them status, and declining status to the balance.

The European League Against Rheumatism (EULAR) remarked on this dilemma shortly after the American College criteria were published, as have others who wanted to know how to classify the patients with widespread pain who did not match up with the ACR's spotty ladies, or those who had the spots but had less than a five-fifths regional distribution of their severe pain.

Advocatus concludes: "Pain is pain."

Pain and distress go hand in hand. There is no place for an Orwellian. "Some pains are more equal than others." The severity of the condition known as fibromyalgia has justified it being named. Other conditions of lesser severity of expressed pain and distress should not be excluded from that name.

WHAT TO DO?

Fully established fibromyalgia is the tip of the iceberg. The patient whose life revolves around her symptoms, who seeks on a regular basis the numerous non-traditional therapies, who has her own Internet blog describing in detail her daily travails and obscenely abuses the doctors who don't give her everything she demands, who after many rejections has now obtained permanent disability status supported by a pension—she is not going to be rehabilitated into functioning society.

On the other hand, the patient diagnosed with fibromyalgia who has remained as active as she could be, in her home and in her job, may well be benefited by the type of program outlined in previous chapters.

But in this, our last chapter, we give attention to how it all happened, to how the flood of disabilities attributable to conditions distinguished by "symptoms without signs" can be slowed, stayed, or possibly even turned around. This will require more than an analysis of the individual patient. It will require an analysis, a rethinking, and a reworking of our entire health system, which as so many have observed, is directed at ill health and not good health.

The physician's education has always been to learn about disease, to be compassionate certainly, but to be compassionate to the people who have a recognizable disease, people she can help, that's why she's there. But the profession has been too clever for it's own good. There isn't much traditional disease left. Many young doctors have experienced the pleasure of working in less wealthy countries, otherwise known as the "third world," or euphemistically, "developing world." There they find all their patients have "real" diseases, they're interesting medically, they can be helped, which gives an ego boost to the doctor. That's what she always wanted to do, why she spent those soul-destroying years in medical school.

Then when she returns to the "first world" and opens her practice, she finds traditional diseases are hard to come by. There's lots of obesity and degeneration accompanied by age, worn-out joints, clogged arteries, tired hearts, but not much in the way of other forms of disease. There are lots of complainers, most of her office time is taken up searching for an explanation for their pains and problems, what at one time in New York was called the *und hier* patients— *schmerz hier, und hier, und hier.* It pays for the baby's booties, but it's not much fun. Her thoughts begin to turn to how soon could she retire.

Some will blame the poor physician for not having an interest in "nondisease," but she didn't spend all those years in medical school with nondisease in mind. Nondisease just isn't in her job description.

We'll focus on fibromyalgia. How did all this come about? What to do?

There was a time when a plaintiff could attribute her nonphysical problems to an accident or some "happening," and the defense was not permitted to inquire into her prior history. Every jurisdiction has its own set of rules, but in some at least it became obvious that history is relevant to current complaints, and on examining the court-ordered doctors' notes it was revealed the patient suffering undoubtedly from a depression disorder had the same disorder for many years prior to her accident. In this way, defense counsel were able to obtain a complete medical history on the plaintiff, dating back a certain number of years, with copies of the records of all the physicians, therapists, and so on, whose advice she had sought. These are the only type of documents the author has seen that allow the reader to follow the progression of patients' symptoms. It is commonly found that the symptoms multiply and grow in severity, coincident with the questions posed and the negative results of repeated exhaustive tests, usually with negative results.

Research into the development and magnification of symptoms in fibromyalgia would be rewarding, but when patients report the large number of doctors they've seen before they reach the one who gives them the satisfaction of this fibromyalgia diagnosis, it will be difficult to assemble all their documents without a court order.

As has been discussed in other chapters, Yunus makes a distinction between *sensitivity* and *sensitization*. This may seem picky, and it seems it's often glossed over or the words used interchangeably. The difference lies in the presumption of a character with prior "sensitivity" that is acted on by circumstances, as opposed to just any person; statistics already recounted suggest that there is in fact such a person, with genetic and environmental history, nature plus nurture, who might be susceptible to this condition—initially *sensitive* and later *sensitized*.

The drama starts with the first medical contact at which time the patient enters into the doctor's world, variously called the therapeutic domain (Hazemeijer 2003), or Foucault's medical *regard*, or Hacking's matrix—all of them terms to describe the patient's surrender of herself to the physician, "the setting where the hunt for a diagnosis can be harmful to health" (Hadler 1996) and "where people can label their internal sensations as illness or disease" (Pennebaker 1982). She tells her primary care physician, "I hurt," and then, in the current jargon, comes the tipping point.

One doctor, after listening to her and examining her, will reassure her the pain is recent, not severe, probably of no consequence, and she should return if it persists. Another doctor will do the same in terms of history and examination but will order "tests." The tests are negative, which inevitably engenders more tests. The patient talks to her friends who make suggestions about CAT scans or MRIs or endoscopies. The doctor is obliged to conform to the suggestions. The doctor loses nothing by ordering them. She has an angry patient, and possibly her attorney to contend with, if she won't order them. And anyway, the baby's booties have to be paid for. And down the slippery slope goes the cart. Into the slough of despond, and on from there to the door of the rheumatologist's office.

Fibromyalgia Must Be Prevented

Once established, experience has shown that fibromyalgia is difficult to eliminate or to minimize. The patient is not born with fibromyalgia. She doesn't catch it like chickenpox. It doesn't come suddenly. There's a tipping point at which her sensitive nature could either be sensitized and made fibromyalgic, or could be handled gently and kept in balance. Physicians learn about diseases, yet half or more of the persons they see in their offices have sensations that only become symptoms when the physician treats them as such. Every sensation reported must be assessed cautiously, but caution does not require exhaustive testing. It is not usual for the student to be taught most of the persons she sees with sensations will not be in need of physical treatment, and their sensations will surely turn into more-severe and deep-rooted symptoms if they are subjected to serial tests with predictable negative results, serial investigations by x-ray, MRI and ultrasound, and serial consultations. If they're fortunate these will all be reported as "nothing untoward found," but the statistical likelihood is some variation of normal will be exposed, resulting in more tests or even surgery. The tipping point is whether the physician embarks on this in the first place. That will depend on the physician's training, her confidence in her decision, and her support against medico-legal bullying.

The patient has a role to play. If the patient does not have confidence in her doctor or if she is determined to have that test she read about on the Internet or in the magazine, or her friends insist she has a "right" to receive, almost certainly she'll have it. It will be inconclusive. Then there'll be more. Then she'll seek out her own therapists and set up in control of her own treatment program. She'll find the "right" doctors who prescribe according to the Internet, she may even have found them from the Internet. She won't be happy. Her symptoms will magnify and multiply the more she reads and the more different forms of treatment she experiences, but she'll persuade herself she's "taken charge" of her pain. It won't be easy to stop this, but fibromyalgia will be alive and well as long as there are Internet sites, magazines, and therapists whose *raison d'être* lies in promotion and not prevention.

The Richard Gordon Solution

Many years ago, Richard Gordon (pen name) wrote a series of humorous books about young doctors' antics in a British medical school. One such innocent, in a moment of passion, proposed marriage to a nurse, only to regret his offer in the cold light of dawn. He knew he couldn't undo what was done but found his exit strategy by hastily proposing marriage to all the other nurses.

The ACR criteria have "married" the profession to fibromyalgia. The diagnosis is recognized by WHO, AMA, ACR, EULAR, and all the other alphabet soups. What is done is done. Now we have to find an exit strategy to deal with the *law of unforeseen consequences.*

It is incontestable that the "tender points" have become a nonsense as a diagnostic test, separating the *haves* from the *have-nots.* Separating fibromyalgia from other forms of chronic widespread pain. It is too late to abolish the diagnostic term "fibromyalgia," so I suggest retention of the term and extension of its application to all those distressed by pain who would qualify for the diagnosis except for failing the five-fifths distribution of pain or not matching up with the spotty ladies. In fact, these are probably the honest ones who haven't arranged their symptoms to match the well-known diagnostic requirements.

The suggestions are:

- Diagnose as "fibromyalgia" all those distressed with chronic widespread pain.
- Pick up the hidden part of the iceberg.

- Arrange appropriate treatment based on distress.
- Give up the sporadic symptom chasing treatment that is the norm today.
- Rethink primary contact medicine so such persons receive early appropriate care.
- In this way they will be prevented from reaching that irredeemable tip of the iceberg.
- Such care will be based on an understanding of neuropathic pain.
- Its prime direction will be to keep the patient functioning in her community.

REFERENCES

Aakerlund, L. P., and J. Rosenberg. 1994. Postoperative delirium: Treatment with supplementary oxygen. *British Journal of Anaesthesia* 72: 286–90.

Aanonsen, L. M., and G. L. Wilcox. 1987. Nociceptive action of excitatory amino acids in the mouse: Effects of spinally administered opioids, phencyclidine and sigma agonists. *Journal of Pharmacology and Experimental Therapeutics* 243: 9–19.

Aanonsen, L. M., S. Lei, and G. L. Wilcox. 1990. Excitatory amino acid receptors and nociceptive neurotransmission in rat spinal cord. *Pain* 41: 309–21.

Aaron, L. A., L. A. Bradley, G. S. Alarcón, R. W. Alexander, M. Triana-Alexander, M. Y. Martin, and K. R. Alberts. 1996. Psychiatric diagnoses in patients with fibromyalgia are related to health care-seeking behavior rather than to illness. *Arthritis and Rheumatism* 39: 436–45.

Aaron, L. A., and D. Buchwald. 2001. A review of the evidence for overlap among unexplained clinical conditions. *Annals of Internal Medicine* 134: 868–81.

———. 2003. Chronic diffuse musculoskeletal pain, fibromyalgia and co-morbid unexplained clinical conditions. *Best Practice Research Clinical Rheumatology* 17: 563–74.

Adamson, J., Y. Ben-Shlomo, N. Chaturvedi, and J. Donovan. 2003. Ethnicity, socioeconomic position and gender—Do they affect reported health-care seeking behaviour? *Society of Scientific Medicine* 57: 895–904.

Afari, N., and D. Buchwald. 2003. Chronic fatigue syndrome: A review. *American Journal of Psychiatry* 160: 221–36.

Affleck, G., S. Urrows, H. Tennen, P. Higgins, and M. Abeles. 1996. Sequential daily relations of sleep, pain intensity and attention to pain among women with fibromyalgia. *Pain* 68: 363–68.

Agency for Healthcare Research and Quality (AHRQ). 2005. Omega-3 fatty acids, effects on cognitive functions. http://www.ahrq.gov/clinic/tp/o3cogntp.htm (accessed February 17, 2008).

Ahles, T. A., S. A. Khan, M. B. Yunus, D. A. Spiegel, and A. T. Masi. 1991. Psychiatric status of patients with primary fibromyalgia, patients with rheumatoid arthritis, and subjects without pain: a blind comparison of DSM-III diagnoses. *American Journal of Psychiatry* 148: 1721–26.

Ahles, T. A., M. B. Yunus, B. Gaulier, S. D. Riley, and A. T. Masi. 1986. The use of contemporary MMPI norms in the study of chronic pain patients. *Pain* 24: 159–63.

Ahles, T. A., M. B. Yunus, S. D. Riley, J. M. Bradley, and A. T. Masi. 1984. Psychological factors associated with primary fibromyalgia syndrome. *Arthritis and Rheumatism* 27: 1101–1106.

Akkus, S., S. Kutluhan, G. Akhan, E. Tunc, M. Ozturk, and H. R. Koyuncuoglu. 2002. Does fibromyalgia affect the outcomes of local steroid treatment in patients with carpal tunnel syndrome? *Rheumatology International* 22: 112–15.

Al-Allaf, A. W., K. L. Dunbar, N. S. Hallum, B. Nosratzadeh, K. D. Templeton, and T. Pullar. 2002. A case-control study examining the role of physical trauma in the onset of fibromyalgia syndrome. *Rheumatology* 41: 450–53.

Alberts, K. R., et al. 1996. Regional cerebral blood flow [rCBF] in the caudate nucleus and thalamus of fibromyalgia [FM] patients is associated with the cerebrospinal fluid [CSF] levels of substance P [SP]. Abstract. 8th World Congress on Pain. Seattle: IASP Press.

Alexander R. W., L. A. Bradley, G. S. Alarcón, M. Triana-Alexander, L. A. Aaron, K. R. Alberts, M. Y. Martin, and K. E. Stewart. 1998. Sexual and physical abuse in women with fibromyalgia: Association with outpatient health care utilization and pain medication usage. *Arthritis Care Research* 11: 102–15.

Alfano, A. P., A. G. Taylor, P. A. Foresman, P. R. Dunkl, G. G. McConnell, M. R. Conaway, and G. T. Gillies. 2001. Static magnetic fields for treatment of fibromyalgia: A randomized controlled trial. *Journal of Alternative and Complementary Medicine* 7: 53–64.

Alfici, S., M. Sigal, and M. Landau. 1989. Primary fibromyalgia syndrome: A variant of depressive disorder? *Psychotherapy Psychosomatics* 51: 1056–61.

Algeri, M., S. Chottiner, V. Ratner, D. Slade, and P. M. Hanno. 1997. Interstitial cystitis: Unexplained associations with other chronic disease and pain syndromes. *Urology* 49: 52–57.

Allen, G., B. Galer, and L. Schwartz. 1999. Epidemiology of complex regional pain syndrome: A retrospective chart review of 134 patients. *Pain* 80: 539–44.

Alnigenis, M. N. Y., and P. Barland. 2001. Fibromyalgia syndrome and serotonin. *Clinical and Experimental Rheumatology* 19: 205–10.

Alnigenis, M. N. Y., J. D. Bradley, J. Wallick, and C. L. Emsley. 2001. Massage therapy in the management of fibromyalgia: A pilot study. *Journal of Musculoskeletal Pain* 9: 55–67.

Altan, L., U. Bingöl, M. Aykaç, Z. Koç, and M. Yurtkuran. 2003. Investigation of the effects of pool based exercise on fibromyalgia syndrome. *Rheumatology International* 24: 272–77.

Ameis, A., and E. Urovitz. 1988. *Whiplash*. Toronto: Seal Books.

American Medical Association Council on Scientific Affairs. 1992. Clinical ecology. *Journal of the American Medical Association* 268: 3465–67.

Amir, M., L. Fostick, M. L. Polliack, S. Segev, J. Zohar, A. Rubinow, and H. Amital. 1997. Posttraumatic stress disorder, tenderness and fibromyalgia. *Journal of Psychosomatic Research* 42: 607–13.

Anch, A. M., F. A. Lue, A. W. MacLean, and H. Moldofsky. 1991. Sleep physiology and psychological aspects of the fibrositis (fibromyalgia) syndrome. *Canadian Journal of Psychology* 45: 179–84.

Anderson, G. D. 2005. Pharmacokinetics of valerenic acid after administration of valerian in healthy subjects. *Phytotherapy Research* 19: 801–803.

Anderson, W. E. 2007. Periodic limb movement disorder. http://www.emedicine.com/neuro/topic523.htm (accessed February 17, 2008).

Andersson, H. I. 2004. The course of non-malignant chronic pain: A 12-year follow-up of a cohort from the general population. *European Journal of Pain* 8: 47–53.

Andersson, H. I., G. Ejlertsson, and I. Leden. 1996. Characteristics of subjects with chronic pain, in relation to local and widespread pain report. A prospective study of symptoms, clinical findings and blood tests in sub-groups of a geographically defined population. *Scandinavian Journal of Rheumatology* 25: 146–54.

Andine, P., L. Ronnback, and B. Jarvholm. 1997. Successful use of a selective serotonin reuptake inhibitor in a patient with multiple chemical sensitivities. *Acta Psychiatrica Scandinavica* 96: 82–83.

Applegate, K. L., F. J. Keefe, and I. C. Siegler. 2005. Does personality at college entry predict number of reported pain conditions at mid-life? A longitudinal study. *Journal of Pain* 6: 92–97.

Arnett, F. C., et al. 1988. The American Rheumatism Association 1987 revised criteria for the classification of rheumatoid arthritis. *Arthritis and Rheumatism* 31: 315–24.

Arnold, L. M. 2006. Biology and therapy of fibromyalgia. New therapies in fibromyalgia. *Arthritis Research Therapeutics* 8: 212.

Arnold, L. M., P. E. Keck Jr., and J. A. Wedge. 2000. Antidepressant treatment of fibromyalgia. A meta-analysis and review. *Psychosomatics* 41: 104–13.

Arnold, L. M., J. I. Hudson, E. V. Hess, A. E. Ware, D. A. Fritz, M. B. Auchenbach, L. O. Starck, and P. E. Keck Jr. 2004. Family study of fibromyalgia. *Arthritis and Rheumatism* 50: 944–52.

Arthritis Foundation. 2006. *Good Living with Fibromyalgia*. Atlanta: Arthritis Foundation.

Aserinsky, E. 1996. Memories of famous neuropsychologists: The discovery of REM sleep. *Journal of the History of the Neurosciences* 5: 213–27.

Aserinsky, E., and N. Kleitman. 1953. Regularly occurring periods of eye motility, and concomitant phenomena, during sleep. *Science* 118: 273–74.

Askwith, R. 1998. How aspirin turned hero. http://opioids.com/heroin/heroinhistory.html (accessed February 17, 2008).

Assis, M. R., L. E. Silva, and A. Martins Barros. 2006. A randomized controlled trial of deep water running: Clinical effectiveness of aquatic exercise to treat fibromyalgia. *Arthritis Care Research* 55: 57–65.

Astrand, P. O. Exercise physiology and its role in disease prevention and rehabilitation. 1987. *Archives of Physiatry and Medical Rehabilitation* 68: 305–309.

Azzini, M., D. Girelli, O. Olivieri, P. Guarini, A. M. Stanzial, A. Frigo, R. Milanino, L. M. Bambara, and R. Corrocher. 1995. Fatty acids and antioxidant micronutrients in psoriatic arthritis. *Journal of Rheumatology* 22: 103–108.

Bachmann, G. A., R. Rosen, V. W. Pinn, W. H. Utian, C. Ayers, R. Basson, Y. M. Binik, C. Brown, D. C. Foster, J. M. Gibbons Jr., I. Goldstein, A. Graziottin, H. K. Haefner, B. L. Harlow, S. K. Spadt, S. R. Leiblum, R. M. Masheb, B. D. Reed, J. D. Sobel, C. Veasley, U. Wesselmann, and S. S. Witkin. 2006. Vulvodynia: A state-of-the-art consensus on definitions, diagnosis and management. *Journal of Reproductive Medicine* 51: 447–56.

Bailer, J., M. Witthöft, C. Paul, C. Bayerl, and F. Rist. 2005. Evidence for overlap between idiopathic environmental intolerance and somatoform disorders. *Psychosomatic Medicine* 67: 921–29.

Baker, D. G. 1988. Complications of rheumatoid arthritis. In *An Illustrated Guide to Pathology, Diagnosis and Management*, edited by H. R. Schumbacher and E. P. Gall. Philadelphia: Lippincott, 15: 1–18.

Balblanc, J. C., D. Hartmann, D. Noyer, P. Mathieu, T. Conrozier, A. M. Tron, M. Piperno, M. Richard, and E. Vignon. 1993. Serum hyaluronic acid in osteoarthritis. *Revue du Rhumatisme Edition Française* 60: 194–202.

Barclay, L. 2004. ACOG issues new guidelines for chronic pelvic pain. *Obstetrics and Gynecology* 103: 589–605. http://medgenmed.medscape.com/viewarticle/471545 _print (accessed January 29, 2009).

Barkhuizen, A., and R. M. Bennett. 1999. Elevated levels of hyaluronic acid in the sera of women with fibromyalgia. *Journal of Rheumatology* 26: 2063–64.

Barrett, S. 2002. Magnet therapy: A skeptical view. Quackwatch, http://www.quack watch.org/04ConsumerEducation/QA/magnet.html (accessed February 17, 2008).

Barsky, A. J., H. M. Peekna, and J. F. Brus. 2001. Somatic symptom reporting in women and men. *Journal of General and Internal Medicine* 16: 266–75.

Basbaum, A. J., and H. L. Fields. 1984. Endogenous pain control systems. *Annual Review of Neuroscience* 7: 309–21.

Basmajian, J. V. 1962. *Muscles Alive*. Baltimore: Williams & Wilkins.

Bauer, J. A., and R. D. Murray. 1999. Electromyographic patterns of individuals suffering from lateral tennis elbow. *Journal of Electromyography and Kinesiology* 9: 245–52.

Baxter, M. P., and C. Dulberg. 1988. "Growing pains" in childhood—A proposal for treatment. *Journal of Pediatric Orthopaedics* 8: 402–406.

BBC News. 2007. Vitamin D urged in pregnant women. http://news.bbc.co.uk/go/pr/fr/ /1/hi/health/7161458.stm (accessed February 17, 2008).

Beaulieu, P., and J.-S. Walczak. 2007. Pharmacological management of sleep and pain inter-reactions. In *Sleep and Pain*, edited by Gilles Lavigne, Barry J. Sessle, Manon Choiniere, and Peter J. Soja. Seattle: IASP Press, pp. 391–415.

Beck, A. T., and A. Bearmesderfer. 1974. Assessment of depression: The depression inventory. *Modern Problems of Pharmacopsychiatry* 7: 151–69.

Beck, A. T., N. Epstein, G. Brown, and R. A. Steer. 1988. An inventory for measuring clinical anxiety: Psychometric properties. *Journal of Consulting Clinical Psychology* 56: 893–97.

Beck, A. T., R. A. Steer, and G. K. Brown. 1996. *Manual for the Beck Depression Inventory II*. San Antonio: Psychological Corporation.

Beck, A. T., C. H. Ward, M. Mendelson, J. Mock, and J. Erbaugh. 1961. An inventory for measuring depression. *Archives of General Psychiatry* 4: 561–67.

Becker, P. M. 2005. Pharmacologic and nonpharmacologic treatment of insomnia. *Neurologic Clinics* 23: 1149–63.

Beecher, H. K. 1955. The powerful placebo. *Journal of the American Medical Association* 159: 1602–1606.

Bell, D. S., K. Jordan, and M. Robinson. 2001. Thirteen-year follow-up of children and adolescents with chronic fatigue syndrome. *Pediatrics* 107: 994–98.

Bendtsen, L. 2000. Central sensitization in tension-type headache—possible pathophysiological mechanisms. *Cephalalgia* 20: 486–508.

Bendtsen, L., and R. Jensen. 2000. Amitriptyline reduces myofascial tenderness in patients with chronic tension-type headache. *Cephalalgia* 20: 603–10.

Bendtsen, L., R. Jensen, and J. Olesen. 1996. A non-selective (amitriptyline), but not a selective (citalopram), serotonin reuptake inhibitor is effective in the prophylactic treatment of chronic tension-type headache. *Journal of Neurology, Neurosurgery and Psychiatry* 61: 285–90.

————. 1996. Qualitatively altered nociception in chronic myofascial pain. *Pain* 65: 259–64.

Bendtsen, L., J. Nørregaard, R. Jensen, and J. Olesen. 1997. Evidence of qualitatively altered nociception in patients with fibromyalgia. *Arthritis and Rheumatism* 40: 98–104.

Bengtsson, A., and E. Backman. 1992. Long term follow up of fibromyalgia patients. *Scandinavian Journal of Rheumatology* 21 (suppl 94): 98.

Bengtsson, A., K. G. Henriksson, L. Jorfeldt, B. Kågedal, C. Lennmarken, and F. Lindström. 1986. Primary fibromyalgia: A clinical and laboratory study of 55 patients. *Scandinavian Journal of Rheumatology* 15: 340–47.

Bengtsson, A., K. G. Henriksson, and J. Larson. 1986. Reduced high energy phosphate levels in the painful muscles of patients with primary fibromyalgia. *Arthritis and Rheumatism* 29: 817–21.

Bennett, R. M. 1989. Beyond fibromyalgia: Ideas on etiology and treatment. *Journal of Rheumatology* 19 (suppl): 185–91.

———. 1989. Confounding features of the fibromyalgia syndrome: A current perspective of differential diagnosis. *Journal of Rheumatology* 16 (suppl): 19–58.

———. 1993. Disabling fibromyalgia: Appearance versus reality. *Journal of Rheumatology* 20: 1821–24.

———. 1996. Multidisciplinary group programs to treat fibromyalgia patients. *Rheumatic Disease Clinics of North America* 22: 351–60.

———. 1997. Chronic widespread pain and the fibromyalgia construct. Fibromyalgia Information Foundation. http://www.myalgia.com/Pain%20digest.pdf (accessed February 17, 2008).

———. 1998. Fibromyalgia, chronic fatigue syndrome, and myofascial pain. *Current Opinion in Rheumatology* 10: 95–103.

———. 1999. Emerging concepts in the neurobiology of chronic pain: Evidence for abnormal sensory processing in fibromyalgia pain. *Mayo Clinic Proceedings* 74: 385–98.

———. 2005. The Fibromyalgia Impact Questionnaire (FIQ): A review of its development, current version, operating characteristics and uses. *Clinical and Experimental Rheumatology* 23: S154–S162.

———. 2005. Neurologic features of fibromyalgia. In *Fibromyalgia and Other Central Pain Syndromes,* edited by D. J. Wallace and D. J. Clauw. Philadelphia: Lippincott Williams & Wilkins, pp. 133–44.

———. 2007. The scientific basis for understanding pain in fibromyalgia. Oregon Fibromyalgia Foundation. http://www.myalgia.com (accessed February 17, 2008).

Bennett, R. M., C. S. Burckhardt, S. R. Clark, C. A. O'Reilly, A. N. Wiens, and S. M. Campbell. 1996. Group treatment of fibromyalgia: A 6 month outpatient program. *Journal of Rheumatology* 23: 621–28.

Bennett, R. M., S. R. Clark, S. M. Campbell, and C. S. Burckhardt. 1992. Low levels of somatomedin C in patients with the fibromyalgia syndrome: A possible link between sleep and muscle pain. *Arthritis and Rheumatism* 35: 1113–16.

Bennett, R. M., S. R. Clark, S. M. Campbell, S. B. Ingram, C. S. Burckhardt, D. L. Nelson, and J. M. Porter. 1991. Symptoms of Raynaud's syndrome in patients with fibromyalgia. *Arthritis and Rheumatism* 34: 264–69.

Bennett, R. M., D. M. Cook, S. R. Clark, C. S. Burckhardt, and S. M. Campbell. 1997. Hypothalamic-pituitary-insulin-like growth factor-I axis dysfunction in patients with fibromyalgia. *Journal of Rheumatology.* 24: 1384–89.

Bennett, R. M., P. De Garmo, and S. R. Clark. 1996. A 1 year double blind placebo-controlled study of guaifenesin in fibromyalgia. *Arthritis and Rheumatism* 39: S212

Bennett, R. M., M. Kamin, R. Karim, and N. Rosenthal. 2003. Tramadol and aceta-minophen combination tablets in the treatment of fibromyalgia pain. *American Journal of Medicine* 114: 537–45.

Bennett, R. M., J. Schein, M. R. Kosinski, D. J. Hewitt, D. M. Jordan, and N. R. Rosenthal. 2005. Impact of fibromyalgia pain on health-related quality of life before and after treatment with tramadol/acetaminophen. *Arthritis and Rheumatism* 53: 519–27.

Bennett, R. M., et al. 2007. An Internet survey of 2,596 people with fibromyalgia. *BioMed Central Journal of Musculoskeletal Disorders* 8: 1186–471, http://www.biomedcentral.com/1471-2474/8/27 (accessed February 17, 2008).

Bentall, R. P., P. Powell, F. J. Nye, and R. H. Edwards. 2002. Predictors of response to treatment for chronic fatigue syndrome. *British Journal of Psychiatry* 181: 248–52.

Berenson, A. 2008. Drug approved. Is disease real? *New York Times*, http://query.nytimes.com/gst/fullpage.html?res=9F0DEEDA103FF937A25752C0A96E9C8B63&scp=5&sq=berenson&st=nyt (accessed January 28, 2008).

Bergman, S. P. Herrström, K. Högström, I. F. Petersson, B. Svensson, and L. T. Jacobsson. 2001. Chronic musculoskeletal pain, prevalence rates, and sociodemographic associations in a Swedish population study. *Journal of Rheumatology* 28: 1369–77.

Berlach, D. M. 2006. Experience with the synthetic cannabinoid nabilone in chronic noncancer pain. *Pain Medicine* 7: 25–29.

Bernacki, E. J. 2004. Factors influencing the costs of workers' compensation. *Clinical Occupational, and Environmental Medicine* 4: 249–57.

Bhalla, R. N., and S. C. Aronson. 2006. Depression. http://www.emedicine.com/med/TOPIC532.HTM (accessed February 17, 2008).

Binckley, K., and S. Kutcher. 1997. Panic response to sodium lactate infusion in patients with multiple chemical sensitivity syndrome. *Journal of Allergy and Clinical Immunology* 99: 570–75.

Biondi, M., and G. Portuesi. 1994. Tension-type headache: Psychosomatic clinical assessment and treatment. *Psychotherapy and Psychosomatics* 61: 41–64.

Birdsall, T. C. 1998. 5-Hydroxytryptophan: A clinically effective serotonin precursor. *Alternative Medicine Review* 3: 271–80.

Birklein, F. B., B. Riedl, B. Neundörfer, and H. O. Handwerker. 1998. Sympathetic vasoconstriction of reflex pattern in patients with complex regional pain syndrome. *Pain* 75: 93–100.

Birnie, D. J., A. A. Knipping, M. H. van Rijswijk, A. C. de Blécourt, and N. de Voogd. 1991. Psychological aspects of fibromyalgia compared with chronic and nonchronic pain. *Journal of Rheumatology* 18: 1845–48.

Bjelakovic, G. 2007. Mortality in randomized trials of antioxidant supplements for primary and secondary prevention. *Journal of the American Medical Association* 297: 842–57.

Bjelakovic, G., D. Nikolova, and L. L. Gluud. 2007. Mortality in randomized trials of antioxidant supplements for primary and secondary prevention: Systematic review and meta-analysis. 297: 842–57.

Blasberg, B., and A. Chalmers. 1989. Temporomandibular pain and dysfunction syndrome associated with generalized musculosketal pain: A retrospective study. *Journal of Rheumatology* 16 (suppl 19): 87–90.

Bliddal, H., H. J. Møller, M. Schaadt, and B. Danneskiold-Samsøe. 2000. Patients with fibromyalgia have normal serum levels of hyaluronic acid. *Journal of Rheumatology* 27: 26–59.

Bliwise, D. L. 2005. Normal aging. In *Principles and Practices of Sleep Medicine*, 4th edition. Philadelphia: Elsevier Saunders, pp. 24–38.

Block, S. R. 1993. Fibromyalgia and the rheumatisms: Common sense and sensibility. *Rheumatic Disease Clinics of North America* 19: 61–78.

Blotman, F., and J. Branco. 2006. *La Fibromyalgie. La Douleur au Quotidien*. Toulouse: Éditions Privat.

BMJ editorial. 2006. Magnet therapy. *British Medical Journal* 332: 4.

Bodden-Heidrich, R., V. Küppers, M. W. Beckmann, M. H. Ozörnek, I. Rechenberger, and H. G. Bender. 1999. Psychosomatic aspects of vulvodynia. Comparison with the chronic pelvic pain syndrome. *Journal of Reproductive Medicine* 44: 411–16.

Boeckner, L. S., C. H. Pullen, S. N. Walker, G. W. Abbott, and T. Block. 2002. Use and reliability of the World Wide Web version of the Block Health Habits and History Questionnaire with older rural women. *Journal of Nutrition Education and Behaviour* 34 (suppl 1): S20.

Boers, M., P. Brooks, L. S. Simon, V. Strand, and P. Tugwell. 2005. OMERACT: An international initiative to improve outcome measurement in rheumatology. *Clinical and Experimental Rheumatology* 23: S10–S13.

Bohm-Starke, N., M. Hilliges, G. Brodda-Jansen, E. Rylander, and E. Torebjörk. 2001. Psychophysical evidence of nociceptor sensitization in vulvarvestibulitis syndrome. *Pain* 94: 177–83.

Bohr, T. 1996. Problems with myofascial pain syndrome and fibromyalgia syndrome. *Neurology* 46: 593–97.

Bonica, J. J. 1973. Causalgia and other reflex sympathetic dystrophies. *Postgraduate Medicine* 53: 143–48.

Bonica, J. J., J. D. Loeser, C. Richard Chapman, and W. E. Fordyc, eds. 1990. Definitions and taxonomy of pain. In *The Management of Pain*, volume 2, 2nd edition. Philadelphia: Lea & Febiger.

Borenstein, D. G., J. W. O'Mara Jr., S. D. Boden, W. C. Lauerman, A. Jacobson, C. Platenberg, D. Schellinger, and S. W. Wiesel. 2001. The value of magnetic resonance imaging of the lumbar spine to predict low-back pain in asymptomatic subjects: A seven-year follow-up study. *Journal of Bone and Joint Surgery* 83-A: 1306–11.

Boselli, M. L., L. Parrino, A. Smerieri, and M. G. Terzano. 1998. Effects of age on EEG arousals in normal sleep. *Sleep* 21: 351–57.

Bou-Holaigah, I., H. Calkins, J. A. Flynn, C. Tunin, H. C. Chang, J. S. Kan, and P. C. Rowe. 1997. Provocation of hypotension and pain during upright tilt table testing in adults with fibromyalgia. *Clinical and Experimental Rheumatology* 15: 239–46.

Bowyer, S., and P. Roettcher. 1996. Pediatric rheumatology clinic populations in the United States: Results of a 3 year survey. *Journal of Rheumatology* 23: 1968–74.

Bradley, L. A., K. R. Alberts, G. S. Alarcón, M. T. Alexander, J. M. Mountz, D. A. Weigert, H. G. Liu, J. E. Blalock, L. A. Aaron, R. W. Alexander, E. C. San Pedro, M. Y. Martin, and A. C. Morell. 1996. Abnormal brain regional cerebral blood flow [rCBF] and cerebrospinal fluid [CSF] levels of substance P [SP] in patients and non-patients with fibromyalgia [FM]. *Arthritis and Rheumatism* 39 (suppl): S212.

Brattberg, G. 1999. Connective tissue massage in the treatment of fibromyalgia. *European Journal of Pain* 3: 235–44.

Breuhl, S., R. N. Harden, B. S. Galer, S. Saltz, M. Backonja, and M. Stanton-Hicks. 2002. Complex regional pain syndrome: Are there distinct subtypes and sequential stages of the syndrome? *Pain* 95: 119–24.

Brown, C. 2003. The stubborn scientist who unraveled a mystery of the night. *Smithsonian Magazine*. http://www.smithsonianmag.com/science-nature/stubborn.html (accessed February 19, 2008).

Brown, E. M. 1980. An American treatment for the "American nervousness." http://bms.brown.edu/HistoryofPsychiatry/Beard.html (accessed January 31, 2008).

Brown, S. R. 2004. *Scurvy. How a Surgeon, a Mariner, and a Gentleman Solved the Greatest Medical Mystery of the Age of Sail*. New York: Thomas Dunne Books.

Buchanan, W. W. 1982. Assessment of joint tenderness, grip strength, digital joint circumference and morning stiffness in rheumatoid arthritis. *Journal of Rheumatology* 9: 763–66.

Buchwald, D., and D. Garrity. 1994. Comparison of patients with chronic fatigue syndrome, fibromyalgia and multiple chemical sensitivities. *Archives of Internal Medicine* 154: 2049–53.

Burckhardt, C. S., S. R. Clark, and R. M. Bennett. 1991. The fibromyalgia impact questionnaire: Development and validation. *Journal of Rheumatology* 18: 728–33.

Burckhardt, C. S., K. Mannerkorpi, L. Hedenberg, and A. Bjelle. 1994. A randomized controlled clinical trial of education and physical training for women with fibromyalgia. *Journal of Rheumatology* 21: 714–20.

Burks, D. A. Irritable bladder syndrome. http://www.ichelp.com/cgi-bin/search.pl (accessed February 17, 2008).

Bursch, B., G. A. Walco, and L. Zeltzer. 1998. Clinical assessment and management of chronic pain and pain-associated disability syndrome. *Journal of Developmental and Behavioral Pediatrics* 19: 45–53.

Burton, A. K., K. M. Tillotson, C. J. Main, and S. Hollis. 1995. Psychosocial predictors of outcome in acute and subchronic low back trouble. *Spine* 20: 722–28.

Buscemi, N. 2006. Efficacy and safety of exogenous melatonin for secondary sleep disorders and sleep disorders accompanying sleep restriction: Meta-analysis. *British Medical Journal* 332: 385–93.

Busch, A. J., C. L. Schachter, P. M. Peloso, and C. Bombardier. 2007. Exercise for treating fibromyalgia syndrome. *Cochrane Database of Systematic Reviews.* (4):CD003786. PMID:17943797.

Buskila, D. 2001. Fibromyalgia, chronic fatigue syndrome, and myofascial pain syndrome. *Current Opinion on Rheumatology* 13: 117–27.

Buskila, D., G. Abramov, A. Biton, and L. Neumann. 2000. The prevalence of pain complaints in a general population in Israel and its implications for utilization of health services. *Journal of Rheumatology* 27: 1521–25.

Buskila, D., M. Abu-Shakra, and L. Neumann. 2001. Balneotherapy for fibromyalgia in the Dead Sea. *Rheumatology International* 20: 105–108.

Buskila, D., L. Neumann, A. Alhoashle, and M. Abu-Shakra. 2000. Fibromyalgia syndrome in men. *Seminars in Arthritis and Rheumatism* 30: 47–51.

Buskila, D., L. Neumann, I. Hazanov, and R. Carmi. 1996. Familial aggregation in the fibromyalgia syndrome. *Seminars in Arthritis and Rheumatism* 26: 605–11.

Buskila, D., L. Neumann, L. R. Odes, E. Schleifer, R. Depsames, and M. Abu-Shakra. 2001. The prevalence of musculoskeletal pain and fibromyalgia in patients hospitalized on internal medicine wards. *Seminars in Arthritis and Rheumatism* 30: 411–17.

Buskila, D., L. R. Odes, L. Neumann, and H. S. Odes. 1999. Fibromyalgia in inflammatory bowel disease. *Journal of Rheumatology* 26: 1167–71.

Buskila, D., and L. Press. 1993. Assessment of non-particular tenderness and prevalence of fibromyalgia in children. *Journal of Rheumatology* 20: 368–70.

Buskila, D., et al. 1997. Increased rate of fibromyalgia following cervical spine injury. A controlled study of 1612 cases of traumatic injury. *Arthritis and Rheumatism* 40: 446–54.

Butler, C. C., M. Evans, D. Greaves, and S. Simpson. 2004. Medically unexplained symptoms: the biopsychosocial model found wanting. *Journal of the Royal Society of Medicine* 97: 219–21.

Cabot, W. Significant soft tissue syndromes. 2007. http://64.233.169.104/search?q =cache:ansOEzjutNoJ:www.orthopedictechreview.com/issues/marapr01/pg26.htm +%22significant+soft+tissue+syndromes%22&hl=en&ct=clnk&cd=1&gl=us&ie =UTF-8 (accessed December 4, 2007).

Cairns, B. E. 2007. Alteration of sleep quality by pain medication: An overview. In *Sleep and Pain*, edited by Gilles Lavigne, Barry J. Sessle, Manon Choiniere, and Peter J. Soja. Seattle: IASP Press, pp. 371–90.

Campbell, S. M., S. Clark, E. A. Tindall, M. E. Forehand, and R. M. Bennett. 1983. Clinical characteristics of fibrositis. I. A "blinded," controlled study of symptoms and tender points. *Arthritis and Rheumatism* 26: 817–24.

Carey, B. 2005. Watching new love as it sears the brain. *New York Times*, May 31, 2005, http://www.sensualism.com/love/brain.html (accessed February 17, 2008).

Cardiel, M. H., and J. Rojas-Serrano. 2002. Community based study to estimate prevalence, burden of illness and help seeking behavior in rheumatic diseases in Mexico City. A COPCORD study. *Clinical and Experimental Rheumatology* 20: 617–24.

Carette, S., G. Oakson, C. Guimont, and M. Steriade. 1995. Sleep electroencephalography and the clinical response to amitriptyline in patients with fibromyalgia. *Arthritis and Rheumatology* 38: 1211–17.

Carlson, E. T. 1970. The nerve weakness of the 19th century. *International Journal of Psychiatry* 9: 50–54.

Carpenter, K. J. 2002. *Beriberi, White Rice and Vitamin B*. Berkeley: University of California Press.

Carragee, E. J., T. F. Alamin, J. L. Miller, and J. M. Carragee. 2005. Discographic, MRI and psychosocial determinants of low back pain disability and remission: A prospective study in subjects with benign persistent back pain. *Spine Journal* 5: 24–35.

Carskadon, M. A., and W. C. Dement. 2005. Normal human sleep: An overview. In *Principles and Practices of Sleep Medicine*, volume 4, edited by F. Kryger. Philadelphia: Elsevier Saunders, pp. 13–23.

Carville, S. F., S. Arendt-Nielsen, H. Bliddal, F. Blotman, J. C. Branco, D. Buskila, J. A. Da Silva, B. Danneskiold-Samsøe, F. Dincer, C. Henriksson, K. G. Henriksson, E. Kosek, K. Longley, G. M. McCarthy, S. Perrot, M. Puszczewicz, P. Sarzi-Puttini, A. Silman, M. Späth, and E. H. Choy. 2007. EULAR evidence-based recommendations for the management of fibromyalgia syndrome. http://www.myalgia.com/ Treatment/EULAR%20revommendations%20for%20treatment%202007.pdf (accessed February 17, 2008).

Cathey, M. A., F. Wolfe, and S. M. Kleinheksel. 1988. Functional ability and work status in patients with fibromyalgia. *Arthritis Care Research* 1: 85–98.

Cathey, M. A., F. Wolfe, S. M. Kleinheksel, and D. J. Hawley. 1986. Socioeconomic impact of fibrositis: A study of 81 patients with primary fibrositis. *American Journal of Medicine* 81: 78–84.

Cathey, M. A., et al. 1990. Demographic, work disability, service utilization and treatment characteristics of 620 fibromyalgia patients in rheumatologic practice (abstract). *Arthritis and Rheumatism* 33: S10.

Catholic Encyclopedia. http://www.newadvent.org/cathen/index.html (accessed February 17, 2008).

CDC. 2006. A chronic multisystem illness affecting Air Force veterans of the Persian Gulf War. http://www.cdc.gov/cfs/publications/cluster_2.htm (accessed January 28, 2008).

Cedraschi, C., J. Desmeules, and E. Rapiti. 2004. Fibromyalgia: A randomized controlled trial of a treatment programme based on self-management. *Annals of Rheumatic Diseases* 63: 290–96.

Cedraschi, C., J. Desmeules, E. Rapiti, E. Baumgartner, P. Cohen, A. Finckh, A. F. Allaz, and T. L. Vischer. 2004. Fibromyalgia: A randomised, controlled trial of a treatment programme based on self management. *Annals of Rheumatic Diseases* 63: 290–96.

Cetin, A., and S. Sivri. 2001. Respiratory function and dyspnea in fibromyalgia syndrome. *Journal of Musculoskeletal Pain* 9: 7–16.

Chalder, T. G. Berelowitz, T. Pawlikowska, L. Watts, S. Wessely, D. Wright, and E. P. Wallace. 1993. Development of a fatigue scale. *Journal of Psychosomatic Medicine* 37: 147–53.

Chen, G., and C. Guilleminault. 2007. Sleep disorders that can exacerbate pain. In *Sleep and Pain*, edited by Gilles Lavigne, Barry J. Sessle, Manon Choiniere, and Peter J. Soja. Seattle: IASP Press, pp. 311–40.

Chen, L., J. Goldman-Knaub, and S. Pullman-Mooar. 2005. Local therapy for fibromyalgia and nonneuropathic pain. In *Fibromyalgia and Other Central Pain Syndromes*, edited by D. J. Wallace and D. J. Clauw. Philadelphia: Lippincott Williams & Wilkins, pp. 353–68.

Chertok, L., O. Bourguignon, F. Guillon, and P. Aboulker. 1977. Urethral syndrome in the female ("irritable bladder"): The expression of fantasies about the urogenital area. *Psychosomatic Medicine* 39: 1–10.

Chesterton, L. S., P. Barlas, N. E. Foster, G. D. Baxter, and C. C. Wright. 2003. Gender differences in pressure pain threshold in healthy humans. *Pain* 101: 259–66.

Childs, S. J. 1994. Dimethyl sulfone (DMSO2) in the treatment of interstitial cystitis. *Urological Clinics of North America* 21: 85–88.

Ciccone, D. S., D. K. Elliott, H. K. Chandler, S. Nayak, and K. G. Raphael. 2005. Sexual and physical abuse in women with fibromyalgia syndrome: A test of the trauma hypothesis. *Clinical Journal of Pain* 21: 378–86.

Clark, P., R. Burgos-Vargas, C. Medina-Palma, P. Lavielle, and F. F. Marina. 1998. Prevalence of fibromyalgia in children: A clinical study of Mexican children. *Journal of Rheumatology* 25: 2009–14.

Clark, S. R. 1994. Prescribing exercise for fibromyalgia patients. *Arthritis Care and Research* 7: 221.

Clark, S. R., S. M. Campbell, M. E. Forehand, E. A. Tindall, and R. M. Bennett. 1985. Clinical characteristics of fibrositis. II. A "blinded," controlled study using standard psychological tests. *Arthritis and Rheumatism* 28: 132–37.

Clark, S. R., K. D. Jones, C. S. Burckhardt, and R. Bennett. 2001. Exercise for patients with fibromyalgia: Risks versus benefits. *Current Rheumatology Reports* 3: 135–46.

Clauw, D. J. 1995. Fibromyalgia: More than just a musculoskeletal disease. *American Family Physician* 52: 843–53.

———. 1995. The pathogenesis of chronic pain and fatigue syndromes, with special reference to fibromyalgia. *Medical Hypotheses* 44: 369–78.

Clauw, D. J., and L. J. Crofford. 1993. Chronic widespread pain and fibromyalgia: What we know, and what we need to know. *Best Practice and Research in Clinical Rheumatology* 17: 685–701.

Clauw, D. J., M. Schmidt, D. Radulovic, A. Singer, P. Katz, and J. Bresette. 1997. The relationship between fibromyalgia and interstitial cystitis. *Journal of Psychiatric Research* 31: 125–31.

Clegg, D. O., D. J. Reda, C. L. Harris, M. A. Klein, J. R. O'Dell, M. M. Hooper, J. D. Bradley, C. O. Bingham III, M. H. Weisman, C. G. Jackson, N. E. Lane, J. J. Cush, L. W. Moreland, H. R. Schumacher Jr., C. V. Oddis, F. Wolfe, J. A. Molitor, D. E. Yocum, T. J. Schnitzer, D. E. Furst, A. D. Sawitzke, H. Shi, K. D. Brandt, R. W. Moskowitz, and H. J. Williams. 2006. Glucosamine, chondroitin sulfate, and the two in combination for painful knee osteoarthritis. *New England Journal of Medicine* 23: 795–808.

Cleveland Clinic. 2007. Myofascial pain syndrome. http://www.webmd.com/pain -management/guide/myofascial-pain-syndrome (accessed February 17, 2008).

Cocchiarella, L., and G. B. Andersson. 2000. *Guides to the Evaluation of Permanent Impairment*, 5th edition. Chicago: American Medical Association Press.

Cochrane Review. 2007. Lecithin for dementia and cognitive impairment. http:// www.medscape.com/viewarticle/485434 (accessed February 16, 2008).

Cohen, H., L. Neumann, M. Shore, M. Amir, Y. Cassuto, and D. Buskila. 2000. Autonomic dysfunction in patients with fibromyalgia: Application of power spectral analysis of heart rate variability. *Seminars in Arthritis and Rheumatism* 29: 217–27.

Colbert, A. P., M. Banerji, and A. A. Pilla. 1999. Magnetic mattress pad use in patients with fibromyalgia: A randomized double-blind pilot study. *Journal of Back and Musculoskeletal Rehabilitation* 13: 19–31.

Cole, J. A., K. J. Rothman, H. J. Cabral, Y. Zhang, and F. A. Farraye. 2006. Migraine, fibromyalgia, and depression among people with IBS: A prevalence study. *BioMed-Central Gastroenterology* 6: 26–34.

College of Physicians and Surgeons Ontario (CPSO). Evidence-based recommendations for medical management of chronic non-malignant pain. http://www.cpso.on.ca/ publications/Opioid_Therapy_Meta_analysis.pdf (accessed February 17, 2008).

Colloca, L., and F. Benedetti. 2007. Nocebo hyperalgesia: How anxiety is turned into pain. *Current Opinion in Anaesthesiology* 20: 435–39.

Colquhoun, W. P. Accidents, injuries and shift work. In *Department of Health and Human Services, Shift Work and Health*. Washington, DC: Government Printing Office.

Conte, P. M., G. A. Walco, Y. Kimura. 2003. Temperament and stress response in children with juvenile primary fibromyalgia syndrome. *Arthritis and Rheumatism* 48: 2923–30.

Corbett, A. D., G. Henderson, A. T. McKnight, and S. J. Paterson. 75 years of opioid research: The exciting but vain quest for the holy grail. *British Journal of Pharmacology* 147: S153–S162.

Cöster, L., S. Kendall, B. Gerdle, C. Henriksson, K. G. Henriksson, and A. Bengtsson. 2008. Chronic widespread musculoskeletal pain—A comparison of those who meet criteria for fibromyalgia and those who do not. *European Journal of Pain* 12(5): 600–10.

Cote, K. A., and H. Moldofsky. 1997. Sleep, daytime symptoms, and cognitive perfor-mance in patients with fibromyalgia. *Journal of Rheumatology* 24: 2014–23.

Cotman, C. W., and L. L. Iversen. 1987. Excitatory amino acids in the brain-focus on NMDA receptors. *Trends in Neuro-Sciences* 10: 263–65.

Crofford, L. J. 2005. Future research directions. In *Fibromyalgia and Other Central Pain Syndromes*, edited by D. J. Wallace and D. J. Clauw. Philadelphia: Lippincott Williams & Wilkins.

Crofford, L. J., S. R. Pillemer, K. T. Kalogeras, J. M. Cash, D. Michelson, M. A. Kling, E. M. Sternberg, P. W. Gold, G. P. Chrousos, and R. L. Wilder. 1994. Hypothalamic-pituitary-adrenal axis perturbations in patients with fibromyalgia. *Arthritis and Rheumatism* 37: 1583–92.

Crofford, L. J., M. C. Rowbotham, P. J. Mease, I. J. Russell, R. H. Dworkin, A. E. Corbin, J. P. Young Jr., L. K. LaMoreaux, S. A. Martin, and U. Sharma. 2005. Pre-gabalin for the treatment of fibromyalgia syndrome. Results of a randomized, double blind, placebo-controlled trial. *Arthritis and Rheumatism* 52: 1264–73.

Croft, P. J. 2004. Pushing pain up the agenda: Tender points and fibromyalgia. Arthritis Research Campaign, http://www.arc.org.uk/news/arthritistoday/124_4.asp (accessed February 5, 2008).

Croft, P., A. S. Rigby, R. Boswell, J. Schollum, and A. Silman. 1993. The prevalence of chronic widespread pain in the general population. *Journal of Rheumatology* 20: 710–13.

Croft, P., J. Schollum, and A. Silman. 1994. Population study of tender point counts and pain as evidence of fibromyalgia. *British Medical Journal* 309: 696–99.

Crook, J., R. Weir, and E. Tunks. 1989. An epidemiological follow-up survey of persistent pain sufferers in a group family practice and specialty pain clinic. *Pain* 36: 49–61.

Cronin, A. 1995. Opioid inhibition of rapid eye movement sleep by a specific mu receptor antagonist. *British Journal of Anaesthesiology* 74: 188–92.

Cudworth, R. 1678. The true intellectual system of the universe. In *Oxford Dictionary of Quotations*, edited by Elizabeth Knowles. Oxford: Oxford University Press.

Cunha, B. A. 2008. Chronic fatigue syndrome. http://www.emedicine.com/ped/TOPIC 2795.HTM (accessed February 17, 2008).

Dadabhoy, D., and D. J. Clauw. 2006. Therapy insight: Fibromyalgia—a different type of pain needing a different type of treatment. *Nature Clinical Practice Rheuma-tology* 2: 364–72.

Dailey, P. A., G. D. Bishop, I. J. Russell, and E. M. Fletcher. 1990. Psychological stress and the fibrositis/fibromyalgia syndrome. *Journal of Rheumatology* 17: 1380–85.

Dalton, R., N. Sabate, and N. A. Forman. 1996. Psychosomatic illness. In *Nelson Text-book of Pediatrics*, 15th edition, edited by Richard E. Behrman, Robert M. Klieg-man, Ann M. Arvin, and Waldo E. Nelson. Philadelphia: W. B. Saunders, pp. 77–78.

Dao, T. T., and L. LeResche. 2000. Gender differences in pain. *Journal of Orofacial Pain* 14: 169–84.

Dauvilliers, Y., and J. Touchon. 2001. Sleep in fibromyalgia: Review of clinical and polysomnographic data. *Neurophysiology Clinic* 31: 18–33.

Dauvilliers, Y., and B. Carlander. 2007. Sleep and pain interactions in medical disorders: The examples of fibromyalgia and headache. In *Sleep and Pain*, edited by Gilles Lavigne, Barry J. Sessle, Manon Choiniere, and Peter J. Soja. Seattle: IASP Press, pp. 285–309.

de Blécourt, A. C., A. A. Knipping, N. de Voogd, and M. H. van Rijswijk. 1993. Weather conditions and complaints in fibromyalgia. *Journal of Rheumatology* 20: 1932–34.

Deloukas, P., et al. 1998. A physical map of 30,000 human genes. *Science* 282: 744–46.

Deodhar, A. 2005. Chronic fatigue syndrome. In *Fibromyalgia and Other Central Pain Syndromes,* edited by D. J. Wallace and D. J. Clauw. Philadelphia: Lippincott Williams & Wilkins, pp. 197–208.

Deodhar, A. A., R. A. Fisher, C. V. Blacker, and A. D. Woolf. Fluid retention syndrome and fibromyalgia. *British Journal of Rheumatology* 33: 576–82.

Department of Health and Human Services. 2005. Dietary guidelines for Americans. http://www.health.gov/dietaryguidelines/dga2005/document/default.htm (accessed February 17, 2008).

Dietz, F. R. K. D. Mathews, and W. J. Montgomery. 1990. Reflex sympathetic dystrophy in children. *Clinical Orthopaedics* 258: 225–31.

Dionne, C. E. 2005. Psychological distress confirmed as predictor of long-term back-related functional limitations in primary care settings. *Journal of Clinical Epidemiology* 58: 714–18.

Dobkin, P. L., M. Abrahamowicz, M. A. Fitzcharles, M. Dritsa, and D. da Costa. 2005. Maintenance of exercise in women with fibromyalgia. *Arthritis Care Research* 53: 724–31.

Dobkin, P. L., D. Da Costa, M. Abrahamowicz, M. Dritsa, R. Du Berger, M. A. Fitzcharles, and I. Lowensteyn. 2006. Adherence during an individualized home based 12-week exercise program in women with fibromyalgia. *Journal of Rheumatology* 33: 333–41.

Dobkin, P. L., A. Sita, and M. J. Sewitch. 2006. Predictors of adherence to treatment in women with fibromyalgia. *Clinical Journal of Pain* 22: 286–94.

Dohrenbusch, R., R. Gruterich, and M. Genth. 1996. Fibromyalgia and Sjörgren's Syndrome: Clinical and methodological aspects. *Zeitschrift für Rheumatologie* 55: 19–27.

Dommerholt, J. 2006. Myofascial trigger points: An evidence based review. *Journal of Manual and Manipulative Therapy* 14: 203–21.

Donaldson, C. C. S., G. E. Sella, and H. H. Mueller. 1998. Fibromyalgia: A retrospective study of 252 consecutive referrals. *Canadian Journal of Clinical Medicine* 5: 116–27.

Doron, Y., R. Peleg, A. Peleg, L. Neumann, and D. Buskila. 2004. The clinical and economic burden of fibromyalgia compared with diabetes mellitus and hypertension among Bedouin women in the Negev. *Family Practice* 21: 415–19.

Drossman, D. A. 2006. Rome III, the functional gastrointestinal disorders. http://www .romecriteria.org/assets/pdf/JClinGastro.pdf (accessed February 17, 2008).

Durmer, J. S., and D. F. Dinges. 2005. Neurocognitive consequences of sleep deprivation. *Seminars in Neurology* 25: 117–29.

Ehrlich, G. E. 2003. Pain is real; fibromyalgia isn't. *Journal of Rheumatology* 30: 1666–67.

Eisenberg, E., and E. Melamed. 2003. Can complex regional pain syndrome be painless? *Pain* 106: 263–67.

Elert, J., and B. Gerdle. 1989. The relationship between contraction and relaxation during fatiguing isokinetic shoulder flexions. An electromyographic study. *European Journal of Applied Physiotherapy and Occupational Physiology* 59: 303–309.

Elert, J. E., S. B. Rantapää-Dahlqvist, K. Henriksson-Larsén, R. Lorentzon, and B. U. Gerdlé. 1992. Muscle performance, electromyography and fibre type composition in fibromyalgia and work-related myalgia. *Scandinavian Journal of Rheumatology* 21: 28–34.

Eliav, E., and R. Benoliel. 2005. Myofascial pain syndromes of the head and face. In *Fibromyalgia and Other Central Pain Syndromes*, edited by D. J. Wallace and D. J. Clauw. Philadelphia: Lippincott Williams & Wilkins, pp. 145–64.

Engel, G. L. 1997. From biomedical to biopsychosocial. *Psychotherapy and Psychosomatics* 66: 57–62.

Engstrom-Laurent, A., and R. Hallgren. 1987. Circulating hyaluronic acid levels vary with physical activity in healthy subjects and in rheumatoid arthritis patients. Relationship to synovitis mass and morning stiffness. *Arthritis and Rheumatism* 30: 1333–38.

Enig, M. G., and S. Fallon. 1999. Tripping lightly down the prostaglandin pathways. http://www.westonaprice.org/knowyourfats/tripping.html (accessed January 13, 2008).

Eraso, R. M., N. J. Bradford, C. N. Fontenot, L. R. Espinoza, and A. Gedalia. 2007. Fibromyalgia syndrome in young children: Onset at age 10 years and younger. *Clinical and Experimental Rheumatology* 25: 639–44.

Erhardt, C. C., P. A. Mumford, P. J. Venables, and R. N. Maini. 1989. Factors predicting a poor life prognosis in rheumatoid arthritis: An eight year prospective study. *Annals of Rheumatic Diseases* 48: 7–13.

Eriksson, P. O. 1988. Symptoms and signs of mandibular dysfunction in primary fibromyalgia syndrome (PSF) patients. *Swedish Dental Journal* 12: 141–49.

Escobar, J. I., M. A. Gara, A. M. Diaz-Martinez, A. Interian, M. Warman, L. A. Allen, R. L. Woolfolk, E. Jahn, and D. Rodgers. 2007. Effectiveness of a time-limited cognitive behavior therapy type intervention among primary care patients with medically unexplained symptoms. *Annals of Family Medicine* 5: 328–35.

Evans, J. A. 1946. Reflex sympathetic dystrophy. *Surgical Clinics of North America* 26: 780–90.

Evaskus, D. S., and D. M. Lasskin. 1972. A biochemical measure of stress in patients with myofascial pain dysfunction syndrome. *Journal of Dental Research* 51: 1464–66.

Eysenbach, G., and J. Wyatt. 2002. Using the Internet for surveys and health research. *Journal of Medical Internet Research* 4: E13.

Fass, R., S. Fullerton, B. Naliboff, T. Hirsh, and E. A. Mayer. 1998. Sexual dysfunction in patients with irritable bowel syndrome and non-ulcer dyspepsia. *Digestion* 59: 79–85.

Fass, R., S. Fullerton, S. Tung, and E. A. Mayer. 2000. Sleep disturbances in clinic patients with functional bowel disorders. *American Journal of Gastroenterology* 95: 1195–2000.

Fass, R., G. F. Longstreth, M. Pimentel, S. Fullerton, S. M. Russak, C. F. Chiou, E. Reyes, P. Crane, G. Eisen, B. McCarberg, and J. Ofman. 2001. Evidence- and consensus-based practice guidelines for the diagnosis of irritable bowel syndrome. *Archives of Internal Medicine* 161: 2081–88.

FDA. 2007. Statement on magnets as medical devices. http://www.fda.gov/cdrh/consumer/magnets.html (accessed February 17, 2008).

FDA News. 2007. FDA approves first drug for treating fibromyalgia. http://www.fda.gov/bbs/topics/NEWS/2007/NEW01656.html (accessed February 17, 2008).

Felson, D. T., and D. L. Goldenberg. 1986. The natural history of fibromyalgia. *Arthritis and Rheumatism* 29: 1522–26.

Feskanich, D., V. Singh, W. C. Willett, and G. A. Colditz. 2002. Vitamin A intake and hip fractures among postmenopausal women. *Journal of the American Medical Association* 287: 47–54.

Fibromyalgia Network. Guaifenesin—Is one placebo better than another? http://www.fmnetnews.com/resources-alert-product6.php (accessed November 6, 2007).

Fibromyalgia often overlooked during pregnancy. Aphrodite Women's Health. http://www.aphroditewomenshealth.com/news/20060605210450_health_news.shtml (accessed December 1, 2007).

Fibromyalgia symptoms. http://www.fibromyalgia-symptoms.org/fibromyalgia_pregnancy.html (accessed February 17, 2008).

Field, H. L. 1997. The future of pain treatment. In *Molecular Neurobiology of Pain*, edited by D. Borsook. Seattle: IASP Press, pp. 307–37.

Field, T., M. A. Diego, M. Hernandez-Reif, S. Schanberg, and C. Kuhn. 2004. Massage therapy effects on depressed pregnant women. *Journal of Psychosomatic Obstetrics and Gynaecology* 25: 115–22.

Field, T., N. Grizzle, F. Scafidi, and S. Schanberg. 1996. Massage and relaxation therapies' effects on depressed adolescent mothers. *Adolescence* 31: 903–11.

Field, T., M. Hernandez-Reif, M. Diego, S. Schanberg, and C. Kuhn. 2005. Cortisol decreases and serotonin and dopamine increase following massage therapy. *International Journal of Neuroscience* 115: 1397–413.

Fietta, P., P. Fietta, and P. Manganelli. 2007. Fibromyalgia and psychiatric disorders. *Acta Biomedica* 78: 88–95.

Finestone, H. M., P. Stenn, F. Davies, C. Stalker, R. Fry, and J. Koumanis. 2000. Chronic pain and health care utilization in women with a history of childhood sexual abuse. *Child Abuse and Neglect* 24: 547–56.

Finley, J. E. 2006. Myofascial pain. http://www.emedicine.com/pmr/TOPIC84.HTM (accessed February 17, 2008).

Fischer, H. P., et al. (quoted Russell 2004).

Fitzcharles, M. A., and P. Boulos. 2003. Inaccuracy in the diagnosis of fibromyalgia. *Rheumatology* 42: 263–67.

Fitzhenry, R. I. 1986. *The Fitzhenry and Whiteside Book of Quotations.* Toronto: Fitzhenry & Whiteside.

Folkard, S., and T. H. Monk. 1979. Shiftwork and performance. *Human Factors* 21: 483–92.

Foreman, S. M., and A. C. Croft, eds. 1995. *Whiplash Injuries,* 2nd edition. Baltimore: Williams & Wilkins.

Fors, E. A., and H. Sexton. 2002. Weather and the pain in fibromyalgia: Are they related? *Annals of Rheumatic Diseases* 61: 247–50.

Forseth, K. O., and J. T. Gran. 1992. The prevalence of fibromyalgia among women aged 20–49 years in Arendal, Norway. *Scandinavian Journal of Rheumatology* 21: 74–78.

Frey, L. D., J. T. Locher, P. Hrycaj, T. Stratz, C. Kovac, P. Mennet, and W. Müller. 1992. Determination of regional rate of glucose metabolism in lumbar muscles in patients with generalized tendomyopathy using dynamic 18F-FDG PET. *Zeitschrift für Rheumatologie* 51: 238–42.

Fricton, J. R., R. Kroening, and D. Haley. 1985. Myofascial pain syndrome of the head and neck: A review of clinical characteristics of 164 patients. *Oral Surgery, Oral Medicine, Oral Pathology* 60: 615–23.

Frissora, C. L., and K. L. Koch. 2005. Symptom overlap and comorbidity of irritable bowel syndrome with other conditions. *Current Gastroenterology Reports* 7: 264–71.

Fukuda, K., R. Nisenbaum, G. Stewart, W. W. Thompson, L. Robin, R. M. Washko, D. L. Noah, D. H. Barrett, B. Randall, B. L. Herwaldt, A. C. Mawle, and W. C. Reeves. 1998. A chronic multisymptom illness affecting Air Force veterans of the Persian Gulf War. *Journal of the American Medical Association* 280: 981–88.

Fukuda, K., S. E. Straus, I. Hickie, M. C. Sharpe, J. G. Dobbins, and A. Komaroff. 1994. The chronic fatigue syndrome: A comprehensive approach to its definition and study. International Chronic Fatigue Syndrome Study Group. *Annals of Internal Medicine* 121: 953–59.

Furlan, A. D., J. A. Sandoval, A. Mailis-Gagnon, and E. Tunks. 2006. Opioids for chronic noncancer pain: A meta-analysis of effectiveness and side effects. *Canadian Medical Association Journal* 174: 1589–94.

Galer, B. S., S. Bruhl, and R. N. Harden. 1998. IASP diagnostic criteria for complex regional pain syndrome: A preliminary empirical validation study. *Clinical Journal of Pain* 14: 48–54.

Galer, B. S., S. Butler, and M. P. Jensen. 1995. Case reports and hypothesis: a neglect-like syndrome may be responsible for the motor disturbance in reflex sympathetic dystrophy (complex regional pain syndrome-one). *Journal of Pain Symptom Management* 10: 385–91.

Galloway, J. 1990. Maintaining serenity in chronic illness. *New York State Medical Journal* 90: 366–67.

García-Rodríguez, L. A., A. Ruigómez, M. A. Wallander, S. Johansson, and L. Olbe. 2000. Detection of colorectal tumor and inflammatory bowel disease during follow-up of patients with initial diagnosis of irritable bowel syndrome. *Scandinavian Journal of Gastroenterology* 35: 306–11.

Garrison, F. H. 1929. *An Introduction to the History of Medicine*, 4th edition. Philadelphia: Saunders.

Gedalia, A., C. O. García, J. F. Molina, N. J. Bradford, and L. R. Espinoza. 2000. Fibromyalgia syndrome: Experience in a pediatric rheumatology clinic. *Clinical and Experimental Rheumatology* 18: 415–19.

Gedalia, A., D. A. Person, E. J. Brewer Jr., and E. H. Giannini. 1985. Hypermobility of the joints in juvenile episodic arthritis/arthralgia. *Journal of Pediatrics* 107: 873–76.

Gedalia, A., J. Press, M. Klein, and D. Buskila. 1993. Joint hypermobility and fibromyalgia in schoolchildren. *Annals of Rheumatic Diseases* 52: 494–96.

Geenen, R., J. W. Jacobs, and J. W. Bijlsma. 2002. Evaluation and management of endocrine dysfunction in fibromyalgia. *Rheumatic Disease Clinics of North America* 28: 389–404.

Geer, R. T., et al. 1997. Incidence of automobile accidents involving anaesthesia residents after on-call duty cycles. *Anaesthesiology* 87: A938.

Gendreau, R. M., M. D. Thorn, J. F. Gendreau, J. D. Kranzler, S. Ribeiro, R. H. Gracely, D. A. Williams, P. J. Mease, S. A. McLean, and D. J. Clauw. 2005. Efficacy of milnacipran in patients with fibromyalgia. *Journal of Rheumatology* 32: 1975–85.

Gerber, S., A. M. Bongiovanni, W. J. Ledger, and S. S. Witkin. 2003. Interleukin-1beta gene polymorphism in women with vulvar vestibulitis syndrome. *European Journal of Obstetrics Gynaecology and Reproductive Biology* 107: 4–77.

Giardino, A. 2006. Fibromyalgia in childhood. http://www.emedicine.com/ped/TOPIC 777.HTM (accessed February 17, 2008).

Gibson, P. R., A. N. Elms, and L. A. Ruding. 2003. Perceived treatment efficacy for conventional and alternative therapies reported by persons with multiple chemical sensitivity. *Environmental Health Perspectives* 111: 1498–504.

Giesecke, T., R. H. Gracely, M. A. Grant, A. Nachemson, F. Petzke, D. A. Williams, and D. J. Clauw. 2004. Evidence of augmented central pain processing in idiopathic chronic low back pain. *Arthritis and Rheumatism* 50: 613–23.

Giesecke, T., D. A. Williams, R. E. Harris, T. R. Cupps, X. Tian, T. X. Tian, R. H. Gracely, and D. J. Clauw. 2003. Subgrouping of fibromyalgia patients on the basis of pressure-pain thresholds and psychological factors. *Arthritis and Rheumatism* 48: 2916–22.

Gilliland, R. P. 2007. Fibromyalgia. http://www.emedicine.com/pmr/topic47.htm (accessed February 17, 2008).

Gilron, I., and S. J. L. Flatters. 2006. Gabapentin and pregabalin for the treatment of neuropathic pain: A review of laboratory and clinical evidence. *Pain Research Management* 11 (suppl A): 16A–29A.

Giovengo, S. L., I. J. Russell, and A. A. Larson. 1999. Increased concentrations of nerve growth factor in cerebrospinal fluid of patients with fibromyalgia. *Journal of Rheumatology* 26: 1564–69.

Gladman, D. F., M. B. Urowitz, J. Gough, and A. MacKinnon. 1997. Fibromyalgia as a major contributor of quality of life and lupus. *Journal of Rheumatology* 24: 2145–48.

Glass, J. M., and D. C. Park. 2001. Cognitive dysfunction in fibromyalgia. *Current Rheumatology Reports* 3: 123–27.

Glenn, W. 2002. Idiopathic environmental intolerance. *Occupational Health & Safety Magazine*, January/February.

Goldberg, M. E., R. Domsky, D. Scaringe, R. Hirsh, J. Dotson, I. Sharaf, M. C. Torjman, and R. J. Schwartzman. 2005. Multi-day low dose ketamine infusion for the treatment of complex regional pain syndrome. *Pain Physician* 8: 17–79.

Goldberg, R. T., W. N. Pachas, and D. Keith. 1999. Relationship between traumatic events in childhood and chronic pain. *Disability Rehabilitation* 21: 23–30.

Goldenberg, D. L. 1986. Psychologic studies in fibrositis. *American Journal of Medicine* 81: 67–70.

———. 1987. Fibromyalgia syndrome: An emerging but controversial condition. *Journal of the American Medical Association* 257: 2782–87.

———. 1989. Fibromyalgia and its relation to chronic fatigue syndrome, viral illness and immune abnormalities. *Journal of Rheumatology* 9: 91–93.

———. 1989. Psychological symptoms and psychiatric diagnosis in patients with fibromyalgia. *Journal of Rheumatology Supplement* 19: 127–30.

———. 1992. Fibromyalgia, chronic fatigue and myofascial pain syndromes. *Current Opinion in Rheumatology* 4: 247–57.

Goldenberg, D. L., K. H. Kaplan, and M. Galvin-Nadeau. 1994. A controlled study of a stress-reduction, cognitive-behavioral treatment program in fibromyalgia. *Journal of Musculoskeletal Pain* 2: 53–59.

Goldenberg, D. L., M. Mayskiy, C. Mossey, R. Ruthazer, and C. Schmid. 1996. A randomized double-blind crossover trial of fluoxetine and amitriptyline in the treatment of fibromyalgia. *Arthritis and Rheumatism* 39: 182–88.

Goldenberg, D. L., R. W. Simms, A. Geiger, and A. L. Komaroff. 1990. High frequency of fibromyalgia in patients with chronic fatigue seen in primary care practice. *Arthritis and Rheumatism* 33: 381–89.

Goldstein, J. A. 1993. *Chronic Fatigue Syndromes: The Limbic Hypothesis.* Binghamton: Haworth Medical Press.

Gonsalkorale, W. M., V. Miller, A. Afzal, and P. J. Whorwell. 2003. Long term benefits of hypnotherapy for irritable bowel syndrome. *Gut* 52: 1623–29.

Goodman, J. E., and P. J. McGrath. 1991. The epidemiology of pain in children and adolescents: A review. *Pain* 46: 247–64.

Gordon, A. S., M. Panahian-Jand, F. Mccomb, C. Melegari, and S. Sharp. 2003. Characteristics of women with vulvar pain disorders: Responses to a Web-based survey. *Journal of Sexual and Marital Therapy* 29 (suppl 1): 45–48.

Gordon, D. A. 2003. Fibromyalgia—Real or imagined? *Journal of Rheumatolgy* 30: 1665.

Gots, R. E. 1993. Multiple chemical sensitivities: What is it? *Risk Communication International,* March 31.

———. 1995. Multiple chemical sensitivities—Public policy. *Journal of Toxicology and Clinical Toxicology* 33: 111–13.

Gowans, S. E., A. deHueck, and S. E. Abbey. 2002. Measuring exercise induced mood changes in fibromyalgia: A comparison of several measures. *Arthritis Care Research* 47: 603–609.

Gowans, S. E., A. deHueck, S. Voss, A. Silaj, S. E. Abbey, and W. J. Reynolds. 2001. Effect of a randomized, control trial of exercise on mood and physical function in individuals with fibromyalgia. *Arthritis and Rheumatology* 45: 519–29.

Gowans, S. E., and A. DeHueck. 2004. Effectiveness of exercise in management of fibromyalgia. *Current Opinion in Rheumatology* 16: 138–42.

Gowers, W. R. 1904. Lumbago: Its lessons and analogues. *British Medical Journal* 1: 117–21.

Grace, G. M., W. R. Nielson, M. Hopkins, and M. A. Berg. 1999. Concentration and memory deficits in patients with fibromyalgia syndrome. *Journal of Clinical and Experimental Neuropsychology* 21: 477–87.

Gracely, R. H. 2007. A pain psychologist's view of tenderness in fibromyalgia. *Journal of Rheumatology* 34: 912–14.

Gracely, R. H., F. Petzke, J. M. Wolf, and D. J. Clauw. 2002. Functional magnetic resonance imaging evidence of augmented pain processing in fibromyalgia. *Arthritis and Rheumatism* 46: 1333–43.

Grahame, R., and A. J. Hakim. 2008. Systemic disorders with rheumatic manifestations. *Current Opinion in Rheumatolgy* 20: 106–10.

Granges, G., and G. O. Littlejohn. 1993. A comparative study of clinical signs in fibromyalgia/fibrositis syndrome, healthy and exercising subjects. *Journal of Rheumatology* 20: 344–51.

————. 1993. Prevalence of myofascial pain syndrome in fibromyalgia syndrome and regional pain syndrome: A comparative study. *Journal of Musculoskeletal Pain* 1: 19–36.

Granges, G., P. Zilko, and G. O. Littlejohn. 1994. Fibromyalgia syndrome: Assessment of the severity of the condition 2 years after diagnosis. *Journal of Rheumatology* 21: 523–29.

Green, J. R., and S. Shah. 1993. Power comparison of various sibship tests of association. *Annals of Human Genetics* 57: 151–58.

Greenfield, S., M. A. Fitzcharles, and J. M. Esdaile. 1992. Reactive fibromyalgia syndrome. *Arthritis and Rheumatism* 35: 678–81.

Greenhalgh, S. 2001. *Under the Medical Gaze. Facts and Fictions of Chronic Pain.* Berkeley: University of California Press.

Griep, E. N., J. W. Boersma, and E. R. de Kloet. 1993. Altered reactivity of the hypothalamic-pituitaty-adrenal axis in the primary fibromyalgia syndrome. *Journal of Rheumatology* 20: 469–74.

Grönblad, M., J. Nykänen, Y. Konttinen, E. Järvinen, and T. Helve. 1993. Effect of zopiclone on sleep quality, morning stiffness, widespread tenderness and pain and general discomfort in primary fibromyalgia patients. A double-blind randomized trial. *Clinical Rheumatology* 12: 186–91.

Gunzburg, R., and M. Szpalski, eds. 1998. *Whiplash Injuries.* Philadelphia: Lippincott-Raven.

Gupta, A., J. McBeth, G. J. Macfarlane, R. Morriss, C. Dickens, D. Ray, Y. H. Chiu, and A. J. Silman. 2007. Pressure pain thresholds and tender points count as predictors of new chronic widespread pain in somatising subjects. *Annals of Rheumatic Diseases* 66: 517–21.

Gupta, A., A. J. Silman, D. Ray, R. Morriss, C. Dickens, G. J. MacFarlane, Y. H. Chiu, B. Nicholl, and J. McBeth. 2007. The role of psychosocial factors in predicting the onset of chronic widespread pain: Results from a prospective population-based study. *Rheumatology* 46: 666–71.

Gureje, et al., cited in F. Blotman and J. Branco. 2006. *La Fibromyalgie. La Douleur au Quotidien.* Toulouse: Éditions Privat.

Gusi, N., P. Thomas-Carus, and A. Hakkinen. 2006. Exercise in waist-high warm water decreases pain and improves health-related quality of life and strength in the lower extremities in women with fibromyalgia. *Arthritis Care Research* 55: 66–73.

Hadler, N. M. 1996. If you have to prove you are ill, you can't get well. The objective lesson of fibromyalgia. *Spine* 21: 2397–400.

————. 2003. "Fibromyalgia" and the medicalization of misery. *Journal of Rheumatology* 30: 1668–70.

Hadler, N. M., and S. Greenhalgh. 2004. Labeling woefulness: The social construction of fibromyalgia. *Spine* 30: 1–4.

Hagglund, K. J., W. E. Deuser, S. P. Buckelew, J. Hewett, and D. R. Kay. 1994. Weather, beliefs about weather, and disease severity among patients with fibromyalgia. *Arthritis Care Research* 7: 130–35.

Halberg, F. Introduction to chronobiology. http://www.msi.umn.edu/~halberg/introd/for.html (accessed February 17, 2008).

Hall, M. C. 1961. *The Ground Substance of Loose Connective Tissue.* Thesis. University of Toronto.

———. 1965. *The Locomotor System. Functional Anatomy.* Springfield: Thomas.

———. 1965. *Luschka's Joint.* Springfield: Thomas.

———. 1996. *IME. The Word Book.* Toronto: Indemed.

———. 1998. *Independent Medical Examinations for Insurance and Legal Reports.* Toronto: Butterworth.

Halpert, A. D., A. C. Thomas, Y. Hu, C. B. Morris, S. I. Bangdiwala, and D. A. Drossman. 2006. A survey on patient educational needs in irritable bowel syndrome and attitudes toward participation in clinical research. *Journal of Clinical Gastroenterology* 40: 37–43.

Hamilton, H. 1960. A rating scale for depression. *Journal of Neurology and Neurosurgery and Psychiatry* 23: 56–62.

Hänsel, R., et al. 1998. In *Rational Phytotherapy*, edited by Volker Schulz, Rudolf Hansel, and Varro E. Tyler. Berlin: Springer, pp. 87–97.

Haraldsson, B. G., A. R. Gross, and C. D. Myers. 2006. Massage for mechanical neck disorders. *Cochrane Database of Systematic Reviews* 3: CD004871.

Harding, S. M. 1998. Sleep in fibromyalgia patients: Subjective and objective findings. *American Journal of Medical Science* 315: 367–76.

Harlow, B. L., and E. G. Stewart. 2003. A population-based assessment of chronic unexplained vulvar pain: Have we underestimated the prevalence of vulvodynia? *Journal of the American Medical Womens Association* 58: 82–88.

———. 2005. Adult-onset vulvodynia in relation to childhood violence victimization. *American Journal of Epidemiology.* 161: 871–80.

Harris, L. A., and L. Chang. 2005. The functional bowel disorder spectrum. In *Fibromyalgia and Other Central Pain Syndromes*, edited by D. J. Wallace and D. J. Clauw. Philadelphia: Lippincott Williams & Wilkins, pp. 209–34.

Harth, M., and W. R. Nielson. 2007. The fibromyalgia tender points: Use them or lose them? A brief review of the controversy. *Journal of Rheumatology* 34: 914–22.

Hartz, A., and E. Kirchdoerfer. 1987. Undetected fibrositis in primary care practice. *Journal of Family Practice* 25: 365–69.

Hasselstrom, et al., cited in F. Blotman and J. Branco. 2006. *La Fibromyalgie. La Douleur au Quotidien.* Toulouse: Éditions Privat.

Hauri, P., and D. R. Hawkins. 1973. Alpha delta sleep. *Electoencephalography and Clinical Neurophysiology* 34: 233–37.

Hawley, D. J., and F. Wolfe. 1991. Pain disability and pain/disability relationships in seven rheumatic disorders: A study of 1522 patients. *Journal of Rheumatology* 18: 1552–57.

———. 1993. Depression is not more common in rheumatoid arthritis: A 10-year longitudinal study of 6,153 rheumatic disease patients. *Journal of Rheumatology* 20: 2025–31.

Hawley, D. J., F. Wolfe, and M. A. Cathey. 1988. Pain, functional disability, and psychological status: A 12-month study of severity in fibromyalgia. *Journal of Rheumatology* 15: 1551–56.

Hazelton, L., and C. Hickey. 2003. Cinderology: The Cinderella of academic medicine. *Canadian Medical Association Journal* 171: 1495–96.

Hazemeijer, I., and J. J. Rasker. 2003. Fibromyalgia and the therapeutic domain. A philosophical study on the origins of fibromyalgia in a specific social setting. *Rheumatology* 42: 507–15.

Hazes, J. M. W., R. Hayton, and A. J. Stilman. 1993. A reevaluation of the symptom of morning stiffness. *Journal of Rheumatology* 20: 1138–42.

Head, H. 1922. An address on certain aspects of pain. *British Medical Journal* 1: 1–5.

Helthoff, K. B., and C. V. Burton. 1985. CT evaluation of the failed back surgery syndrome. *Orthopaedic Clinics of North America* 16: 417–44.

Henriksson, C., I. Gundmark, A. Bengtsson, and A. C. Ek. 1992. Living with fibromyalgia: Consequences for everyday life. *Clinical Journal of Pain* 8: 138–44.

Henry, M. 2007. Doctor jailed for trafficking in painkillers. *Toronto Star*, November 14. http://www.thestar.com/printArticle/276283 (accessed February 17, 2008).

Hentschel, H. D., and J. Schneider. 2004. The history of massage in the ways of life and health in India. *Wurzburg Medizinhistorich Mitteilungen* 23: 179–203.

Hester, G., A. E. Grant, and I. J. Russell. 1982. Psychological evaluation and behavioural treatments with fibrositis. *Arthritis and Rheumatism* 25: S148.

Heymann-Mönnikes, I., R. Arnold, I. Florin, C. Herda, S. Melfsen, and H. Mönnikes. 2000. The combination of medical treatment plus multicomponent behavioral therapy is superior to medical treatment alone in the therapy of irritable bowel syndrome. *American Journal of Gastroenterology* 95: 981–94.

Hills, E. C. 2006. Adult physiatric history and examination. http://www.emedicine.com/pmr/TOPIC146.HTM (accessed February 17, 2008).

Hoheisel, U., S. Mense, and M. Ratkai. 1995. Effects of spinal cord superfusion with substance P on the excitability of rat dorsal horn neurons processing input from deep tissues. *Journal of Musculoskeletal Pain* 3: 23–43.

Holbrook, A. M. 2000. The diagnosis and management of insomnia in clinical practice. *Canadian Medical Association Journal* 162: 216–38.

Holman, A. J., and R. R. Myers. 2005. A randomized, double-blind, placebo-controlled trial of pramipexole, a dopamine agonist, in patients with fibromyalgia receiving concomitant medications. *Arthritis and Rheumatism* 52: 2495–505.

Holmes, E. B. 2007. Impairment rating and disability evaluation. http://www.emedicine .com/pmr/TOPIC170.HTM (accessed January 15, 2008).

Holmes, G. P., et al. 1988. Chronic fatigue syndrome: A working case definition. *Annals of Internal Medicine* 108: 387–89.

Holroyd, K. A., F. J. O'Donnell, M. Stensland, G. L. Lipchik, G. E. Cordingley, and B. W. Carlson. 2001. Management of chronic tension-type headache with tricyclic antidepressant medication, stress management therapy, and their combination: A randomized controlled trial. *Journal of the American Medical Association* 285: 2208–215.

Holstege, G. 2003. Orgasm akin to a shot of heroin. *Expatica.* http://www.sensualism .com/sex/orgasm.html (accessed February 17, 2008).

Hong, C.-Z., T.-C. Hsueh, and D. G. Simons. 1995. Difference in pain relief after trigger point injections in myofascial pain patients with and without fibromyalgia. *Journal of Musculoskeletal Pain* 3 (suppl 1): 60.

Hord, E.-D., and S. Mueed. 2006. Reflex sympathetic dystrophy. http://www.emedicine .com/neuro/TOPIC627.HTM (accessed December 15, 2007).

Horizon, A. H., and M. H. Weisman. 2005. Prognosis. In *Fibromyalgia and Other Central Pain Syndromes*, edited by D. J. Wallace and D. J. Clauw. Philadelphia: Lippincott Williams & Wilkins.

Horne, J. 2006. *Sleepfaring.* Oxford: Oxford University Press.

Hudson, J. I., L. M. Arnold, and P. E. Keck Jr. 2004. Family study of fibromyalgia and affective spectrum disorder. *Biological Psychiatry* 56: 884–91.

Hudson, J. I., D. L. Goldenberg, H. G. Pope Jr., P. E. Keck Jr., and L. Schlesinger. 1992. Comorbidity of fibromyalgia with medical and psychiatric disorders. *American Journal of Medicine* 92: 363–67.

Hudson, J. I., M. S. Hudson, L. F. Pliner, D. L. Goldenberg, and H. G. Pope Jr. 1985. Fibromyalgia and major affective disorder: A controlled phenomenology and family history study. *American Journal of Psychiatry* 142: 441–46.

Hudson, J. I., B. Mangweth, H. G. Pope Jr., C. De Col, A. Hausmann, S. Gutweniger, N. M. Laird, W. Biebl, M. T. Tsuang. 2003. Family study of affective spectrum disorder. *Archives of General Psychiatry* 60: 170–77.

Hudson, J. I., L. F. Pliner, M. S. Hudson, D. L. Goldenberg, and J. C. Melby. 1984. The dexamethasone suppression test in fibrositis. *Biological Psychiatry* 19: 1489–93.

Hudson, J. I., and H. G. Pope Jr. 1995. Does childhood sexual abuse cause fibromyalgia? *Arthritis and Rheumatism* 38: 161–63.

Hughes, G., et al. 2006. The impact of a diagnosis of fibromyalgia on health care resource use by primary care patients in the UK: An observational study based on clinical practice. *Arthritis and Rheumatism* 54: 177–83.

Hulisz, D. 2004. The burden of illness of irritable bowel syndrome: Current challenges and hope for the future. *Journal of Managed Care Pharmacy* 10: 299–309.

Hunt, I. M., A. J. Silman, S. Benjamin, J. McBeth, and G. J. Macfarlane. 1999. The prevalence and associated features of chronic widespread pain in the community using the "Manchester" definition of chronic widespread pain. *Rheumatology* 38: 275–79.

Hurwitz, E. L., H. Morgenstern, F. Yu. 2003. Cross-sectional and longitudinal associations of low-back pain and related disability with psychological distress among patients enrolled in the UCLA Low-Back Pain Study. *Journal of Clinical Epidemiology* 56: 463–71.

Hutchins, M. O., and H. S. Skjonsby. 1990. Microtrauma to rat superficial masseter muscles following lengthening contractions. *Journal of Dental Research* 69: 1580–85.

Iadarola, M. J., M. B. Max, K. F. Berman, M. G. Byas-Smith, R. C. Coghill, R. H. Gracely, and G. J. Bennett. 1995. Unilateral decrease in thalamic activity observed with positron emission tomography in patients with chronic neuropathic pain. *Pain* 63: 55–64.

IMS Health. National Prescription Audit Plus. http://www.imshealth.com (accessed January 20, 2008).

Inanici, F., et al. 1998. Prognosis of regional fibromyalgia: Comparison with fibromyalgia syndrome. *Journal of Musculoskeletal Pain* 6: 97–103.

Inanici, F., M. B. Yunus, and J. C. Aldag. 1999. Clinical features and psychological factors in regional soft tissue pain: Comparison with fibromyalgia syndrome. *Journal of Musculoskeletal Pain* 7: 293–301.

Institute of Medicine. 2007. Dietary reference intake research synthesis. http://www.iom.edu/ (accessed February 17, 2008).

International Foundation for Functional Gastro-Intestinal Disorders. Facts about IBS. http://www.iffgd.org/site/gi-disorders/adults/functional-gi-disorders (accessed January 20, 2008).

International Headache Society. Classification. http://www.ihs-classification.org/en/02_klassifikation/02_teil1/ (accessed February 17, 2008).

Ironson, G., T. Field, F. Scafidi, M. Hashimoto, M. Kumar, A. Kumar, A. Price, A. Goncalves, I. Burman, C. Tetenman, R. Patarca, and M. A. Fletcher. 1996. Massage therapy is associated with enhancement of the immune system's cytotoxic capacity. *International Journal of Neuroscience* 84: 205–17.

Jacob, S. W., and J. Appleton. 2003. *MSM: The Definitive Guide. A Comprehensive Review of the Science and Therapeutics of Methylsulfonylmethane.* Topanga: Freedom Press, pp. 107–21.

Jacobsen, S., and B. Holm. 1992. Muscle strength and endurance compared to aerobic capacity in primary fibromyalgia syndrome. *Clinical and Experimental Rheumatology* 10: 419–27.

Jacobsen, S., and O. J. Hoydalsmo. 1993. Experiment or research on muscle physiology during work and exercise. Progress in fibromyalgia and myofascial pain. *Pain Research and Clinical Management 6.* Amsterdam: Elsevier.

Jacobsen, S., et al. 1993. Consensus document on fibromyalgia: The Copenhagen Declaration. *Journal of Musculoskeletal Pain* 1: 295–312.

Jacobsson, L., F. Lindgärde, and R. Manthorpe. 1989. The commonest rheumatic complaints of over six weeks' duration in a twelve-month period in a defined Swedish population. Prevalences and relationships. *Scandinavian Journal of Rheumatology* 18: 353–60.

Jain, A. K., et al. 2003. Fibromyalgia syndrome: Canadian clinical working case definition, diagnostic and treatment protocols—a consensus document. *Journal of Musculoskeletal Pain* 11: 3–107.

James, S. D. 2007. People need both drugs and faith to get rid of pain. http://abcnews .go.com/Health/Technology/story?id=3433101&page=1 (accessed February 17, 2008).

Jamieson, D. J., and J. F. Steege. 1996. The prevalence of dysmenorrhoea, dyspareunia, pelvic pain and irritable bowel syndrome in primary care practice. *Obstetrics and Gynecology* 87: 55–58.

Jänig, W., and M. Stanton-Hicks, eds. 1996. *Reflex Sympathetic Dystrophy: A Reappraisal.* Seattle: IASP Press.

Jantos, M. 2007. Understanding chronic pelvic pain. *Pelviperineology* 26: 66–69.

Jason, L. A., J. A. Richman, A. W. Rademaker, K. M. Jordan, A. V. Plioplys, R. R. Taylor, W. McCready, C. F. Huang, S. Plioplys. 1999. A community-based study of chronic fatigue syndrome. *Archives of Internal Medicine* 159: 2129–37.

Jeffrey, S. 2007. Gene variant found for periodic limb movements in sleep. *New England Journal of Medicine.* http://www.medscape.com/viewarticle/560145 (accessed February 17, 2008).

Jeffreys, D. 2004. *Aspirin: The Remarkable Story of a Wonder Drug.* London: Bloomsbury.

Jensen, M. C. 1994. Magnetic resonance imaging of the lumbar spine in people without back pain. *New England Journal of Medicine* 331: 69–73.

Jensen, R. 1999. Pathophysiological mechanisms of tension-type headache: A review of epidemiological and experimental studies. *Cephalalgia* 19: 602–21.

———. 2001. Tension-type headache. *Current Treatment Options in Neurology* 3: 169–80.

Jensen, R., and J. Olesen. 1996. Initiating mechanisms of experimentally induced tension-type headache. *Cephalalgia* 16: 175–82.

———. 2000. Tension-type headache: An update on mechanisms and treatment. *Current Opinion in Neurology* 13: 285–89.

Jentoft, E. S., A. G. Kvalik, and A. M. Mengshoel. 2001. Effects of pool-based and land-based aerobic exercise on women with fibromyalgia / chronic widespread muscle pain. *Arthritis Care Research* 45: 42–47.

Jones, K. D., C. Burckhardt, and J. A. Bennett. 2004. Motivational interviewing may encourage exercise in persons with fibromyalgia by enhancing self efficacy. *Arthritis Care Research* 51: 864–67.

Jones, K. D., C. Burckhardt, and S. R. Clark. 2002. A randomized controlled trial of muscle strengthening versus flexibility training in fibromyalgia. *Journal of Rheumatology* 29: 1041–48.

Jones, K. D., and S. R. Clark. 2002. Individualizing the exercise prescription for persons with fibromyalgia. *Rheumatic Disease Clinics of North America* 28: 1–18.

Jones, K. D., S. R. Clark, and R. M. Bennett. 2002. Prescribing exercise for people with fibromyalgia. *American Association of Colleges of Nursing Clinical Issues* 13: 277–93.

Joyce, J., M. Hotopf, and S. Wessely. 1997. The prognosis of chronic fatigue syndrome: A systematic review. *Quarterly Journal of Medicine* 90: 223–33.

KAHC. 2007. Ayurvedic treatments. http://www.kahc.co.uk/treatments.html (accessed February 17, 2008).

Kang, Y-K, I. J. Russell, G. A. Vipraio, and I. N. Acworth. 1998. Low urinary 5-hydroxyindole acetic acid in fibromyalgia syndrome: Evidence in support of a serotonin-deficiency pathogenesis. *Myalgia* 1: 14–21.

Karjalainen, K., A. Malmivaara, M. W. van Tulder, R. Roine, M. Jauhiainen, H. Hurri, and B. W. Koes. 2000. Multi-disciplinary rehabilitation for fibromyalgia and musculoskeletal pain in working age adults. *Cochrane Database of Systematic Reviews* 2:CD001984.

Katon, W., M. Sullivan, and E. Walker. 2001. Medical symptoms without identified pathology: Relationship to psychiatric disorders, childhood and adult trauma, and personality traits. *Annals of Internal Medicine* 11: 917–25.

Katz, R. S., and H. M. Kravitz. 1996. Fibromyalgia, depression, and alcoholism: A family history study. *Journal of Rheumatology* 23: 149–54.

Katz, R. S., F. Wolfe, and K. Michaud. 2006. Fibromyalgia diagnosis: A comparison of clinical, survey, and American College of Rheumatology criteria. *Arthritis and Rheumatism.* 54: 169–76.

Kawakami, N., N. Iwata, S. Fujihara, and T. Kitamura. 1998. Prevalence of chronic fatigue syndrome in a community population in Japan. *Tohoku Journal of Experimental Medicine* 186: 33–41.

Kay, D. C. 1969. Morphine effects on human REM state, waking state and REM sleep. *Psychopharmacologica* 14: 404–16.

Kaye, V., and M. E. Branstater. 2007. Transcutaneous electrical nerve stimulation. http://emedicine.medscape.com/article/325107 (accessed March 31, 2009).

Keifer, J. C. 1992. Sleep disruption and increased apneas following pontine microinjection of morphine. *Anesthesiology* 77: 973–82.

———. 1996. Pontine cholinergic mechanisms modulate the cortical electroencephalographic spindles of halothane anesthesia. *Anesthesiology* 84: 945–54.

Kellgren, J. H. 1938. Observations on referred pain arising from muscle. *British Medical Journal* 1: 325–27.

————. 1939. On the distribution of pain arising from deep somatic structures with charts of segmental pain areas. *Clinical Science* 4: 35–53.

————. 1949. Deep pain sensibility. *Lancet* 1: 943–49.

Kemler, M. A., and C. A. Furnee. 2002. Economic evaluation of spinal cord stimulation for chronic reflex dystrophy. *Neurology* 59: 1203–1209.

Kennedy, T., R. Jones, S. Darnley, P. Seed, S. Wessely, and T. Chalder. 2005. Cognitive behaviour therapy in addition to antispasmodic treatment for irritable bowel syndrome in primary care: Randomised controlled trial. *British Medical Journal* 331: 435–39.

Khostanteen, I., E. R. Tunks, C. H. Goldsmith, and J. Ennis. 2000. Fibromyalgia: Can one distinguish it from simulation? An observer-blind controlled study. *Journal of Rheumatology* 27: 2671–76.

Kieffer, B. 2007. European College of Neuropsychopharmacology. How does the opioid system control pain, reward addictive behavior? http://www.sciencedaily.com/releases/2007/10/071014163647.htm (accessed January 10, 2008).

Kim, C. S. 2002. Musculoskeletal pain in adolescents: Diagnostic criteria are distinct from those of adult forms. *Postgraduate Medicine* 111. http://www.postgradmed.com/issues/2002/04_02/kim.htm (accessed February 17, 2008).

King, A. E., and J. A. Lopez-Garcia. 1993. Excitatory amino acid receptor-mediated neurotransmission from cutaneous afferents in rat dorsal horn in vitro. *Journal of Physiology* 472: 443–57.

Kirmayer, L. J., J. M. Robbins, and M. A. Kapusta. 1988. Somatization and depression in fibromyalgia syndrome. *American Journal of Psychiatry* 14: 950–54.

Kivimäki, M., P. Leino-Arjas, M. Virtanen, M. Elovainio, L. Keltikangas-Järvinen, S. Puttonen, M. Vartia, E. Brunner, and J. Vahtera. 2004. Work stress and incidence of newly diagnosed fibromyalgia: Prospective cohort study. *Journal of Psychosomatic Research* 57: 417–22.

Kleinman, L., N. K. Leidy, J. Crawley, A. Bonomi, and P. Schoenfeld. 2001. A comparative trial of paper-and-pencil versus computer administration of the Quality of Life in Reflux and Dyspepsia (QOLRAD) questionnaire. *Medical Care* 39: 181–89.

Kleinstück, F., J. Dvorak, and A. F. Mannion. 2006. Are "structural abnormalities" on magnetic resonance imaging a contraindication to the successful conservative treatment of chronic nonspecific low back pain? *Spine* 31: 2250–57.

Kleitman, N. 1963. *Sleep and Wakefulness.* Chicago: University of Chicago Press.

Kocsis, J. J., S. Harkaway, and R. Snyder. 1975. Biological effects of the metabolites of dimethyl sulfoxide. *Annals of the New York Academy of Science* 243: 104–109.

Koerber, R. K., R. Torkelson, G. Haven, J. Donaldson, S. M. Cohen, and M. Case. 1984. Increased cerebrospinal fluid 5-HT and 5-HIAA in Kleine-Levin syndrome. *Neurology* 34: 1597–1600.

Kozin, F. Painful shoulder and the reflex sympathetic dystrophy syndrome. In *Arthritis and Allied Conditions*, 13th edition, edited by W. J. Koopman. Philadelphia: Williams & Wilkins.

————. 2005. Reflex sympathetic dystrophy syndrome. In *Fibromyalgia and Other Central Pain Syndromes*, edited by D. J. Wallace and D. J. Clauw. Philadelphia: Lippincott Williams & Wilkins, pp. 259–66.

Krogh-Poulsen, W. G., and A. Olsson. 1966. Occlusal disharmonies and dysfunction of the stomatognathic system. *Dental Clinics of North America* 11: 627–35.

Krolczyk, S. J., M.-C. B. Wilson, L. Benes-Cases, S. Chen, and A. R. Gonzalez-Rodriguez. 2007. Persistent idiopathic facial pain. http://www.emedicine.com/neuro/TOPIC25.HTM (accessed February 17, 2008).

Kryger, M., T. Roth, and W. Dement. 2000. *Principles & Practices of Sleep Medicine*. Philadelphia: W. B. Saunders Company.

Kshatri, A. M. 1998. Cholinomimetics, but not morphine, increase antinociceptive behaviour from pontine reticular regions regulating rapid eye movement sleep. *Sleep* 21: 677–85.

Kurland, J. E., W. J. Coyle, A. Winkler, and E. Zable. 2006. Prevalence of irritable bowel syndrome and depression in fibromyalgia. *Digestive Diseases Sciences* 51: 454–60.

Kwiatek, R., L. Barnden, R. Tedman, R. Jarrett, J. Chew, C. Rowe, and K. Pile. 2000. Regional cerebral blood flow in fibromyalgia: Single photon-emission computed tomography evidence of reduction in the pontine tegmentum and thalami. *Arthritis and Rheumatism* 43: 2823–33.

Lacour, M., T. Zunder, M. Dettenkofer, S. Schönbeck, R. Lüdtke, and C. Scheidt. 2002. An interdisciplinary therapeutic approach for dealing with patients attributing chronic fatigue and functional memory disorders to environmental poisoning—A pilot study. *International Journal of Hygiene and Environmental Health* 204: 339–46.

Lampe, A., E. Solder, and A. Ennemoser. 2000. Chronic pelvic pain and previous sexual abuse. *Obstetrics and Gynecology* 96: 929–33.

Lander, E. S., et al. 2001. International human genome sequencing consortium: Initial sequencing and analysis of the human genome. *Nature* 409: 860–921.

Landro, N. I., T. C. Stiles, and H. Sletvold. 1997. Memory functioning in patients with primary fibromyalgia and major depression and healthy controls. *Journal of Psychosomatic Research* 42: 297–306.

Lápossy, E., R. Maleitzke, P. Hrycaj, W. Mennet, and W. Müller. 1995. The frequency of transition of chronic low back pain to fibromyalgia. *Scandinavian Journal of Rheumatology* 24: 29–33.

Larson, A. A., S. L. Giovengo, I. J. Russell, and J. E. Michalek. 2000. Changes in the concentrations of amino acids in the cerebrospinal fluid that correlate with pain in patients with fibromyalgia: Implications for nitric oxide pathways. *Pain* 87: 201–11.

Lautenbacher, S., G. B. Rollman, and G. A. MacCain. 1994. Multi-method assessment of experimental and clinical pain in patients with fibromyalgia. *Pain* 59: 45–53.

Lavigne, G. Pain and sleep. *In Principles and Practices of Sleep Medicine*, volume 4, edited by M. T. Kryger. Philadelphia: Elsevier Saunders, pp. 1246–55.

————. 2007. Tools and methodological issues in the investigation of sleep and pain interactions. In *Sleep and Pain*, edited by Gilles Lavigne, Barry J. Sessle, Manon Choiniere, and Peter J. Soja. Seattle: IASP Press, pp. 235–63.

Lawrence, R. C., C. G. Helmick, F. C. Arnett, R. A. Deyo, D. T. Felson, E. H. Giannini, S. P. Heyse, R. Hirsch, M. C. Hochberg, G. G. Hunder, M. H. Liang, S. R. Pillemer, V. D. Steen, and F. Wolfe. 2008. Estimates of the prevalence of arthritis and selected musculoskeletal disorders in the United States: Part II. *Arthritis and Rheumatism* 58: 26–35.

Lawton, M. P., and E. M. Brody. 1969. Assessment of older people: Self-maintaining and instrumental activities of daily living. *Gerontologist* 9: 179–86.

Lax, M. B., and P. K. Henneberger. 1995. Patients with multiple chemical sensitivities in an occupational health clinic: Presentation and follow-up. *Archives of Environmental Health* 50: 425–31.

Leavitt, F., and R. S. Katz. 1989. Is the MMPI invalid for assessing psychological disturbance in pain related organic conditions? *Journal of Rheumatology* 16: 521–26.

Leavitt, F., R. S. Katz, H. E. Golden, P. B. Glickman, and L. F. Layfer. 1986. Comparison of pain properties in fibromyalgia patients and rheumatoid arthritis patients. *Arthritis and Rheumatism* 29: 775–81.

Ledingham, J., S. Doherty, and M. Doherty. 1993. Primary fibromyalgia syndrome: An outcome study. *British Journal of Rheumatology* 32: 139–42.

Leger, D. 1994. The cost of sleep-related accidents: A report for the National Commission on Sleep Disorders Research. *Sleep* 17: 84–93.

Lehmkuhl, D. 1987. General anaesthesia and post-narcotic sleep disorders. *Neuropsychobiology* 18: 37–42.

Lehrer, J. 2007. Irritable bowel syndrome. http://www.emedicine.com/med/TOPIC 1190.HTM (accessed February 17, 2008).

Lenznoff, A. 1997. Provocation challenges in patients with multiple chemical sensitivity. *Journal of Allergy and Clinical Immunology* 99: 438–42.

Leong, S. A., V. Barghout, H. G. Birnbaum, C. E. Thibeault, R. Ben-Hamadi, F. Frech, and J. J. Ofman. 2003. The economic consequences of irritable bowel syndrome: A US employer perspective. *Archives of Internal Medicine* 163: 929–35.

Leriche, R. 1916. De la causalgie envisagée comme une névrite du sympathique et de son traitement par la dénudation et l'excision des plexus nerveux périarteriels. *Presse Médicale* 24: 178–280.

————. 1937. *La Chirurgie de la Douleur.* Paris: Masson.

Levy, R. L., M. Von Korff, W. E. Whitehead, P. Stang, K. Saunders, P. Jhingran, V. Barghout, and A. D. Feld. 2001. Costs of care for irritable bowel syndrome patients in a health maintenance organization. *American Journal of Gastroenterology* 96: 3122–29.

Liller, T. K., J. B. Muller, and J. L. Catlett. 1995. *Fibromyalgia: A Multi-dimensional Profile.* Fairfax, VA: Fibromyalgia Association of Greater Washington.

Lim, B., E. Manheimer, L. Lao, E. Ziea, J. Wisniewski, J. Liu, and B. M. Berman. 2004. Acupuncture for treatment of irritable bowel syndrome. *Cochrane Database of Systematic Reviews*: CD005111.

Lind, J. 1980. *Treatise on the Scurvy*. Birmingham: Gryphon Editions Limited.

Lindell, L., S. Bergman, I. F. Petersson, L. T. Jacobsson, and P. Herrström. 2000. Prevalence of fibromyalgia and chronic widespread pain. *Scandinavian Journal of Primary Health Care* 18: 149–53.

Lineker, S. E., E. Badley, C. Charles, L. Hart, and D. Streiner. 1999. Defining morning stiffness in rheumatoid arthritis. *Journal of Rheumatology* 26: 1052–57.

Linton, S. J. 2005. *Understanding Pain for Better Clinical Practice: A Psychologist's Perspective*. London: Elsevier.

Lisse, J. R., and M. Oberto-Medina. 2006. Raynaud phenomenon. http.www.emedicine.com./med/TOPIC1993.HTM (accessed March 31, 2009).

Littlejohn, G. O., C. Weinstein, and R. D. Helme. 1987. Increased neurogenic inflammation in fibrositis syndrome. *Journal of Rheumatology* 14: 1022–25.

Longstreth, G. F., and J. F. Yao. 2004. Irritable bowel syndrome and surgery: A multivariable analysis. *Gastroenterology* 126: 1665–73.

Loomis, A. L., E. N. Harvey, and G. Hobart. 1938. Distribution of disturbance patterns in the human electroencephalogram with special reference to sleep. *Journal of Neurophysiology* 1: 413–30.

Lue, F., A. MacLean, and H. Moldofsky. 1991. Sleep physiology and psychological aspects of the fibrositis (fibromyalgia) syndrome. *Canadian Journal of Psychology* 45: 179–84.

Luetkemeyer, J. 2005. Rheumatologists are NOT the doctors to deal with fibromyalgia. http:www.medscape.com/viewarticle/538164 (accessed February 17, 2008).

Lund, N., A. Bengtsson, and P. Thorberg. 1986. Muscle tissue oxygen pressure in primary fibromyalgia. *Scandinavian Journal of Rheumatology* 15: 165–73.

Lurie, M., K. Caidahl, G. Johansson, and B. Bake. 1990. Respiratory function in chronic primary fibromyalgia. *Scandinavian Journal of Rehabilitation Medicine* 22: 151–55.

Lydell, C. 1992. The prevalence of fibromyalgia in a South African community. *Scandinavian Journal of Rheumatology* 94 (suppl): S143.

Lydic, R., and H. A. Baghdoyan. 2007. Neurochemical mechanisms mediating opioid-induced REM sleep disruption. In *Sleep and Pain*, edited by Gilles Lavigne, Barry J. Sessle, Manon Choiniere, and Peter J. Soja. Seattle: IASP Press, pp. 99–122.

Lyznicki, J. M., T. C. Doege, R. M. Davis, and M. A. Williams. 1998. Sleepiness, driving, and motor vehicle crashes. Council on Scientific Affairs, American Medical Association. *Journal of the American Medical Association* 279: 1908–13.

MacFarlane, G. J., E. Thomas, and A. C. Papageorgiou. 1996. The natural history of chronic pain in the community: A better prognosis than in the clinic? *Journal of Rheumatology* 23: 1617–20.

MacFarlane, J. G., B. Shahal, C. Mously, and H. Moldofsky. 1996. Periodic K-alpha sleep EEG activity and periodic limb movements during sleep: Comparisons of clinical features and sleep parameters. *Sleep* 19: 200–204.

Macnair, T. 2006. Transcutaneous electrical nerve stimulation (TENS). http://www.bbc .co.uk/health/conditions/tens1.shtml (accessed January 14, 2008).

Maes, M., et al. 1998. Increased 24-hour urinary cortisol excretion in patients with post-traumatic stress disorder and patients with major depression, but not in patients with fibromyalgia. *Acta Psychiatrica Scandinavica* 98: 328–35.

Maetzel, A., and L. Li. 2002. The economic burden of low back pain: A review of studies published between 1996 and 2001. *Best Practice and Research Clinical Rheumatology* 16: 23–30.

Magill, M. K., and A. Suruda. 1998. Multiple chemical sensitivity syndrome. http:// www.aafp.org/afp/980901ap/magill.html (accessed February 17, 2008).

Magni, G. 1991. The use of antidepressants in the treatment of chronic pain: A review of the current evidence. *Drugs* 42: 730–48.

Mailis-Gagnon, A., and D. Israelson. 2005. *Beyond Pain: Symptoms, Diagnosis and Treatment Options of Chronic Pain Disorders.* Toronto: Penguin.

Major, R. H. 1945. *Classic Descriptions of Disease*, 3rd edition. Springfield, IL: Thomas.

———. 1954. *A History of Medicine.* Springfield, IL: Thomas.

Mäkelä, W., and M. Heliövaara. 1991. Prevalence of primary fibromyalgia in the Finnish population. *British Medical Journal* 303: 216–19.

Malleson, A. 2002. *Whiplash and Other Useful Illnesses.* Montreal: McGill-Queen's University Press.

———. 2003. The whiplash debate. *Canadian Medical Association Journal* 169: 753–95.

Malleson, P. N., M. al-Matar, and R. E. Petty. 1992. Idiopathic musculoskeletal pain syndromes in children. *Journal of Rheumatology* 19: 1786–89.

Malmberg, A. R., and T. L. Yaksh. 1992. Hyperglycemia mediated by spinal glutamate or substance P receptor blockade by spinal cyclooxygenate inhibition. *Science* 257: 1276–79.

Mannerkorpi, K., and G. Gard. 2003. Physiotherapy group treatment for patients with fibromyalgia: An embodied learning process. *Disability Rehabilitation* 28: 1372–80.

Mannerkorpi, K., and C. Hernelid. 2005. Leisure time physical activity at home and work instrument: Development, face validity, construct validity and test-retest reliability for subjects with fibromyalgia. *Disability Rehabilitation* 27: 695–701.

Manning, A. P., W. G. Thompson, K. W. Heaton, and A. F. Morris. 1978. Towards positive diagnosis of the irritable bowel. *British Medical Journal* 2 (6138): 653–54.

Mantyselka et al. Cited in F. Blotman and J. Branco, *La Fibromyalgie. La Douleur au Quotidien.* Toulouse: Éditions Privat, 2006.

Marcus, C. L., and G. M. Loughlin. 1996. Effect of sleep deprivation on driving safety in housestaff. *Sleep* 19: 763–66.

Marcus, D. A., C. Bernstein, and T. E. Rudy. 2005. Fibromyalgia and headache: An epidemiological study supporting migraine as part of the fibromyalgia syndrome. *Clinical Rheumatology* 24: 595–601.

Marks, G. A. 1995. A functional role for REM sleep in brain maturation. *Behavioural Brain Research* 1–2: 1–11.

Mason, B. A. 2007. Fibromyalgia and high risk pregnancy. http://www.fmaware.org/site/News2?page=NewsArticle&id=5343 (accessed February 17, 2008).

Martensson, B., S. Nyberg, G. Toresson, E. Brodin, and L. Bertilsson. 1989. Fluoxetine treatment of depression: Clinical effects, drug concentrations and monoamine metabolites and N-terminally extended substance P in cerebrospinal fluid. *Acta Psychiatrica Scandinavica* 79: 586–96.

Martin, L., A. Nutting, B. R. MacIntosh, S. M. Edworthy, D. Butterwick, and J. Cook. 1996. An exercise program in the treatment of fibromyalgia. *Journal of Rheumatology* 23: 1050–56.

Martinez-Lavin, M. 2001. Is fibromyalgia a generalized reflex sympathetic dystrophy? *Clinical and Experimental Rheumatology* 19: 1–3.

———. 2002. Management of dysautonomia in fibromyalgia. *Rheumatic Disease Clinics of North America* 28: 379–87.

Martinez-Lavin, M., and A. G. Hermosillo. 2000. Autonomic nervous system dysfunction may explain the multisystem features of fibromyalgia. *Seminars in Arthritis and Rheumatolgy* 29: 197–99.

Martinez-Lavin, M., A. G. Hermosillo, M. Rosas, and M. E. Soto. 1998. Circadian studies of autonomic nervous balance in patients with fibromyalgia: A heart rate variability analysis. *Arthritis and Rheumatology* 41: 1966–71.

Martinez-Lavin, M., O. Infante, and C. Lerma. 2008. Hypothesis: The chaos and complexity theory may help our understanding of fibromyalgia and similar maladies. *Seminars in Arthritis and Rheumatism* 37: 260–64.

Martinez-Mena, J. M., and J. Pastor. 1998. Polyneuropathy in patients with periodic leg movements during sleep. *Revista de Neurologica* 27: 745–49.

Mascherpa, F., F. Bogliatto, P. J. Lynch, L. Micheletti, and C. Benedetto. 2007. Vulvodynia as a possible somatization disorder. *Journal of Reproductive Medicine* 52: 107–10.

Masear, V. R. 1996. Chronic pain syndromes. In *Primary Care Orthopaedics*, edited by Masear. Philadelphia: W. B. Saunders, pp. 258–62.

Mason, J. H., et al. 1989. The impact of fibromyalgia on work: A comparison with RA. *Arthritis and Rheumatism* 32: S197 (abstract).

Mathias, S. D., M. Kuppermann, R. F. Liberman, R. C. Lipschutz, and J. F. Steege. 1996. Chronic pelvic pain: Prevalence, health-related quality of life, and economic correlates. *Obstetrics and Gynecology* 87: 321–27.

Matthes, H. W., R. Maldonado, F. Simonin, O. Valverde, S. Slowe, I. Kitchen, K. Befort, A. Dierich, M. Le Meur, P. Dollé, E. Tzavara, J. Hanoune, B. P. Roques, and B. L.

Kieffer. 1996. Loss of morphine-induced analgesia, reward effect and withdrawal symptoms in mice lacking the mu-opioid-receptor gene. *Nature* 383: 819–23.

Maxton, D. G., J. Morris, and P. J. Whorwell. 1991. More accurate diagnosis of irritable bowel syndrome by the use of "non-colonic" symptomatology. *Gut* 32: 784–86.

May, K. P., S. G. West, M. R. Baker, and D. W. Everett. 1993. Sleep apnea in male patients with the fibromyalgia syndrome. *American Journal of Medicine* 94: 505–508.

Mayers, A. G., and D. S. Baldwin. 2005. Antidepressants and their effect on sleep. *Human Psychopharmacology: Clinical and Experimental* 20: 533–59.

McBeth, J. 2005. The epidemiology of chronic widespread pain and fibromyalgia. In *Fibromyalgia and Other Central Pain Syndromes*, edited by D. J. Wallace and D. J. Clauw. Philadelphia: Lippincott Williams & Wilkins, pp. 17–28.

McBeth, J., G. J. MacFarlane, S. Benjamin, and A. J. Silman. 2001. Features of somatization predict the onset of chronic widespread pain: Results of a large population-based study. *Arthritis and Rheumatism* 44: 940–46.

McBeth, J., G. J. MacFarlane, I. M. Hunt, and A. J. Silman. 2001. Risk factors for persistent chronic widespread pain: A community-based study. *Rheumatology* 40: 95–101.

McCahill, M. E. 1999. Labelling the somatically preoccupied. *American Family Physician* 59. http://www.aafp.org/afp/990600ap/editorials.html (accessed January 28, 2008).

McCain, G. A. 1993. The clinical features of the fibromyalgia syndrome. In *Pain Research and Clinical Management*. Amsterdam: Elsevier.

———. 1996. A cost-effective approach to the diagnosis and treatment of fibromyalgia. *Rheumatic Disease Clinics of North America* 22: 323–49.

McCain, G. A., D. A. Bell, F. M. Mai, and P. D. Halliday. 1988. A controlled study of the effects of a supervised cardiovascular training program on the manifestations of primary fibromyalgia. *Arthritis and Rheumatism* 31: 1135–41.

McCain, G. A., and R. A. Scudds. 1988. The concept of primary fibromyalgia (fibrositis): Clinical value, relation and significance to other musculoskeletal pain syndromes. *Pain* 33: 273–87.

McCartt, A. T., J. W. Rohrbaugh, M. C. Hammer, and S. Z. Fuller. 2000. Factors associated with falling asleep at the wheel among long-distance truck drivers. *Accident Analysis and Prevention* 32: 493–504.

McDermid, A. J., G. B. Rolliman, and G. A. McCain. 1996. Generalized hypervigilance in fibromyalgia: Evidence of perceptual amplification. *Pain* 66: 133–44.

McPartland, J. M. 2004. Travell trigger points—Molecular and osteopathic perspectives. *Journal of the American Osteopathic Association* 104: 244–48.

MCSS Factsheet. United States National Institute of Environmental Health Sciences. http://www.niehs.nih.gov/health/ (accessed March 8, 2009).

Meador, C. K. 1965. The art and science of non-disease. *New England Journal of Medicine* 272: 92–95.

Mease, P. J. 2005. Fibromyalgia syndrome: Review of clinical presentation, pathogenesis, outcome measures, and treatment. *Journal of Rheumatology* 32 (suppl 75): 6–21.

Mease, P. J., et al. 2005. Fibromyalgia syndrome. *Journal of Rheumatology* 32: 2270–77.

Meldrum, M. L. 2003. History of pain management. *Journal of the American Medical Association* 290: 2470–75.

Melhus, H., K. Michaëlsson, A. Kindmark, R. Bergström, L. Holmberg, H. Mallmin, A. Wolk, and S. Ljunghall. 1998. Excessive dietary intake of vitamin A is associated with reduced bone mineral density and increased risk of hip fracture. *Annals of Internal Medicine* 129: 770–78.

Melzak, R. 1987. The short form McGill Pain Questionnaire. *Pain* 30: 191–97.

Mengshoel, A. M., O. Forre, and H. B. Kommaes. 1990. Muscle strength and aerobic capacity in primary fibromyalgia. *Clinical and Experimental Rheumatology* 8: 475–79.

———. 1992. The effects of 20 weeks of physical fitness training in female patients with fibromyalgia. *Clinical and Experimental Rheumatology* 10: 345–49.

Mengshoel, A. M., and M. Haugen. 2001. Health status in fibromyalgia—A followup study. *Journal of Rheumatology* 28: 2085–89.

Merskey, H. 1996. Introduction. Plenary Session on Fibromyalgia. *Pain Research and Management* 1: 41.

———. 1996. Psychological medicine, pain, and musculoskeletal disorders. *Rheumatic Disease Clinics of North America* 22: 623–37.

Merskey, H., and N. Bogduk. 1994. *Classification of Common Pain Syndromes and Definitions of Terms*, 2nd edition. Seattle: IASP Press.

Metts, J. F. 1999. Vulvodynia and vulvar vestibulitis: Challenges in diagnosis and management. *American Family Physician*. http://www.aafp.org/afp/990315ap/1547 .html (accessed February 17, 2008).

Michaëlsson, K., H. Lithell, B. Vessby, and H. Melhus. 2003. Serum retinol levels and the risk of fracture. *New England Journal of Medicine* 348: 287–94.

Michiels, V., R. Chuydts, and B. Fischler. 1998. Attention and verbal learning in patients with chronic fatigue syndrome. *Journal of the International Neuropsychological Society* 4: 456–66.

Micó, J. A. 2006. Antidepressants and pain. *Trends in Pharmacological Science* 27: 348–54.

Miller, R. D., and B. G. Katzung. 2001. Skeletal muscle relaxants. In *Basic and Clinical Pharmacology*, edited by Katzung. San Francisco: McGraw-Hill, pp. 447–62.

Mitchell, S. W. 1965. *Injuries of Nerves and Their Consequences*. New York: Dover Publications. And in "Who Named It?" http://www.whonamedit.com/doctor.cfm/959 .html (accessed January 24, 2008).

Mitler, M. M., M. A. Carskadon, C. A. Czeisler, W. C. Dement, D. F. Dinges, and R. C. Graeber. 1988. Catastrophes, sleep and public policy: Consensus report. *Sleep* 11: 100–109.

————. 1982. Rheumatic pain modulation syndrome: The interrelationships between sleep, central nervous system serotonin, and pain. *Advances in Neurology* 33: 51–57.

————. 1989. Non-restorative sleep and symptoms after a febrile illness in patients with fibrositis and chronic fatigue syndrome. *Journal of Rheumatology Supplement* 19: 1505–38.

————. 1993. Fibromyalgia, sleep disorder and chronic fatigue syndrome. *Ciba Foundation Symposium* 173: 262–79.

————. 2001. Sleep and pain. *Sleep Medicine Revue* 5: 387–98.

————. 2002. Management of sleep disorders in fibromyalgia. *Rheumatic Disease Clinics of North America* 28: 353–65.

Moldofsky, H., and J. G. MacFarlane. 2005. Fibromyalgia and chronic fatigue syndrome. In *Principles and Practices of Sleep Medicine*, volume 4, edited by M. Kryger. Philadelphia: Elsevier Saunders, pp. 1225–36.

————. 2005. Sleep and its potential role in chronic pain and fatigue. In *Fibromyalgia and Other Central Pain Syndromes*, edited by D. J. Wallace and D. J. Clauw. Philadelphia: Lippincott Williams & Wilkins, pp. 115–24.

Moldofsky, H., and P. Scarisbrick. 1976. Induction of neurasthenic musculoskeletal pain syndrome by selective sleep stage deprivation. *Psychosomatic Medicine* 38: 35–44.

Moldofsky, H., P. Scarisbrick, R. England, and H. Smythe. 1975. Musculoskeletal symptoms and non-REM sleep disturbance in patients with "fibrositis syndrome" and healthy subjects. *Psychosomatic Medicine* 37: 341–51.

Moldofsky, H., M. T. Wong, and F. A. Lue. 1993. Litigation, sleep, symptoms and disabilities in post accident pain (fibromyalgia). *Journal of Rheumatology* 20: 1821–24.

Monga, A. K., J. M. Marrero, S. L. Stanton, M. C. Lemieux, and J. D. Maxwell. 1997. Is there an irritable bladder in the irritable bowel syndrome? *British Journal of Obstetrics and Gynaecology* 104: 1409–12.

Moore, P., and J. E. Dimsdale. 2002. Opioids, sleep and cancer-related fatigue. *Medical Hypotheses* 58: 77–82.

Morris, A. Idiopathic Environmental Intolerance (IEI). http://www.allergyclinic.co .uk/chemical_sensitivity.htm (accessed February 17, 2008).

Morrissey, M. J., S. P. Duntley, A. M. Anch, and R. Nonneman. 2004. Active sleep and its role in the prevention of apoptosis in the developing brain. *Medical Hypotheses* 62: 876–79.

Morton, J. I., and B. V. Siegel. 1986. Effects of oral dimethyl sulfoxide and dimethyl sulfone on murine autoimmune lymphoproliferative disease. *Proceedings of the Society of Experimental Biology and Medicine* 182: 227–30.

Mountz, J. M., L. A. Bradley, and G. S. Alarcon. 1998. Abnormal functional activity of the central nervous system in fibromyalgia syndrome. *American Journal of Medical Science* 315: 385–96.

Mountz, J. M., L. A. Bradley, J. G. Modell, R. W. Alexander, M. Triana-Alexander, L. A. Aaron, K. E. Stewart, G. S. Alarcón, and J. D. Mountz. 1995. Fibromyalgia in women. Abnormalities of regional cerebral blood flow in the thalamus and the caudate nucleus are associated with low pain thresholds. *Arthritis and Rheumatism* 38: 926–38.

Moyal-Barracco, M., and P. J. Lynch. 2004. 2003 ISSVD terminology and classification of vulvodynia: A historical perspective. *Journal of Reproductive Medicine* 49: 772–77.

Mueller, H. H., et al. 2001. Treatment of fibromyalgia incorporating EEG-driven stimulation: A clinical outcomes study. *Journal of Clinical Psychology* 57: 933–52.

Muller, D. 2007. Non-articular rheumatism/regional pain syndrome. http://www .emedicine.com/med/TOPIC2934.HTM (accessed February 17, 2008).

Müller, W. 1991. Der Verlauf der primarin generalisierten Tendomyopathie (GTM). In *Generalisierte Tendomyopathie (Fibromyalgie)*, edited by Müller. Darmstadt: Springer Verlag, pp. 29–43.

Müller, W., E. M. Schneider, and T. Stratz. 2007. The cassification of fibromyalgia syndrome. *Rheumatology International* 27: 1005–10.

Murav'ev, I. V., M. S. Venikova, G. N. Pleskovskaia, T. A. Riazantseva, and I. A. Sigidin. 1991. Effect of dimethyl sulfoxide and dimethyl sulfone on a destructive process in the joints of mice with spontaneous arthritis. Pub Med 1881708.

Murthy, S. N., et al. 1991. Acute effect of substance P in immunological vasculitis in the rat colon. *Peptides* 12: 1337–45.

National Commission on Sleep Disorder Research. 1993. *Wake Up America. Report of the National Commission on Sleep Disorders Research.* Palo Alto: Department of Health and Human Services.

National Fibromyalgia Association. NFA Internet survey questionnaire. http:// fmawareorg0.web120.discountasp.net/survey/2005/epidemological/emailBlast.htm (accessed January 24, 2008).

National Fibromyalgia Association response to *New York Times* article, January 14, 2008. http://www.fmaware.org/site/News2?page=NewsArticle&id=6835 (accessed March 8, 2009).

NCCAM. National Center for Complementary and Alternative Medicine. 2006. Publication No. D341. Evening primrose oil. http://nccam.nih.gov/health/eveningprimrose/ (accessed February 17, 2008).

———. 2007. Massage therapy as CAM. http://nccam.nih.gov/health/massage/ (accessed December 4, 2007).

———. 2008. An introduction to acupuncture. http://nccam.nih.gov/health/acupuncture/ (accessed January 15, 2008).

Neeck, G., and W. Riedel. 1999. Hormonal perturbations in fibromyalgia syndrome. *Annals of the New York Academy of Science* 876: 325–38.

Neinstein, L. S., and F. R. Kaufman. 1996. Normal physical growth and development. In *Adolescent Health Care: A Practical Guide*, 3rd edition, edited by Neinstein. Baltimore: Williams & Wilkins.

Nicassio, P. M., V. Radojevic, and M. H. Weisman. 1997. A comparison of behavioral and educational intervention for fibromyalgia. *Journal of Rheumatology* 24: 2000–2007.

Nicolson, A. 2003. God's Secretaries. New York: HarperCollins.

NIH. Office of Dietary Supplements. http://health.nih.gov/result.asp?terms=dietary%20supplements&disease_id=1103 (accessed March 8, 2009).

———. Vulvodynia. http://orwh.od.nih.gov/health/VulvodyniaFS.pdf (accessed February 17, 2008).

Nyberg, F., Z. Liu, and C. Lind. 1995. Enhanced CSF levels of substance P in patients with painful arthroses but not in patients with pain from herniated discs. *Journal of Musculoskeletal Pain* 3 (suppl 1): 2.

Offenbacher, M., and G. Stucki. 2000. Physical therapy in the treatment of fibromyalgia. *Scandinavian Journal of Rheumatology* 29 (suppl 113): 78–85.

Okano, K., Y. Kuraishi, and M. Satoh. 1993. Pharmacological evidence for involvement of excitatory amino acids in aversive responses induced by intrathecal substance P in rats. *Biological and Pharmaceutical Bulletin* 16: 861–65.

———. 1994. Involvement of substance P and excitatory amino acids in aversive behavior elicited by intrathecal capsaicin. *Neuroscience Research* 19: 125–30.

O'Malley, P. G., et al. 2000. Treatment of fibromyalgia with anti-depressants. *Journal of General Internal Medicine* 15: 659–66.

Onen, S. H. 2005. How pain and analgesics disturb sleep. *Clinical Journal of Pain* 21: 422–31.

Orr, W. C., et al. 1997. Sleep and gastric function in irritable bowel syndrome: Derailing the brain-gut axis. *Gut* 41: 390–93.

Pack, A. L., et al. 1995. Characteristics of crashes attributed to the driver having fallen asleep. *Accident Analysis and Prevention* 27: 769–75.

Pai, S., and L. J. Sundaram. 2004. Low back pain: An economic assessment in the United States. *Orthopaedic Clinics of North America* 35: 1–5.

Paiva, T., et al. 1997. Chronic headaches and sleep disorders. *Archives of Internal Medicine* 157: 1701–1705.

Palm, O., et al. 2001. Fibromyalgia and chronic widespread pain in patients with inflammatory bowel disease: A cross-sectional population survey. *Journal of Rheumatology* 28: 590–94.

Panter, S. S., S. W. Yun, and A. I. Faden. 1990. Alteration in extracellular amino acids after traumatic spinal cord injury. *Annals of Neurology* 27: 96–99.

Papageorgiou, A. C., A. J. Silman, G. J. MacFarlane. 2002. Chronic widespread pain in the population: A seven year follow-up study. *Annals of Rheumatic Diseases* 61: 1071–74.

Paré, P., et al. 2006. Health-related quality of life, work productivity, and health care resource utilization of subjects with irritable bowel syndrome: Baseline results from LOGIC (Longitudinal Outcomes Study of Gastrointestinal Symptoms in Canada), a naturalistic study. *Clinical Therapeutics* 28: 1726–35.

Park, D. C., et al. 2001. Cognitive function in fibromyalgia patients. *Arthritis and Rheumatism* 44: 2125–33.

Parnes, J. 2006. Temporomandibular joint syndrome. http://www.emedicine.com/emerg/ TOPIC569.HTM (accessed February 17, 2008).

Pascual, J., R. Colas, and J. Castillo. 2001. Epidemiology of chronic daily headache. *Current Pain and Headache Reports* 5: 529–36.

Passo, M. H. 1982. Aches and limb pain. *Pediatric Clinics of North America* 29: 209–19.

Patucchi, E., et al. 2003. Prevalence of fibromyalgia in diabetes mellitus and obesity. *Recent Progress in Medicine* 94: 163–65.

Pawilowska, T., et al. 1994. Population based study of fatigue and psychological distress. *British Medical Journal* 308: 763–66.

Payne, C. K. Cystitis. The bladder on fire. What should you do? http://urology.stanford .edu/articles/cystitis.html (accessed February 17, 2008).

Payne, T. C., et al. 1982. Fibrositis and psychological disturbance. *Arthritis and Rheumatism* 25: 213–17.

PBS Frontline. Opium throughout history. http://www.pbs.org/wgbh/pages/frontline/ shows/heroin/etc/history.html (accessed February 17, 2008).

Peale, N. V. 2007. *Power of Positive Thinking.* New York: Fireside.

Peever, J. H., and D. McGinty. 2007. Why do we sleep? In *Sleep and Pain*, edited by Gilles Lavigne, Barry J. Sessle, Manon Choiniere, and Peter J. Soja. Seattle: IASP Press, pp. 3–21.

Pellegrino, M. J. 1996. *Post-Traumatic Fibromyalgia: A Medical Perspective.* Columbus: Anadem Press.

———. 2007. http://www.update.fibromyalgia.com (accessed March 8, 2009).

Pennebaker, J. W. 1982. *The Psychology of Physical Symptoms.* New York: Springer.

Peres, M. F. 2003. Fibromyalgia, fatigue and headache disorders. *Current Neurology and Neuroscience Reports* 3: 97–103.

Peres, M. F., et al. 2001. Fibromyalgia is common in patients with transformed migraine. *Neurology* 57: 1326–28.

Perez-Ruiz, F., et al. 1995. High prevalence of undetected carpal tunnel syndrome in patients with fibromyalgia syndrome. *Journal of Rheumatology* 22: 501–504.

Perez-Ruiz, F., et al. 1997. Fibromyalgia and carpal tunnel syndrome. *Annals of Rheumatic Diseases* 56: 438–39.

Peterson, H. 1986. Growing pains. *Pediatric Clinics of North America* 33: 1365–72.

Piergiacomi, G., et al. 1989. Personality pattern in rheumatoid arthritis and fibromyalgic syndrome: Psychological investigation. *Zeitschrift für Rheumatologie* 48: 288–93.

Pinal, R. S., A. T. Massi, and R. A. Larse. 1981. Preliminary criteria for clinical remission of rheumatoid arthritis. *Arthritis and Rheumatism* 24: 1308–15.

Pincus, T. 1995. Why should rheumatologists collect patient self-report questionnaires in routine rheumatologic care? *Rheumatic Disease Clinics of North America* 21: 271–319.

Pincus, T., and F. Wolfe. 2005. Patient questionnaires for clinical research and improved standard patient care: Is it better to have 80% of the information in 100% of patients or 100% of the information in 5% of patients? *Journal of Rheumatology* 32: 575–77.

Pioro-Boisset, M., J. Esdaile, and M. Fitzchaeles. 1996. Alternative medicine use in fibromyalgia syndrome. *Arthritis Care Research* 9: 13–17.

Placidi, F. 2000. Effect of antiepileptic drugs on sleep. *Clinical Neurophysiology* 111 (suppl 2): S115–19.

Plesh, O., F. Wolfe, and N. Lane. 1996. The relationship between fibromyalgia and temporomandibular disorders: Prevalence and symptom severity. *Journal of Rheumatology* 23: 1948–52.

Plewes, L. W. 1956. Sudeck's atrophy in the hand. *Journal of Bone Joint Surgery* 38B: 195–203.

Pollock, B. E. 2005. Comparison of posterior fossa exploration and stereotactic radiosurgery in patients with previously nonsurgically treated idiopathic trigeminal neuralgia. *Neurosurgical Focus* 18: 132–40.

Porter, R. W. 1997. Spinal surgery and alleged medical negligence. *Journal of the Royal College of Surgeons Edinburgh* 42: 376–80.

Poyares, D. R. 2002. Can valerian improve the sleep of insomniacs after benzodiazepine withdrawal? *Progress in Neuro-Psychopharmacology and Biological Psychiatry* 26: 539–45.

Prator, B. C. 2006. Serotonin syndrome. *Journal of Neuroscience Nursing* 38: 102–105. http://www.medscape.com/viewarticle/547426 (accessed January 12, 2008).

Prescott, E., et al. Fibromyalgia in the adult Danish population: 1. A prevalence study. *Scandinavian Journal of Rheumatology* 22: 233–37.

Price, R. K., et al. 1992. Estimating the prevalence of chronic fatigue syndrome and associated symptoms in the community. *Public Health Reports* 107: 514–22.

Prince, A., A. L. Bernard, and A. P. Esdall. 2000. A descriptive analysis of fibromyalgia from the patient's perspective. *Journal of Musculoskeletal Pain* 8: 35–47.

Pukall, C. F., et al. 2002. Vestibular tactile and pain thresholds in women with vulvar vestibulitis syndrome. *Pain* 96: 163–75.

Quigley, E. M. 2005. Irritable bowel syndrome and inflammatory bowel disease: Interrelated diseases? *Chinese Journal of Digestive Diseases* 6: 122–32.

Rammelsberg, P., L. LeResche, and S. Dworkin. 2003. Longitudinal outcome of temporomandibular disorders: A 5-year epidemiologic study of muscle disorders defined by research diagnostic criteria for temporomandibular disorders. *Journal of Orofacial Pain* 17: 9–20.

Rang, H. P. 2003. Anxiolytic and hypnotic drugs. In *Pharmacology*, 5th edition. Edinburgh: Churchill Livingstone.

Raphael, K. G., and J. J. Marbach. 2000. Comorbid fibromyalgia accounts for reduced fecundity in women with myofascial face pain. *Clinical Journal of Pain* 16: 29–36.

————. 2001. Widespread pain and the effectiveness of oral splints in myofascial face pain. *Journal of the American Dental Association* 132: 305–16.

Raphael, K. G., et al. 2004. Familial aggregation of depression in fibromyalgia: A community-based test of alternate hypotheses. *Pain* 112: 409–10.

Rasmussen, B. K. 1993. Migraine and tension-type headache in a general population: Precipitating factors, female hormones, sleep pattern and relation to lifestyle. *Pain* 53: 65–72.

Rasmussen, B. K., R. Jensen, and M. Schroll. 1991. Epidemiology of headache in a general population—A prevalence study. *Journal of Clinical Epidemiology* 44: 1147–57.

Rasmussen, B. K., and J. Olesen. 1994. Epidemiology of migraine and tension-type headache. *Current Opinion in Neurology* 7: 264–71.

Raspe, H., and C. Baumgartner. 1993. The epidemiology of the fibromyalgia syndrome (FMS): Different criteria—Different results. *Journal of Musculoskeletal Pain* 1: 149–52.

Rau, C. L., and I. J. Russell. 2000. Is fibromyalgia distinct clinical syndrome? *Current Review of Pain* 4: 287–94.

Raymond, I. 2004. Sleep disturbances, pain and analgesia in adults hospitalized for burn injuries. *Sleep Medicine* 6: 551–59.

Rea, W. J., et al. 2006. Considerations for the diagnosis of chemical sensitivity. http://www.aehf.com/articles/A55.htm (accessed February 17, 2008).

Rechtschaffen, A., M. A. Gilliland, B. M. Bergman, and J. B. Winter. 1983. Physiological correlates of prolonged sleep deprivation in rats. *Science* 221: 182–84.

Rechstaffen, A., and A. Kales, eds. 1968. *A Manual of Standardized Terminology, Techniques and Scoring System for Sleep Stages of Human Subjects.* Los Angeles: UCLA Brain Information Service/Brain Research Institute.

Reed, B. D. 2006. Reliability and validity of self-reported symptoms for predicting vulvodynia. *Obstetrics and Gynecology* 108: 906–13. http://www.medscape.com/viewarticle/546277 (accessed February 17, 2008).

Reichgott, M. J. Clinical evidence of dysautonomia. http://www.ncbi.nlm.nih.gov/books/bookres.fcgi/cm/ch076pdf.pdf (accessed February 15, 2008).

Reilly, P. A., and G. O. Littlejohn. 1990. Fibromyalgia and chronic fatigue syndrome. *Current Opinion in Rheumatolgy* 2: 282–90.

Reiter, R. C. 1990. A profile of women with chronic pelvic pain. *Clinical Obstetrics and Gynecology* 33: 130–36.

Rhodes, C. 2008. How safe are your daily supplements? http://www.telegraph.co.uk/global/main.jhtml;jsessionid=RY1LIATJFA2XFQFIQMFCFGGAVCBQYIV0?xml=/global/2008/01/21/noindex/hsupp121.xml (accessed January 20, 2008).

Richards, S. C. M., and D. L. Scott. 2002. Prescribed exercise in people with fibromyalgia: Parallel group randomised controlled trial. *British Medical Journal* 325: 185–89.

Richardson, G. S., J. D. Miner, and C. A. Czeisler. 1989. Impaired driving performance in shiftworkers: The role of the circadian system in a multifactorial model. *Alcohol, Drugs and Driving* 5: 265–73.

Riek, S., A. E. Chapman, and T. Miller. 1999. A simulation of muscle force and internal kinematics of extensor carpi radialis brevis during backhand tennis stroke: Implication for injury. *Clinical Biochemistry* 14: 477–83.

Restless Leg Syndrome Medical Bulletin. 2005. http://www.rls.org/NETCOMMUNITY/ Page.aspx?&pid=471&srcid=-2 (accessed February 17, 2008).

Robbins, J. M., I. J. Kinmayer, and M. A. Kapusta. 1990. Illness worry and disability in fibromyalgia syndrome. *International Journal of Psychiatry in Medicine* 20: 49–63.

Robertson, V., and K. Baker. 2001. A review of therapeutic ultrasound: Effectiveness studies. *Physical Therapy* 81: 1339–49.

Robinson, V., et al. 2002. Thermotherapy for treating rheumatoid arthritis. *Cochrane Library Issue 4*. Chichester: John Wiley & Sons.

Roizenblatt, S., et al. 1995. Juvenile fibromyalgia-infant-mother association. *Journal of Musculoskeletal Pain* 3 (suppl 3).

Romano, T. J. 1988. Coexistence of irritable bowel syndrome and fibromyalgia. *West Virginia Medical Journal* 84: 16–18.

———. 1990. Clinical experience with post-traumatic fibromyalgia syndrome. *West Virginia Medical Journal* 86: 198–202.

———. 1999. Presence of nocturnal myoclonus in patients with fibromyalgia syndrome. *American Journal of Pain Management* 9: 85–89.

Rooks, D. S. 2007. Fibromyalgia and exercise. *Archives of Internal Medicine* 167: 2192–200.

Rosenberg, J. 1994. Late postoperative nocturnal episodic hypoxaemia and associated sleep pattern. *British Journal of Anaesthesia* 72: 145–50

———. 2001. Sleep disturbances after non-cardiac surgery. *Sleep Medicine Review* 5: 129–37.

Rosenberg, T. 2007. When is a pain doctor a drug pusher? *New York Times*, June 17. http://www.nytimes.com/2007/06/17/magazine/17pain-t.html?em&ex=1182571200 &en=c8fef3ea2de55654&ei=5070.

Rosenberg-Adamsen, S. 1996. Postoperative sleep disturbances: Mechanisms and clinical implications. *British Journal of Anaesthesia* 76: 552–59.

Rosenbloom, M. 2007. Toxicity, vitamin. http://www.emedicine.com/emerg/TOPIC 638.HTM (accessed February 17, 2008).

Rosomoff, H. L., and R. S. Rosomoff. 1996. A rehabilitation physical medicine perspective. In *Pain Treatment Centers at a Crossroads*, edited by M. J. M. Cohen and J. N. Campbell. Seattle: IASP Press, pp. 47–58.

Rowe, P. C., et al. 1995. Is neurally mediated hypotension an unrecognised cause of chronic fatigue? *Lancet* 345 (8950): 623–24.

RTT News (Real Time Traders). 2007. Forest Labs and Cypress announce submission of NDA for milnacipran for treatment of fibromyalgia syndrome. http://www.rttnews.com/sp/breakingnews.asp?date=12/31/2007&item=26&vid=0 (accessed January 1, 2008).

Russell, A. S., and S. L. Aaron. 2003. Opioids and chronic pain. *Canadian Medical Association Journal* 169: 902.

Russell, I. J. 1992. Fibrositis/Fibromyalgia. In *The Clinical and Scientific Basis of Myalgic Encephalomyelitis / Chronic Fatigue Syndrome*, edited by B. M. Hyde, J. Goldstein, and P. Levine. Ottawa: Nightingale Research Foundation, chapter 23.

———. 1996. Neurochemical pathogenesis of fibromyalgia syndrome. *Journal of Musculoskeletal Pain* 1: 61–92.

———. 1998. Advances in fibromyalgia: Possible role for central neurochemicals. *American Journal of Medical Science* 315: 377–84.

———. 1999. Is fibromyalgia distinct clinical entity? The clinical investigator's evidence. *Best Practice & Research Clinical Rheumatology* 13: 445–54.

———. 2004. *The Fibromyalgia Syndrome: A Clinical Case Definition for Practitioners*. Binghampton: Haworth Press.

———. 2005. Neurotransmitters, cytokines, hormones, and the immune system in chronic nonneuropathic pain. In *Fibromyalgia and Other Central Pain Syndromes*, edited by D. J. Wallace and D. J. Clauw. Philadelphia: Lippincott Williams & Wilkins, pp. 63–80.

Russell, I. J., et al. 1991. Treatment of primary fibrositis/fibromyalgia syndrome with ibuprofen and alprazolam: A double-blind, placebo-controlled study. *Arthritis and Rheumatism* 34: 552–60.

Russell, I. J., et al. 1992. Cerebrospinal fluid biogenic amine metabolites in fibromyalgia/fibrositis syndrome and rheumatoid arthritis. *Arthritis and Rheumatism* 35: 550–56.

Russell, I. J., et al. 1992. Early life traumas and confiding in fibromyalgia syndrome. *Scandinavian Journal of Rheumatology* 94: S14.

Russell, I. J., et al. 1994. Elevated cerebrospinal levels of substance P in patients with the fibromyalgia syndrome. *Arthritis and Rheumatism* 37: 1593–601.

Russell, I. J., et al. 1998. Cerebrospinal fluid [CSF] substance P[SP] in fibromyalgia: Changes in CSF SP over time parallel changes in clinical activity. *Journal of Musculoskeletal Pain* 6 (suppl 2): 77.

Russell, I. J., et al. 1999. Reduction of morning stiffness and improvement in physical function in fibromyalgia syndrome patients treated sublingually with low doses of human interferon-alpha. *Journal of Interferon and Cytokine Research* 19: 961–68.

Ryan, M., and J. T. Slevin. 2006. Restless legs syndrome. *American Journal of Health-System Pharmacy* 63: 1599–612.

Saarto, T., and P. J. Wiffen. 2005. Antidepressants for neuropathic pain. *Cochrane Database Systematics Review* 3: CD005454.

Saito, M. 2005. Symptom profile of multiple chemical sensitivity in actual life. *Psychosomatic Medicine* 67: 318–25.

Salaffi, F., A. R. De, and W. Grassi. 2005. Prevalence of musculoskeletal conditions in an Italian population sample: Results of a regional community-based study. I. The MAPPING study. *Clinical and Experimental Rheumatology* 23: 819–28.

Salvarani, C., et al. 2004. Polymyalgia rheumatica. *Best Practice and Research Clinical Rheumatology* 18: 705–22.

Samborski, W., et al. 1991. Comparative studies of the incidence of vegetative and functional disorders in backache and generalized tendomyopathies. *Zeitschrift für Rheumatologie* 50: 378–81.

Sammaritano, M., and A. Sherwin. 2000. Effects of anticonvulsants on sleep. *Neurology* 54: S16–24.

Sandler, R. S., et al. 2002. The burden of selected digestive diseases in the United States. *Gastroenterology* 122: 1500–511.

Sandroni, P., et al. 1998. Complex regional pain syndrome I (CRPS I): Prospective study and laboratory evaluation. *Clinical Journal of Pain* 14: 282–89.

Saper, C. B., T. B. Scammell, and J. Lu. 2005. Hypothalamic regulation of sleep and circadian rhythms. *Nature* 437: 1257–263.

Saper, J. R. 1996. Health care reform and access to pain treatment: A challenge to managed care concepts. In *Pain Treatment at a Crossroads: A Practical and Conceptual Reappraisal*, edited by M. J. M. Cohen and J. N. Campbell. Seattle: IASP Press, pp. 275–86.

Saper, J. R., S. D. Silberstein, and A. E. Lake. 1994. Double-blind trial of fluoxetine: Chronic daily headache and migraine. *Headache* 34: 497–502.

Saper, J. R., P. K. Winner, and A. E. Lake. 2001. An open-label dose-titration study of the efficacy and tolerability of tizanidine hydrochloride tablets in the prophylaxis of chronic daily headache. *Headache* 41: 357–68.

Sarmer, S., et al. 2002. Prevalence of carpal tunnel syndrome in patients with fibromyalgia. *Rheumatology International* 22: 68–70.

Sarnoch, H., F. Adler, and O. B. Scholz. 1997. Relevance of muscular sensitivity, muscular activity, and cognitive variables for pain reduction associated with EMG biofeedback in fibromyalgia. *Perceptual and Motor Skills* 84: 1043–50.

Sasaki, Y., et al. 2000. Sleep onset REM period appearance rate is affected by REM propensity in circadian rhythm in normal nocturnal sleep. *Clinical Neurophysiology* 111: 428–33.

Saskin, P., H. Moldofsky, and F. A. Lue. 1986. Sleep and post-traumatic rheumatic pain modulation disorder (fibrositis syndrome). *Psychosomatic Medicine* 48: 319–23.

Sateia, M., and P. D. Nowell. 2004. Insomnia. *Lancet* 364: 1959–973.

Saxon, L., C. Finch, and S. Bass. 1999. Sports participation, sports injuries and osteoarthritis: Implications for prevention. *Sports Medicine* 28: 123–35.

Scheuler, W., et al. 1988. The alpha-sleep pattern: Quantitative analysis and functional aspects. In *Sleep*, edited by W. P. Koella et al. Stuttgart: Gustav Fischer, pp. 284–86.

Schley, M. 2006. Delta-9-THC based monotherapy in fibromyalgia patients on experimentally induced pain, axon reflex flare, and pain relief. *Current Medical Research and Opinion* 22: 1269–76.

Schochat, T., and H. Raspe. 2003. Elements of fibromyalgia in an open population. *Rheumatology* 42: 829–35.

Schrader, H., G. Bovim, and T. Sand. 2003. The whiplash debate. *Canadian Medical Association Journal* 169: 754–55.

Schrader, H., et al. 1996. Natural evolution of late whiplash syndrome outside the medicolegal context. *Lancet* 347: 1207–11.

Schwarcz, J. 2008. What works? A tale of two treatments. *Montreal Gazette*, January 12. http://www.canada.com/montrealgazette/news/books/story.html?id=e008fb1e-2ce8 -495e-8abb-07a3f358afc8 (accessed January 25, 2008).

Schwartzman, R. J., and T. L. McLellan. 1987. Reflex sympathetic dystrophy: A review. *Archives of Neurology* 44: 555–61.

Schwarz, M. J., et al. 1999. Relationship of substance P.5-hydroxyindole acetic acid and tryptophan in serum of fibromyalgia patients. *Neuroscience Letter* 259: 196–98.

Scudds, R. A., and V. Janzen. 1995. The use of topical 4% lidocaine in spheno-palatine ganglion blocks for the treatment of chronic muscle pain syndrome: A randomized controlled trial. *Pain* 62: 69–77.

Scudds, R. A., et al. 1987. Pain perception and personality measures as discriminators in the classification of fibrositis. *Journal of Rheumatology* 14: 563–69.

Sessle, B. J. 2007. What is pain, and why and how do we experience pain? In *Sleep and Pain*, edited by G. Lavigne et al. Seattle: IASP Press, pp. 23–44.

Sewitch, M. J., et al. 2004. Medication non-adherence in women with fibromyalgia. *Rheumatology* 43: 648–54.

Shapiro, J. R., D. A. Anderson, and S. Burg. 2005. A pilot study of the effects of behavioral weight loss treatment on fibromyalgia symptoms. *Journal of Psychosomatic Research* 59: 275–82.

Shaw, P. J. 2000. Correlates of sleep and waking in *Drosophilia melanogaster*. *Science* 287: 1834–37.

Shaw, P. J. 2002. Stress response genes protect against lethal effects of sleep deprivation in *Drosophilia*. *Nature* 417: 287–91.

Shepherd, C. 2001. Pacing and exercise in chronic fatigue syndrome. *Physiotherapy* 87: 395–96.

Sherkey, J. 1997. The neurological basis of chronic fatigue syndrome and fibromyalgia. Reported in I. J. Russell, *The Fibromyalgia Syndrome: A Clinical Case Definition for Practitioners*, Binghamton: Haworth Press, 2004.

Sherry, D. D. 2005. Fibromyalgia in children. In *Fibromyalgia and Other Central Pain Syndromes*, edited by D. J. Wallace and D. J. Clauw. Philadelphia: Lippincott Williams & Wilkins, pp. 177–86.

Shorter, E. 1992. *From Paralysis to Fatigue. A History of Psychosomatic Illness in the Modern Era*. New York: Free Press.

Sieben, K. J. M., et al. 2002. Pain-related fear in acute low back pain: The first two weeks of a new episode. *European Journal of Pain* 6: 229–37.

Siegel, D. M., D. Janeway, and J. Baum. 1998. Fibromyalgia syndrome in children and adolescents: Clinical features at presentation and status at follow-up. *Pediatrics* 101: 377–82.

Silverman, S. L., and S. A. Martin. 2005. Assessment tools and outcome measures used in the investigation of fibromyalgia. In *Fibromyalgia and Other Central Pain Syndromes*, edited by D. J. Wallace and D. J. Clauw. Philadelphia: Lippincott Williams & Wilkins, pp. 309–20.

Sim, J., and N. Adams. 2002. Systemic review of randomized controlled trials of nonpharmacological interventions for fibromyalgia. *Clinical Journal of Pain* 18: 324–36.

Simmons, D. G. 1981. Myofascial trigger points: A need for understanding. *Archives of Physical Medicine and Rehabilitation* 62: 97–99.

Simms, R. W. 1996. Is there muscle pathology in fibromyalgia syndrome? *Rheumatic Disease Clinics of North America* 22: 245–66.

Simpson, L. O. 1989. Nondiscocytic erythrocytes in myalgic encephalomyelitis. *New Zealand Medical Journal* 102: 126–27.

Singh, M. K. 2005. Chronic pain syndrome. http://www.emedicine.com/pmr/TOPIC 32.HTM (accessed January 10, 2008).

———. 2007. Muscle contraction tension headache. http://www.emedicine.com/neuro/TOPIC231.HTM (accessed February 17, 2008).

Singh, M. K., and P. Jashvant. 2006. Chronic pelvic pain. http://www.emedicine.com/med/topic2939.htm (accessed February 17, 2008).

Sivri, A., et al. 1996. Bowel dysfunction and irritable bowel syndrome in fibromyalgia patients. *Clinical Rheumatology* 15: 283–86.

Skinner, H. A., 1961. *The Origin of Medical Terms*, 2nd edition. Baltimore: Williams & Wilkins.

Sletvold, H., T. C. Stiles, and N. I. Landrø. 1995. Information processing in primary fibromyalgia, major depression and healthy controls. *Journal of Rheumatology* 22: 137–42.

Slotkoff, A. T., D. A. Radulovic, and D. J. Clauw. 1997. The relationship between fibromyalgia and multiple chemical sensitivity syndrome. *Scandinavian Journal of Rheumatology* 26: 364–67.

Smets, E. M. A., et al. 1995. The multidimensional fatigue inventory (MFI): Psychometric qualities of an instrument to assess fatigue. *Journal of Psychosomatic Medicine* 39: 315–25.

Smith, M. T. 2002. Comparative meta-analysis of pharmacotherapy and behavior therapy for persistent insomnia. *American Journal of Psychiatry* 150: 5–11.

Smith, M. T., and J. A. Haythornthwaite. 2007. Cognitive-behavioural treatment for insomnia and pain. In *Sleep and Pain*, edited by G. Lavigne et al. Seattle: IASP Press, pp. 439–58.

Smullin, D. H., S. R. Skilling, and A. A. Larson. 1990. Interactions between substance P, calcitonin gene-related peptide, taurine and excitatory amino acids in the spinal cord. *Pain* 42: 93–101.

Smythe, H. A. 1979. "Fibrositis" as a disorder of pain modulation. *Clinics in Rheumatic Diseases* 5: 823–32.

———. 1985. "Fibrositis" and other diffuse musculoskeletal syndromes. In *Textbook of Rheumatology Volume Two*, edited by W. N. Kelley, E. D. Harris Jr., S. Ruddy, and C. B. Sledge. Philadelphia: W. B. Saunders, pp. 481–89.

Smythe, H. A., and H. Moldofsky. 1977. Two contributions to understanding of the "fibrositis" syndrome. *Bulletin of the Rheumatic Diseases* 28: 928–31.

Smythe, H., et al. 1997. Strategies for accessing pain and pain exaggeration: Controlled studies. *Journal of Rheumatology* 24: 1622–29.

Sorkin, L. S., D. J. McAdoo, and W. D. Willis. 1993. Raphe magnus stimulation-induced antinociception in the cat is associated with release of amino acids as well as serotonin in the lumbar dorsal horn. *Brain Research* 618: 95–108.

Spaeth, M., T. Straz, and L. Farber. 2004. The treatment of fibromyalgia with tropisetron; dose and efficacy correlations. *Scandinavian Journal of Rheumatology* 33: 63–66.

Spiegel, B. M., et al. 2004. Testing for celiac sprue in irritable bowel syndrome with predominant diarrhea: A cost-effectiveness analysis. *Gastroenterology* 126: 1721–32.

Spitzer, M. 2006. ACOG guidelines for treatment of vulvodynia. *Obstetrics and Gynecology* 108: 1049–52. http://www.medscape.com/viewarticle/545473 (accessed February 17, 2008).

Staats, P. S. 1996. Pain is pain: Why the dichotomy of approach to cancer and non-cancer pain? In *Pain Treatment at a Crossroads: A Practical and Conceptual Reappraisal*, edited by M. J. M. Cohen and J. N. Campbell. Seattle: IASP Press, pp. 117–24.

Stanton-Hicks, M. 2000. Reflex sympathetic dystrophy syndrome: A sympathetically mediated pain syndrome or not? *Current Review of Pain* 4: 269–75.

Stanton-Hicks, M., et al. 1994. Reflex sympathetic dystrophy: Changing concepts and taxonomy. *Pain* 63: 127–33.

Stanton-Hicks, M., et al. 1998. Complex regional pain syndromes: Guidelines for therapy. *Clinical Journal of Pain* 14: 156–66.

Starlanyl, D. 2006. http://www.fibromyalgia.com (accessed February 17, 2008).

Starlanyl, D., and M. E. Copeland. 2001. *Fibromyalgia & Chronic Myofascial Pain*, 2nd edition. Oakland: New Harbinger Publications.

Staud, R. 2005. The neurobiology of chronic musculoskeletal pain (including chronic regional pain). In *Fibromyalgia and Other Central Pain Syndromes*, edited by D. J. Wallace and D. J. Clauw. Philadelphia: Lippincott Williams & Wilkins, pp. 45–62.

Staud, R., and C. Adamec. 2007. *Fibromyalgia for Dummies*, 2nd edition. Hoboken: Wiley.

Staudenmayer, H. 1997. Multiple chemical sensitivities or idiopathic environmental intolerances: Psychophysiologic foundation of knowledge for a psychogenic explanation. *Journal of Allergy and Clinical Immunology* 99: 434–37.

Staudenmayer, H., and S. Phillips. 2007. MMPI-2 validity, clinical and content scales, and the Fake Bad Scale for personal injury litigants claiming idiopathic environmental intolerance. *Journal of Psychosomatic Research* 62: 61–72.

Staudenmayer, H., and J. C. Selner. 1995. Failure to assess psychopathology in patients presenting with chemical sensitivities. *Journal of Occupational Medicine* 37: 704–709.

Steele, J. 1969. The hysteria and psychasthenia constructs as an alternative to manifest anxiety and conflict-free ego functions. *Journal of Abnormal Psychology* 74: 79–85.

Steele, M. T., et al. 1999. The occupational risk of motor vehicle collisions for emergency medicine residents. *Academic Emergency Medicine* 6: 1050–53.

Steinberg, A. D. 1978. On morning stiffness. *Journal of Rheumatology* 5: 3–6.

Stetvold, H., H. Stiles, and N. I. Landro. 1995. Information processing in primary fibromyalgia, major depression and healthy controls. *Journal of Rheumatology* 22: 137–43.

Stiefel, F., and D. Stagno. 2004. Management of insomnia in patients with chronic pain conditions. *CNS Drugs* 18: 285–96.

Stoohs, R. A., et al. 1994. Traffic accidents in commercial long-haul truck drivers: The influence of sleep-disordered breathing and obesity. *Sleep* 17: 619–23.

Straus, S. E. 1991. History of chronic fatigue syndrome. *Review of Infectious Diseases* 13 (suppl 1): S2–S7.

Strusberg, I., et al. 2002. Influence of weather conditions on rheumatic pain. *Journal of Rheumatology* 29: 335–38.

Stutts, J. C., et al. 2003. Driver risk factors for sleep-related crashes. *Accident Analysis and Prevention* 35: 321–31.

Subbarao, J., and G. K. Stillwell. 1981. Reflex sympathetic dystrophy syndrome of the upper extremity: Analysis of total outcome of management. *Archives of Physical Medicine and Rehabilitation* 62: 549–54.

Sudeck, P. H. M. 1900. Über die akute entzündliche Knockenatrophie. *Verhandlungen der Deutschen Gesellschaft für Chirurgie* 29: 673–82.

Sumpton, J. 2007. Fibromyalgia for pharmacists. http://fm-cfs.ca/pharmacists.pdf (accessed February 17, 2008).

Sun, J. S., et al. 1996. Ultrastructural studies on myobrillogenesis and neogenesis of skeletal muscles after prolonged traction in rabbits. *Histology and Histopathology* 11: 285–92.

Talbot, L. Failed back surgery syndrome. *British Medical Journal* 327: 985–86.

Talley, N. J. 2006. A unifying hypothesis for the functional gastrointestinal disorders: Really multiple diseases or one irritable gut? *Reviews in Gastroenterological Disorders* 6: 72–78.

Talley, N. J., et al. 1995. Medical costs in community subjects with irritable bowel syndrome. *Gastroenterology* 109: 1736–41.

Tayag-Kier, C. E., G. F. Keenan, and L. V. Scalzi. 2000. Sleep and periodic limb movement in sleep in juvenile fibromyalgia. *Pediatrics* 106: E70.

Terman, G. W., and J. J. Bonica. 2001. Spinal mechanisms and their modalities. In *Bonica's Management of Pain*, 3rd edition, edited by J. D. Loeser et al. Philadelphia: Lippincott Williams & Wilkins.

Thompson, S., et al. 1989. Abnormally fucosylated seum haptoglobins in patients with inflammatory joint disease. *Clinica Chimica Acta* 184: 251–58.

Tishler, M., et al. 2006. Neck injury and fibromyalgia—Are they really associated? *Journal of Rheumatology* 33: 1183–85.

Tofferl, J. K., J. L. Jackson, and P. G. O'Malley. 2004. Treatment of fibromyalgia with cyclobenzaprine: A meta-analysis. *Arthritis and Rheumatism* 51: 9–13.

Tolan, R. W. 2007. Chronic fatigue syndrome. http://www.emedicine.com/ped/TOPIC 2795.HTM (accessed February 17, 2008).

Topbas, M., et al. 2005. The prevalence of fibromyalgia in women aged 20–64 in Turkey. *Scandinavian Journal of Rheumatology* 34: 140–44.

Traut, E. F. 1968. Fibrositis. *Journal of the American Geriatric Society* 16: 531–38.

Travell, J. G. 1968. *Office Hours: Day and Night. The Autobiography of Janet Travell, MD.* New York: World Publishing.

Travell, J. G., and D. G. Simons. 1983. *Myofascial Pain and Dysfunction. The Trigger Point Manual*, volume 1: *The Upper Extremities.* Baltimore: Williams & Wilkins.

Travell, J. G., D. Simons, and L. Simons. 1999. *Myofascial Pain and Dysfunction. The Trigger Point Manual*, vols. 1–2, 2nd edition. Baltimore: Lippincott Williams & Wilkins.

Triadafilopoulos, G., R. W. Simms, and D. L. Goldenberg. 1991. Bowel dysfunction in fibromyalgia syndrome. *Digestive Disease Science* 36: 59–64.

Tsuno, N. 2005. Sleep and depression. *Journal of Clinical Psychiatry* 66: 1254–69.

Turk, D. C., and A. Okifuji. 1997. Evaluating the role of physical, operant, cognitive and affective factors in the pain behaviors of chronic pain patients. *Behaviour Modification* 21: 259–80.

Turk, D. C., et al. 1998. Interdisciplinary treatment for fibromyalgia syndrome: Clinical and statistical significance. *Arthritis Care and Research* 11: 186–92.

Ulrich, V., M. B. Russell, R. Jensen R. 1996. A comparison of tension-type headache in migraineurs and in non-migraineurs: A population-based study. *Pain* 67: 501–506.

Undeland, M., and K. Malterud. 2007. The fibromyalgia diagnosis—Hardly helpful for the patients. *Scandinavian Journal of Primary Health Care* 25: 250–55.

United States Census Bureau. United States Census 2000. http://www.census.gov/main/ www/cen2000.html (accessed January 25, 2008).

University of California Drug Industry Document Archive. http://dida.library.ucsf.edu (accessed January 12, 2008).

University of Michigan Health System. 2008. Chronic multisystem illness. http://www .med.umich.edu/painresearch/pro/cmi.htm (accessed January 28, 2008).

Unruh, A. M., J. Ritchie, and H. Merskey. 1999. Does gender affect appraisal of pain and pain coping strategies? *Clinical Journal of Pain* 15: 31–40.

Ursin, R. 2002. Serotonin and sleep. *Sleep Medicine Review* 6: 57–69.

Uveges, J. M., et al. 1990. Psychological symptoms in primary fibromyalgia syndrome: Relationship to pain, life stress, and sleep disturbance. *Arthritis and Rheumatism* 33: 1279–83.

Vaeroy, H., F. Nyberg, and L. Terenius. 1991. No evidence for endorphin deficiency in fibromyalgia following investigation of cerebrospinal fluid [CSF] dynorphin A and Met-enkephalin-Arg6-Phe7. *Pain* 46: 139–43.

Vaeroy, H., et al. 1988. Elevated CSF levels of substance P and high incidence of Raynaud's phenomenon in patients with fibromyalgia: New features for diagnosis. *Pain* 32: 21–26.

Van den Bosch, M. A., et al. 2004. Evidence against the use of lumbar spine radiography for low back pain. *Clinical Radiology* 59: 69–76.

Vanderah, T. W., et al. 1996. Single intrathecal injections of dynorphin A or des-tyr-dynorphins produce long-lasting allodynia in rats: Blockade by MK-801 but not naloxone. *Pain* 68: 275–81.

Van Houdenhove, B., et al. 2002. Daily hassles reported by chronic fatigue syndrome and fibromyalgia patients in tertiary care: A controlled quantitative and qualitative study. *Psychotherapy and Psychosomatics* 71: 207–13.

Van Tulder, M., B. Koes, and C. Bombardier. 2002. Low back pain. *Best Practice and Research in Clinical Rheumatology* 16: 761–75.

Veale, D., et al. 1991. Primary fibromyalgia and the irritable bowel syndrome: Different expressions of a common pathogenetic process. *British Journal of Rheumatology* 30: 220–22.

Veldman, P. H., H. M. Reynen, and I. E. Arnz. 1993. Signs and symptoms of reflex sympathetic dystrophy: Prospective study of 829 patients. *Lancet* 342: 1012–16.

Venuturupalli, S., and D. J. Wallace. 2005. Controversial syndromes and their relationship to fibromyalgia. In *Fibromyalgia and Other Central Pain Syndromes*, edited by D. J. Wallace and D. J. Clauw. Philadelphia: Lippincott Williams & Wilkins, pp. 281–92.

Vernia, P., et al. 1995. Lactose malabsorption and irritable bowel syndrome. Effect of a long-term lactose-free diet. *Italian Journal of Gastroenterology* 27: 117–21.

Vertrugno, R., R. D'Angelo, and P. Montagna. 2007. Periodic limb movements in sleep and periodic limb movement disorder. *Neurologic Science* 28: S9–S14.

Vestergaard-Poulsen, P., et al. 1995. ^{31}P NMR specrtroscopy and electromyography during exercise and recovery in patients with fibromyalgia. *Journal of Rheumatology* 22: 1544–51.

Viner, R., and M. Hotopf. 2004 Childhood predictors of self reported chronic fatigue syndrome / myalgic encephalomyelitis in adults: National birth cohort study. *British Medical Journal* 329: 941–51.

Viner, R., and D. Russell. 2005. ABC of adolescence. Fatigue and somatic symptoms. *British Medical Journal* 330: 1012–15.

Vlaeyen, J. W., N. J. Teeken-Gruben, and M. E. Goosens. 1996. Cognitive-educational treatment of fibromyalgia: A randomized clinical trial. Clinical effects. *Journal of Rheumatology* 23: 1237–45.

Waddell, G., et al. 1980. Non-organic physical signs in low-back pain. *Spine* 5: 117–25.

Wager, T. D., et al. 2004. Placebo-induced changes in fMRI in the anticipation and experience of pain. *Science* 303: 1162–67.

Walewski, W., and L. Szcepanski. 1992. Epidemiological studies of fibromyalgia syndrome morbidity. *Scandinavian Journal of Rheumatology* 94: S138.

Walker, L. S., et al. 1995. Long-term health outcomes in patients with recurrent abdominal pain. *Journal of Pediatric Psychology* 20: 233–45.

Wallace, D. J. 1990. Genitourinary manifestations of fibrositis: An increased association with the female urethral syndrome. *Journal of Rheumatology* 17: 238–39.

———. 2004. To fibromyalgia nihilists: Stop pontificating and test your hypothesis. *Journal of Rheumatology* 31: 632.

———. 2005. The economic impact of fibromyalgia on society and disability issues. In *Fibromyalgia and Other Central Pain Syndromes*, edited by D. J. Wallace and D. J. Clauw. Philadelphia: Lippincott Williams & Wilkins, pp. 399–404.

———. 2005. Genitourinary associations with fibromyalgia. In *Fibromyalgia and Other Central Pain Syndromes*, edited by D. J. Wallace and D. J. Clauw. Philadelphia: Lippincott Williams & Wilkins, pp. 235–40.

———. 2005. The history of fibromyalgia. In *Fibromyalgia and Other Central Pain Syndromes*, edited by D. J. Wallace and D. J. Clauw. Philadelphia: Lippincott Williams & Wilkins, pp. 1–8.

Wallace, D. J., and J. Gotto. 2008. Hypothesis: Bipolar illness with complaints of chronic musculoskeletal pain is a form of pseudofibromyalgia. *Seminars in Arthritis and Rheumatism* 37: 256–59.

Wallace, D. J., and J. B. Wallace. 2003. *Fibromyalgia: An Essential Guide for Patients and Their Families.* New York: Oxford University Press.

Ward, M. M. 1994. Are patient self-report measures of arthritis activity confounded by mood? A longitudinal study of patients with rheumatoid arthritis. *Journal of Rheumatology* 21: 1046–50.

Ware, J. C. 1985. Nocturnal myoclonus: Possible mediation by the sympathetic nervous system. *Sleep Research* 14: 24.

Ware, J. E., M. Kosinski, and S. D. Keller. 1994. *SF-36 Physical and Mental Health Summary Scales: A User's Manual.* Boston: Health Assessment Lab.

Warner, J. 2007. A hole in the head. *New York Times*, November 22. http://warner.blogs.nytimes.com/2007/11/22/ (accessed January 25, 2008).

Waylonis, G. W., and R. H. Perkins. 1994. Post-traumatic fibromyalgia. A long term follow-up. *American Journal of Physical Medicine and Rehabilitation* 73: 403–12.

Weigert, D. A., et al. 1998. Current concepts in the pathophysiology of abnormal pain perception in fibromyalgia. *American Journal of Medical Science* 315: 405–12.

Weinberger, L. M. 1977. Traumatic fibromyositis: A critical review of an enigmatic concept. *Western Journal of Medicine* 127: 99–102.

Welin, M., et al. 1995. Elevated substance P levels are contrasted by a decrease in met-enkephalin-arg-phe levels in CSF from fibromyalgia patients. *Journal of Musculoskeletal Pain* 3 (suppl 1): 4.

Werle, E., et al. 2005. Serum hyaluronic acid levels are elevated in arthritis patients, but normal and not associated with clinical data in patients with fibromyalgia syndrome. *Clinical Laboratory* 51: 11–19.

Wessely, S. 2001. Chronic fatigue: Symptoms and syndrome. *Annals of Internal Medicine* 134: 838–43.

Westlund, K. N., D. L. McNeill, and R. E. Coggeshall. 1998. Glutamate immunoactivity in rat dorsal root axons. *Neuroscience Letter* 96: 13–17.

Wheatley, D. 2001. Kava and valerian in the treatment of stress-induced insomnia. *Phytotherapy Research* 15: 549–51.

White, A. A., and S. L. Gordon. 1982. Synopsis: Workshop on idiopathic low-back pain. *Spine* 7: 141–49.

White, K. P., and J. Thompson. 2003. Fibromyalgia syndrome in an Amish community: A controlled study to determine disease and symptom prevalence. *Journal of Rheumatology* 30: 1835–40.

White, K. P., et al. 1995. Fibromyalgia in rheumatology practice: A survey of Canadian rheumatologists. *Journal of Rheumatology* 22: 722–26.

White, K. P., et al. 1999. The London fibromyalgia epidemiology study: Direct health care costs of fibromyalgia syndrome in London, Canada. *Journal of Rheumatology* 26: 884–89.

White, K. P., et al. 1999. The London fibromyalgia epidemiology study: The prevalence of fibromyalgia syndrome in London, Ontario. *Journal of Rheumatology* 26: 1570–76.

White, K. P., et al. 1999. The London fibromyalgia epidemiology study: Comparing the demographic and clinical characteristics in 100 random community cases of fibromyalgia versus controls. *Journal of Rheumatology* 26: 1577–85.

White, K. P., et al. 2002. Does the label "fibromyalgia" alter health status, function, and health service utilization? A prospective, within-group comparison in a community cohort of adults with chronic widespread pain. *Arthritis and Rheumatism* 47: 260–65.

Whitehead, W. E., O. Palsson, and K. R. Jones. 2002. Systemic review of the comorbidity of irritable bowel syndrome with other disorders: What are the causes and implications? *Gastroenterology* 122: 1140–56.

Whitehead, W. E., et al. 1982. Learned illness behaviour in patients with irritable bowel syndrome and peptic ulcer. *Digestive Disease Science* 27: 202–208.

Whitney, C. W., and M. VonKorff. 1992. Regression to the mean in treated versus untreated chronic pain. *Pain* 50: 281–85.

Whorwell, P. J., et al. 1986. Bladder smooth muscle dysfunction in patients with irritable bowel syndrome. *Gut* 27: 1014–17.

Whorwell, P. J., et al. 1986. Non-colonic features of irritable bowel syndrome. *Gut* 27: 37–40.

Wieting, J. M., and A. P. Cugalj. 2007. Massage, traction, and manipulation. http://www.emedicine.com/pmr/TOPIC200.HTM (accessed February 17, 2008).

Wigers, S. H., T. C. Stiles, and P. A. Vogel. 1996. Effects of aerobic exercise versus stress management in fibromyalgia. A 4.5 year prospective study. *Scandinavian Journal of Rheumatology* 25: 77–86.

Williams, D. A., et al. 2004. Pain assessment in patients with fibromyalgia syndrome: A consideration of methods for clinical trials. *Clinical Journal of Pain* 20: 348–56.

Williams, K. I., S. H. Burstein, and D. S. Layne. 1966. Metabolism of dimethyl sulfide, dimethyl sulfoxide, and dimethyl sulfone in the rabbit. *Archives of Biochemistry and Biophysics* 117: 84–87.

Willweber-Strumpf cited F. Blotman, and J. Branco. 2006. *La Fibromyalgie. La Douleur au Quotidien*. Toulouse: Éditions Privat.

Winfield, J. 2007. Fibromyalgia. http://www.emedicine.com/med/topic790.htm (accessed February 17, 2008).

Woda, A. S., et al. 2005. Towards a taxonomy of idiopathic orofacial pain. *Pain* 116: 396–406.

Wolfe, F. 1982. Non-articular symptoms of fibrositis, rheumatoid arthritis, osteoarthritis and arthralgia syndromes. *Arthritis and Rheumatism* 25: S146.

———. 1986. The clinical syndrome of fibrositis. *American Journal of Medicine* 8 (suppl 3A): 7–14.

———. 1993. The epidemiology of fibromyalgia. *Journal of Musculoskeletal Medicine* 1: 137–48.

———. 1993. Fibromyalgia and problems in classification of musculoskeletal disorders. In *Progress in Fibromyalgia and Myofascial Pain*, edited by H. Vaeroy and H. Merskey. Amsterdam: Elsevier, pp. 217–35.

———. 1994. Post-traumatic fibromyalgia: A case narrated by the patient. *Arthitis Care and Research* 7: 161–65.

———. 1995. Fibromyalgia. In *Temporomandibular Disorders and Related Pain Conditions*, edited by B. J. Sessle et al. Seattle: IASP Press, pp. 31–46.

————. 1997. The fibromyalgia problem. *Journal of Rheumatology* 24: 1247–49.

————. 1997. The relation between tender points and fibromyalgia symptom variables: Evidence that fibromyalgia is not a discrete disorder in the clinic. *Annals of Rheumatic Diseases* 56: 268–71.

————. 1998. What use are fibromyalgia control points? *Journal of Rheumatology* 25: 2476.

————. 2003. Stop using the American College of Rheumatology Criteria in the clinic. *Journal of Rheumatology* 30: 1671–72.

Wolfe, F., and M. A. Cathey. 1983. Prevalence of primary and secondary fibrositis. *Journal of Rheumatology* 10: 965–68.

Wolfe, F., and D. J. Hawley. 1993. Fibromyalgia. In *Textbook of Rheumatology*, edited by W. N. Kelley et al. Philadelphia: Saunders.

Wolfe, F., and T. Pincus. 1991. Standard self-report questionnaires in routine clinical and research practice—An opportunity for patients and rheumatologists. *Journal of Rheumatology* 18: 643–46.

Wolfe, J., and J. J. Rasker. 2006. The Symptom Intensity Scale, fibromyalgia, and the meaning of fibromyalgia-like symptoms. *Journal of Rheumatology* 33: 2113–14.

Wolfe, F., et al. 1984. Psychological status in primary fibrositis and fibrositis associated with rheumatoid arthritis. *Journal of Rheumatology* 11: 500–506.

Wolfe, F., et al. 1985. Fibrositis: Symptom frequency and criteria for diagnosis. An evaluation of 291 rheumatic disease patients and 58 normal individuals. *Journal of Rheumatology* 12: 1159–63.

Wolfe, F., et al. 1990. The American College of Rheumatology 1990 Criteria for the Classification of Fibromyalgia: Report of the Multicenter Criteria Committee. *Arthritis and Rheumatism* 33: 160–72.

Wolfe, F., et al. 1992. The fibromyalgia and myofascial pain syndromes: A preliminary study of tender points and trigger points in persons with fibromyalgia, myofascial pain syndrome and no disease. *Journal of Rheumatology* 19: 944–51.

Wolfe, F., et al. 1995: The prevalence and characteristics of fibromyalgia in the general population. *Arthritis and Rheumatism* 38: 19–28.

Wolfe, F., et al. 1996. The prevalence and meaning of fatigue in rheumatic disease. *Journal of Rheumatology* 23: 1407–17.

Wolfe, F., et al. 1997. Health status and disease severity in fibromyalgia: Results of a six center longitudinal study. *Arthritis and Rheumatism* 40: 1571–79.

Wolfe, F., et al. 1997. A prospective, longitudinal, multicenter study of service utilization and costs in fibromyalgia. *Arthritis and Rheumatism* 40: 1560–70.

Wolfe, F., et al. 1997. Work and disability status of persons with fibromyalgia. *Journal of Rheumatology* 24: 1171–78.

Wong, C. S., et al. 2007. Collateral meridian therapy dramatically attenuates pain and improves functional activity of a patient with complex regional pain syndrome. *Anesthesia and Analgesia* 104: 452.

Wood, P. B. 2004. Stress and dopamine: Implications for the pathophysiology of chronic widespread pain. *Medical Hypotheses* 62: 420–24.

———. 2006. Mesolimbic dopaminergic mechanisms and pain control. *Pain* 120: 230–34.

Woolf, C. J., G. J. Bennett, and M. Doherty. 1999. Towards a mechanism-based classification of pain? *Pain* 77: 227–29.

World Health Organization. 1980. *International Classification of Impairments, Disabilities, and Handicaps.* Geneva.

Yaron, I., et al. 1997. Elevated levels of hyaluronic acid in the sera of women with fibromyalgia. *Journal of Rheumatology* 24: 2221–24.

Yawn, B. P., et al. 2001. Do published guidelines for evaluation of irritable bowel syndrome reflect practice? *BioMed Central Gastroenterology* 1: 11.

Yazici, Y., et al. 2004. Morning stiffness in patients with early rheumatoid arthritis is associated more strongly with functional disability than with joint swelling and erythrocyte sedimentation rate. *Journal of Rheumatology* 31: 1723–26.

Young, L. 2004. Reward mechanism involved in addiction likely regulates pair bonds between monogamous animals. Emory University Health Sciences Center. http://www.sensualism.com/love/addiction.html (accessed February 17, 2008).

Yule, H., and A. C. Burnell. 1994. *Hobson-Jobson.* Sittingbourne: Linguasia.

Yunus, M. B. 1984. Primary fibromyalgia syndrome: Current concepts. *Comprehensive Therapy* 10: 21–28.

———. 1994. Fibromyalgia syndrome: Clinical features and spectrum. *Journal of Musculoskeletal Pain* 1: 5–21.

———. 1994. Psychological aspects of fibromyalgia syndrome: A component of the dysfunctional spectrum syndrome. *Baillieres Clinical Rheumatology* 9: 811–37.

———. 2000. Central sensitivity syndromes: A unified concept for fibromyalgia and other similar maladies. *Journal of the Indian Rheumatology Association* 8: 27–33.

———. 2005. The concept of central sensitivity syndromes. In *Fibromyalgia and Other Central Pain Syndromes*, edited by D. J. Wallace and D. J. Clauw. Philadelphia: Lippincott Williams & Wilkins, pp. 29–44.

———. 2005. Symptoms and signs of fibromyalgia syndrome: An overview. In *Fibromyalgia and Other Central Pain Syndromes*, edited by D. J. Wallace and D. J. Clauw. Philadelphia: Lippincott Williams & Wilkins, pp. 125–32.

———. 2007. Fibromyalgia and overlapping disorders: The unifying concept of central sensitivity syndromes. *Seminars in Arthritis and Rheumatism* 36: 339–56.

———. 2007. Quoted in Overlapping Syndrome. Fibromyalgia network. http://www.fmnetnews.com/basics-overlap.php (accessed January 25, 2008).

———. 2008. Central sensitivity syndromes: a new paradigm and group nosology for fibromyalgia and overlapping conditions, and the related issue of disease versus illness. Seminars in Arthritis and Rheumatism. http://www.ncbi.nlm.nih.gov/pubmed/18191990 (accessed February 4, 2008).

Yunus, M. B., and J. C. Aldag. 1996. Restless leg syndrome and leg cramps in fibromyalgia syndrome: A controlled study. *British Medical Journal* 312: 1336–39.

Yunus, M. B., S. Arslan, and J. C. Aldag. 2002. Relationship between body mass index and fibromyalgia features. *Scandinavian Journal of Rheumatology* 31:27–31.

———. 2002. Relationship between fibromyalgia features and smoking. *Scandinavian Journal of Rheumatology* 31: 301–305.

Yunus, M. B., F. Inanici, and J. C. Aldag. 1998. Incomplete fibromyalgia syndrome: Clinical and psychological comparison with fibromyalgia syndrome. *Arthritis and Rheumatism* 41 (suppl 9): S528.

Yunus, M. B., et al. 1981. Primary fibromyalgia (fibrositis): Clinical study of 50 patients with matched normal controls. *Seminars in Arthritis and Rheumatism* 11: 151–71.

Yunus, M. B., et al. 1997. Fibromyalgia consensus report: Additional comments. *Journal of Clinical Rheumatism* 3: 3324–27.

Yunus, M. B., et al. 1999. Genetic linkage analysis of multicase families with fibromyalgia syndrome. *Journal of Rheumatology* 26: 408–12.

Yunus, M. B., et al. 2000. Fibromyalgia in men: Comparison of clinical features with women. *Journal of Rheumatology* 27: 485–90.

Zagaria, M. A. E. 2007. Serotonin Syndrome. Identification, Resolution, and Prevention. http://www.uspharmacist.com/index.asp?show=article&page=8_2153.htm (accessed January 12, 2008).

Zamula, E. Interstitial cystitis. Progress against disabling bladder condition. FDA Home Page. http://www.fda.gov/fdac/features/995_cystitis.html (accessed February 17, 2008).

Zeltzer, L. K., et al. 1997. A psychobiologic approach to pediatric pain: Part I. History, physiology, and assessment strategies. Part II. Prevention and treatment. *Current Problems in Pediatrics* 27: 223–84.

Zepelin, H. 2005. Mammalian sleep. In *Principles and Practices of Sleep Medicine*, volume 4. Philadelphia: Elsevier Saunders, pp. 91–100.

Zidar, J., et al. 1990. Quantitative EMG and muscle tension in painful muscles in fibromyalgia. *Pain* 40: 249–54.

Zollinger, P. E., et al. 2007. Can vitamin C prevent complex regional pain syndrome in patients with wrist fractures? A randomised controlled multicenter dose response study. *Journal of Bone and Joint Surgery* 89A: 1424–31.

Zondervan, K. T., et al. 1999. Prevalence and incidence of chronic pelvic pain in primary care: Evidence from a national general practice database. *British Journal of Obstetrics and Gynaecology* 106: 1149–55.

Zubieta, J.-K., et al. 2007. Why don't painkillers work for people with fibromyalgia? *Journal of Neuroscience* 27: 10000–10006. http://www.sciencedaily.com/releases/2007/ 09/070927131357.htm (accessed March 8, 2009).

Zwaigenbaum, L., et al. 1999. Highly somatizing young adolescents and the risk of depression. *Pediatrics* 103: 1203–1209.

INDEX